MATERNAL INFANT HEALTH
CARE PLANNING

SECOND EDITION

Kathryn A. Melson, RN, MSN

Marie S. Jaffe, RN, MS

MATERNAL INFANT HEALTH CARE PLANNING

SECOND EDITION

Kathryn A. Melson, RN, MSN

Marie S. Jaffe, RN, MS

Springhouse Corporation
Springhouse, Pennsylvania

Staff

PUBLICATION STAFF

Executive Director, Editorial
Stanley Loeb

Senior Publisher, Trade and Textbooks
Minnie B. Rose, RN, BSN, MEd

Art Director
John Hubbard

Clinical Consultant
Maryann Foley, RN, BSN

Associate Acquisitions Editor
Caroline Lemoine

Copy Editors
Mary Hohenhaus Hardy, Barbara Hodgson

Designers
Stephanie Peters (associate art director),
Laurie Mirijanian (book designer)

Permissions Coordinator
Betsy K. Snyder

Typography
Diane Paluba (manager), Elizabeth Bergman,
Joyce Rossi Biletz, Phyllis Marron, Robin
Mayer, Valerie Rosenberger

Manufacturing
Deborah Meiris (manager), T.A. Landis, Anna
Brindisi, Kate Davis

℞ A member of the Reed Elsevier plc group

Library of Congress Cataloging-in-Publication Data

Jaffe, Marie S.
  Maternal-infant health care planning/Marie S. Jaffe, Kathryn A. Melson.—2nd ed.
    p.   cm.
  Rev. ed. of: Maternal iInfant health care plans. c1989.
  Includes bibliographical references and index.
  1. Maternity nursing.   2. Infants (Newborn)—Diseases—Nursing.   3. Nursing care plans.
  I. Melson, Kathryn A.   II. Jaffe, Marie S.   III. Title.
  [DNLM: 1. Maternal-Child Nursing.   2. Patient Care Planning.   WY 157.3 1994]
  RG951.J34 1994
  610.73'678—dc20
  DNLM/DLC
  for Library of Congress   94-16947
  ISBN 0-87434-739-4   CIP

Acknowledgments

The authors wish to thank the following individuals whose contributions to the preparation of this book have been invaluable:

Sister Sharon Becker, RN, MSN, CNM, Clinical Coordinator, Nurse-Midwifery Program, Texas Tech Regional Academic Health Science Center, El Paso, Texas

Carolyn H. Routledge, RN, MSN, CNM, Director, Nurse-Midwifery Program, Texas Tech Regional Academic Health Science Center, El Paso, Texas

Margaret T. Steinbach, RN, MSN, RNC, Neonatal Clinician, West Texas Neonatal Associates, El Paso, Texas

Contents

Introduction   ix

Section I: Antepartum
Normal Antepartum   2
Abortion   14
Abruptio Placentae   20
Acquired Immunodeficiency Syndrome (AIDS) — Maternal   24
Ectopic Pregnancy   30
Hydatidiform Mole (Molar Pregnancy)   34
Hyperemesis Gravidarum   37
Multiple Gestation   41
Placenta Previa   44
Pregnancy Complicated by Cardiac Disease   48
Pregnancy Complicated by Diabetes Mellitus   53
Pregnancy-Induced Hypertension   58
Premature Rupture of Membranes   64
Preterm or Premature Labor   67
Prolapsed Umbilical Cord   71
Rh Isoimmunization   74
Sexually Transmitted Diseases/TORCH   77
Vaginal and Urinary Infections   80

Section II: Intrapartum
Cesarean Section Birth   85
Labor and Vaginal Birth   92
Oxytocin-Induced or Oxytocin-Augmented Labor   103

Section III: Postpartum
Puerperium   108
Hemorrhage   116
Puerperal Infection   119
Thromboembolic Disease   123

Section IV: Newborn Infant Assessment Guides
Ballard Gestational-Age Assesment Tool   127
Newborn Infant Postdelivery Assessment   128
Major Neonatal Reflexes   129
Newborn Infant Nursery Assessment   130

Section V: Infant
Acquired Immunodeficiency Syndrome — Infant   134
Air Leak Syndromes   139
Anemia   142
Birth Trauma   146
Bowel Obstruction, Small or Large   150
Bronchopulmonary Dysplasia   154
Choanal Atresia   158
Circumcision   160
Cleft Lip and Cleft Palate   164
Congenital Heart Disease   170
Congestive Heart Failure   177

Drug Addiction and Withdrawal 183
Fetal Alcohol Syndrome 190
Full-Term Infant, 38 to 42 Weeks 194
Hip Dysplasia 201
Hyaline Membrane Disease—Respiratory Distress Syndrome (RDS I) 205
Hyperbilirubinemia 213
Hypocalcemia 221
Hypoglycemia 225
Hypothermia and Hyperthermia 229
Inappropriate Size or Weight for Gestational Age, Large 235
Inappropriate Size or Weight for Gestational Age, Small 239
Intracranial Hemorrhage 243
Meconium Aspiration Syndrome 247
Necrotizing Enterocolitis 251
Postoperative Care 257
Preoperative Care 263
Preterm Infant, Less Than 37 Weeks 268
Sepsis Neonatorum and Infectious Disorders 276
Skin Disorders 283
Spinal Cord Defects and Hydrocephalus 287
Talipes Deformity 293
Tracheoesophageal Fistula or Esophageal Atresia 297
Transient Tachypnea (RDS II) 303

Appendices

1. NANDA Taxonomy of Nursing Diagnoses 307
2. Selected Daily Dietary Allowances—Maternal 309
3. Selected Substances and Fetal Abnormalities 310
4. Aspects of Psychological Care—Maternal 312
5. Preparing for Nonemergency Surgery 317
6. Selected Methods of Family Planning 318
7. The Family and Home Assessment 321
8. Fluid and Nutritional Needs in Infancy 322
9. Assessing Vital Signs in the Infant 323
10. Normal Lab Values for the Newborn Infant 324
11. Transporting an Infant to Another Hospital 327
12. Parent Teaching Guides 328
    How to Bathe Your Infant 328
    Breast-feeding the Infant 330
    Bottle-feeding the Infant 333
    How to Hold the Infant 333
    Postpartum Exercises 334
13. 1993 CDC Revised Classification System for
    HIV Infection/AIDS Surveillance Case Definition 336
14. CDC Guidelines for Preventing HIV Transmission
    in Health Care Settings 337

Selected References 338

Index 339

Introduction

These plans of care are designed to serve as a tool to guide nurses in providing safe and effective perinatal and infant care.

The maternal section of this book covers antepartum, intrapartum, and postpartum care; the infant section covers preterm and full-term conditions, with care provided in the newborn nursery or neonatal intensive care nursery. These sections address normal and common abnormal conditions.

Each plan uses these organizational headings:
- **Definition** of the condition and the focus of the plan.
- **Etiology and Precipitating Factors**—causes or predisposing or contributing factors—that place the mother or infant at risk.
- **Physical Findings** organized by body system; in the maternal plans, the findings begin in the signs and symptoms; in the infant plans, the findings include maternal history, infant status at birth, and signs and symptoms.
- **Diagnostic Studies and Laboratory Data** assist in formulating nursing diagnoses.
- **Nursing Diagnoses and Collaborative Problems** focus primarily on nursing functions but include independent and interdependent actions. The former are exclusive to nursing, whereas the latter are nursing and medically oriented.
- **Goals** state nurse- or patient-oriented expectations (or both) as outcomes from the nursing diagnoses.
- **Interventions and Rationales** give specific patient or nurse activities with appropriate physiologic or descriptive explanations for their use.
- **Additional Individualized Interventions** provide for specific patient interventions related to aspects of care not included in the plan.
- **Associated Plans and Appendices** cross-reference to other plans and to the appendices and related resources.
- **Additional Nursing Diagnoses** identify other problems that may need to be addressed and integrated into the care.

Nursing diagnoses are derived from the North American Nursing Diagnosis Association (NANDA) system of classification following the 1994 Eleventh National Conference. (See Appendix 1 for NANDA-approved diagnoses.) Collaborative problems are included and may or may not reflect the approved NANDA statements.

Although these guidelines for nursing interventions are specific, they serve only as guidelines for care and do not override or replace safe alternatives based on patient condition or profile, physician order, drug information inserts, agency policy or protocol, position papers, or official standards of care.

In this book, please interpret parents *to mean both parents or a single parent or* guardian.

SECTION I
ANTEPARTUM

Normal Antepartum	**2**
Abortion	**14**
Abruptio Placentae	**20**
Acquired Immunodeficiency Syndrome (AIDS) — Maternal	**24**
Ectopic Pregnancy	**30**
Hydatidiform Mole (Molar Pregnancy)	**34**
Hyperemesis Gravidarum	**37**
Multiple Gestation	**41**
Placenta Previa	**44**
Pregnancy Complicated by Cardiac Disease	**48**
Pregnancy Complicated by Diabetes Mellitus	**53**
Pregnancy-Induced Hypertension	**58**
Premature Rupture of Membranes	**64**
Preterm or Premature Labor	**67**
Prolapsed Umbilical Cord	**71**
Rh Isoimmunization	**74**
Sexually Transmitted Diseases/TORCH	**77**
Vaginal and Urinary Infections	**80**

Normal Antepartum

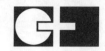

DEFINITION
The antepartum or prenatal period of pregnancy begins with the fertilization of the ovum and ends before the onset of labor. Pregnancy imposes marked anatomic, physiologic, and biochemical changes in the woman. The nurse must be aware of these normal adaptations and be able to differentiate between them and any deviations. This plan of care focuses on identification of the pregnant patient, promotion of health measures to ensure good maternal and fetal outcomes, and prevention and recognition of the discomforts associated with pregnancy.

ETIOLOGY AND PRECIPITATING FACTORS
Conjoining of an ovum and sperm results in fertilization; ovulatory function is one of the requisites and, without contraception, an 85% pregnancy rate will occur within 1 year.

PHYSICAL FINDINGS
Cardiovascular
• arterial blood pressure essentially unchanged from baseline values; slight decrease in diastolic pressure during second trimester
• increased resting pulse of 10 to 15 beats/minute
• shift of apex and apical pulse (point of maximal intensity) upward and 3/8″ to 5/8″ (1.0 to 1.5 cm) left, dependent on degree of uterine displacement; usually heard in fourth rather than fifth intercostal space; ECG reflects displacement along with increased size of cardiac silhouette
• S_1 — exaggerated splitting and loudness
• physiologic S_3
• systolic murmurs that intensify with respiratory activity are commonly observed; soft, diastolic, or continuous murmurs are less commonly observed

Genitourinary
• amenorrhea
• progressive uterine enlargement, with an ultimate 500- to 1,000-fold increase in capacity and eventual dextroversion
• irregular, painless uterine contractions (Braxton Hicks contractions)
• cervical softening, with bluish discoloration
• leukorrhea (profuse, thick white vaginal discharge)
• vaginal discoloration and lengthening
• breast tenderness and tingling; enlargement and nodularity; increased pigmentation of nipple and areola; colostrum secretion near term
• presence of fetal heart tones (FHT), uterine souffle, and funic or umbilical souffle

Integumentary
• chloasma (mask of pregnancy)
• linea nigra from top of fundus to symphysis pubis
• striae gravidarum (stretch marks)
• vascular spiders (nevi)
• palmar erythema
• epulis; bleeding gums

Musculoskeletal
• progressive lordosis
• waddle gait
• integrity of teeth unchanged

Renal
• glycosuria

Respiratory
• respiratory rate essentially unchanged; depth increased
• shortness of breath, near term
• thoracic breathing pattern as pregnancy progresses
• flaring of rib cage and elevated diaphragm as pregnancy progresses
• nasal congestion, occasional epistaxis

Subjective
• "morning sickness"
• fatigue
• increased appetite
• complaints of urinary frequency in first and third trimesters
• backache
• quickening (perception of fetal life)

DIAGNOSTIC STUDIES
• Accurate and complete history and physical examination may render a diagnosis of presumptive, probable, or positive pregnancy.

Laboratory data
• Radioimmunoassay reveals human chorionic gonodotropin in maternal plasma or urine.

EVIDENCE OF PREGNANCY

Presumptive	Probable	Positive
• Amenorrhea • Increased breast size; nodularity; tenderness and tingling; colostrum secretion; increased pigmentation of nipple and areola • Chadwick's sign: blue-purple discoloration of cervix and vaginal mucosa (at 6 weeks) • Increased skin pigmentation; abdominal striae • Subjective accounts of fatigue; "morning sickness"; increased appetite; urinary frequency; quickening	• Progressive increase in uterine size and abdominal palpation by 20 weeks • Progressive uterine shape change from pear to globular to ovoid • Hegar's signs: softening of uterine isthmus (at 6 to 8 weeks) • Goodell's sign: softening of cervix (at 6 to 8 weeks) • Braxton Hicks contractions in second and third trimesters • Ballottement: fetal rebound after release of uterine pressure (at midpregnancy) • Positive pregnancy test (human chorionic gonadotropin present in maternal plasma or urine)	• Fetal heart tones distinct from gravida's at 12 weeks (with Doppler device), at 20 weeks (with fetoscope) • Fetal activity (at 20 weeks) • Sonographic identification (at 5 to 8 weeks) or radiographic identification (after 16 weeks)

Nursing diagnosis: *Anxiety related to anatomic and physiologic changes associated with pregnancy*

GOAL: Minimize anxiety and bolster patient's support systems.

Interventions

1. Introduce self to patient. Refer to her as Ms. if marital status is unknown.

2. Be nonjudgmental. If pregnancy is probable, do not assume it is welcome.

3. Assess progression through psychological tasks of pregnancy.

4. Assess teaching receptivity. Note presence of significant others and allow them to stay with patient before or after examination, according to patient's wishes.

Rationales

1. Establishment of good rapport is essential to a trusting relationship. By assuming patient is married, the nurse implies a personal value that may be destructive to nurse-patient relationship.

2. Reactions to pregnancy vary among prospective mothers and depend on age, parity, marital status, health, financial status, education, culture, ethnic background, and desire for children. Emotional responses to pregnancy may include disbelief, joy, fear, ambivalence, a sense of being intruded upon, egocentrism, introversion, emotional lability, change in decision-making patterns, change in self-image, and altered sexual desires.

3. Tasks include accepting the pregnancy; working through past experiences, expectations, and conflicts related to pregnancy and parenting; working through age-related developmental tasks; and preparing for the practical aspects of parenthood. Progression through tasks may indicate acceptance of pregnancy and readiness for motherhood.

4. Health awareness and teaching assist in preventing or minimizing deviations from normal and in facilitating patient compliance. Incorporation of health teaching facilitates maternal and fetal well-being. Family and friends may reinforce health care information presented.

LANDMARKS IN MEASUREMENT OF FUNDAL HEIGHT

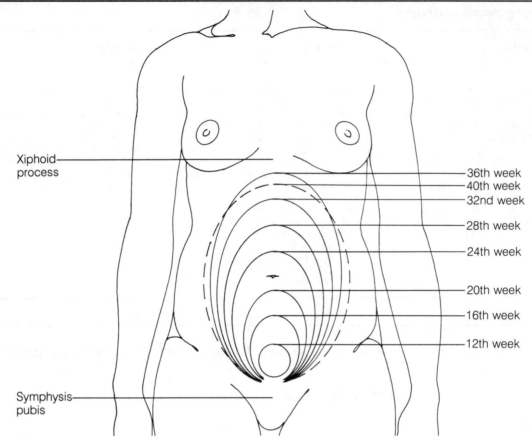

Xiphoid process

36th week
40th week
32nd week
28th week
24th week
20th week
16th week
12th week

Symphysis pubis

Note:
1. Usually, fundal height in centimeters = weeks
2. After week 22, the fundus rises about 1 cm/week
3. Calculation of fundal height during third trimester by McDonald's rule:
   • fundal height (cm) × 2/7 = gestation in lunar months, or
   • fundal height (cm) × 8/7 = gestation in weeks

Interventions

5. Note and document signs and symptoms that suggest past or present sexual or physical abuse:
• bruising anywhere on body
• frequent unexplained or implausible accidents, falls, burns, or fractures; scarring from past incidents
• course of past pregnancies; incidence of spontaneous abortion
• marked resistance to disrobing or undergoing physical examinations and invasive procedures
• ambivalence toward authority figures
• aversion to either all male or all female caregivers
• controlling behaviors regarding all aspects of care
• inability to sleep; nightmares

6. Additional individualized interventions: _____

Rationales

5. Evidence of current abuse warrants referral to appropriate social and psychological services for crisis intervention. Police action might be indicated.
  Pregnancy may trigger suppressed memories of sexual abuse. Confusion about trust, control, authority, self-image, boundary setting, and sexuality are typical. Caregivers must recognize patient's needs, must include patient in decision making, and must allow her to control and direct as much of her care as possible.

6. Rationales: _____

Collaborative problem: *Altered anatomy, physiology, and metabolism related to pregnancy (2 goals)*

GOAL 1: Identify the pregnant patient by alterations imposed by pregnancy, and date the pregnancy.

Interventions

1. Obtain complete history, including obstetric and gynecologic histories.

2. Note regularity of menses, date of last menstrual period (LMP), and use of contraceptives. (See *Evidence of pregnancy,* page 3.) Perform physical examination and correlate data.

3. Estimate the menstrual or gestational age and determine estimated date of confinement (EDC) using Nägele's rule: Add 7 days to the date of the 1st day of the LMP; count back 3 months.

4. Additional individualized interventions: _____

Rationales

1. A complete history and physical examination assist in diagnosis. Amenorrhea and the presumptive and probable signs of pregnancy may suggest various gynecologic or endocrine disorders. Diagnosis is most difficult in early pregnancy, when the uterus is still located in the pelvic cavity. Subsequent examination usually proves more definitive.

2. Estimation of time of ovulation helps determine the time of fertilization and the dating of the pregnancy.

3. Duration of pregnancy is approximately 280 days, 10 lunar months, or 40 weeks. Note that the EDC is only an estimate, and labor may begin 7 to 14 days before or after this date.

4. Rationales: _____

GOAL 2: Promote maternal well-being by identifying alterations of pregnancy.

Interventions

1. Codify the obstetric history, using the four-digit system separated by dashes:
   - digit 1—number of term infants
   - digit 2—number of preterm infants
   - digit 3—number of abortions
   - digit 4—number of living children

For example, 1-1-0-2 would indicate 1 term, 1 preterm, 0 abortions, 2 living children.

2. Coach patient on deep breathing for relaxation during vaginal examination. Have patient void before procedure. Assist with vaginal examination, Papanicolaou smear, and cultures, as indicated. Refer to laboratory for serologic testing.

3. After the 12th week of gestation, assess fundal height. Measure from the superior aspect of the symphysis pubis to the top of the fundus. (See *Landmarks in measurement of fundal height.*)

4. Assess vital signs. Take resting pulse and blood pressure. Allow time for a second reading if patient seems apprehensive or values are outside established norms. Note variations with each visit.

Rationales

1. Various systems may be used, each summarizing the gravida's obstetric history for quick integration into a complete clinical profile.

2. Vaginal examination and testing monitors tissue integrity, presence of lesions, and discharge as well as progressive vaginal and cervical changes associated with pregnancy. In the latter part of pregnancy, another vaginal examination may be performed to estimate pelvic size, capacity, and adequacy.

3. Increasing fundal height indicates advancing pregnancy and fetal growth. Greater than normal height may be attributed to full rectum (bladder should be emptied before examination), multiple pregnancy, obesity, hydramnios, or myomata; less than normal height, to lack of certainty about LMP or to intrauterine growth retardation.

4. Higher values may be attributed to sympathetic reflex action. An accurate resting value is critical in establishing baseline norms and evaluating adaptations associated with pregnancy or maladaption associated with pregnancy-induced hypertension (PIH) or chronic hypertension.

DISCOMFORTS OF PREGNANCY AND THEIR MANAGEMENT

Problem	Management
Nausea and vomiting ("morning sickness")	• Avoid foods that specifically aggravate problem. • Keep dry crackers or other dry carbohydrates at bedside and eat several before arising. • Eat six small meals a day; alternate meal with no liquid with one that is only liquid. • Drink liquids 30 minutes after eating solids. • Avoid greasy, fried, highly spiced, or gas-forming foods. • Avoid eating or preparing highly aromatic foods.
Heartburn	• Take sips of milk over 15-minute period. • Eat smaller meals more frequently. • Avoid greasy, gas-producing foods or those that specifically aggravate symptom. • Avoid lying down after eating; change position if symptom occurs. • Chew gum. • Take low-sodium antacids as a last resort and only if prescribed; do not take any sodium bicarbonate or over-the-counter medicines.
Breast tenderness	• Wear support bra day and night.
Backache	• Avoid excessive or undue lifting, bending, or walking. • Use good body mechanics and perform pelvic tilt exercises regularly.
Leg cramps (muscle spasm)	• Have physician evaluate to rule out phlebitis or thrombosis. • Take adequate dietary calcium or calcium supplementation. • Wear adequate clothing to prevent chilling extremities. • Apply heat to affected muscle. • Exercise regularly, especially with knee flexion and foot dorsiflexion to stretch affected muscle.
Varicosities	• Avoid prolonged standing, sitting, or crossing legs at knee. • Avoid constrictive clothing (such as garters). • Take periodic rests with legs elevated. • Wear elastic stockings.
Foot and ankle edema	• Have regular evaluations to rule out edema of hands, face, or body. • Avoid prolonged standing or sitting and constricting clothing. • Rest in left side-lying position.
Shortness of breath	• For symptoms of malignant cardiovascular or pulmonary disorders, contact physician. • Recognize that shortness of breath is normal during pregnancy. • Maintain good posture. • Use extra pillows in bed. • Avoid large meals.
Vertigo	• Avoid prolonged standing or walking; avoid undue fatigue. • Change position slowly and deliberately. • Eat regular, well-balanced meals.
Constipation	• Ensure adequate hydration and dietary fiber. • Take moderate exercise. • Defecate when urge presents itself. • Schedule for daily bowel movements. • Do not use laxatives, cathartics, or enemas.
Hemorrhoids	• Prevent constipation. • Take warm soaks or sitz or tub baths. • Use local anesthetizing agents. • Manually reinsert protruding hemorrhoids into rectum.

MATERNAL IMPLICATIONS OF CHEMICAL SUBSTANCE USE DURING PREGNANCY

The pregnant patient who uses chemical substances is at risk for a wide range of problems. Drug dilutants and impurities may compound the negative effects of chemical substance use.

Habitual use of chemical substances may be hard to assess; the patient may deny the practice and give an inaccurate or distorted history. Attempts to dissuade a patient from using chemical substances may prove futile and may even cause her to spurn prenatal care.

This chart describes the possible consequences of chemical substance use during pregnancy. Although it addresses only single-substance use, the nurse should keep in mind that multiple-substance use is common. (For fetal and neonatal problems linked with maternal substance use, see Appendix 3: Selected Substances and Fetal Abnormalities.)

Substance	Possible maternal outcome
Alcohol	Spontaneous abortion
Cocaine	Spontaneous abortion, abruptio placentae, preterm or precipitous delivery, stillbirth, sudden death, arrhythmias, myocardial infarction, aortic rupture, cerebrovascular accident, seizures, bowel ischemia, hyperthermia
Opioids	Bacteremia, endocarditis, phlebitis, cellulitis, pneumonia, tetanus, hepatitis, human immunodeficiency virus infection (with I.V. injection)
Tobacco	Spontaneous abortion, abruptio placentae, placenta previa, premature or prolonged rupture of membranes, amnionitis (dose related)

Interventions

5. Aid in laboratory tests as follows:

• Perform finger stick for hemoglobin (Hb) measurement.

• Obtain clean-catch urine specimen for dipstick analysis. Test for glucose, protein, and nitrites.

6. Note weight: actual, ideal, and changes. Monitor for edema and differentiate between benign, dependent, and pathologic types. Chart prepregnant weight and height.

7. Schedule subsequent visits as follows:
• each month for first 7 months
• every 2 weeks for month 8
• every week thereafter until delivery.
Continue to note vital signs, weight, and fundal height. Modify schedule according to patient condition. (See *Discomforts of pregnancy and their management.*)

8. Additional individualized interventions: _____

Rationales

5. Laboratory test results help establish baseline values and allow for ongoing monitoring.

• Hb values of 12 to 16 g/dl are consistent with adequate circulatory volume and iron stores. Anemia is defined as an Hb value below 11 g/dl during the first and third trimesters and an Hb value below 10.5 g/dl during the second trimester. Anemia in pregnancy is associated most commonly with iron deficiency and acute blood loss.

• Mild glycosuria is usually benign; patients with an elevated glucose level or a familial history of diabetes may require further testing because pregnancy is diabetogenic. Proteinuria of +1 or greater is associated with PIH and needs to be investigated further. Sudden weight gain of more than 2 lb/week and significant blood pressure elevation usually precede proteinuria in the classic triad of symptoms. Nitrites may indicate infection.

6. A progressive weight gain of 25 lb or more is expected and indicates maternal adaptation and well-being. Failure to gain weight is associated with poor fetal outcome; sudden gain, with PIH. Careful assessment is essential in distinguishing true weight gain from fluid retention.

7. Systematic appraisal of anticipated changes of pregnancy is necessary to monitor adaptation.

8. Rationales: _____

Nursing diagnosis: *High risk for fetal injury related to dependence on maternal well-being and genetic and environmental factors*

GOAL: Prevent or minimize injury.

Interventions

1. Include a high-risk profile in maternal history, noting:
• maternal weight less than 100 lb (45 kg) or 20% greater than desired body weight; pregnant weight gain less than 15 lb (6.8 kg) or greater than 35 lb (15.8 kg)
• medical history of hypertension, diabetes, cardiovascular disorders, infectious and childhood diseases, and Rh and ABO incompatibilities with partner
• familial history of genetic disorders
• obstetric history of anemia, bleeding, protracted or precipitous labors, preterm deliveries, delivery of macrosomic infant, deliveries by cesarean or extraction, and compromised fetal outcome
• unhealthy life-style patterns, including multiple sexual partners or use of caffeine, nicotine, alcohol, or over-the-counter, prescribed, or illicit drugs (see *Maternal implications of chemical substance use during pregnancy,* page 7, and Appendix 3: Selected Substances and Fetal Abnormalities).
• family history of relationship dysfunction, abuse, or financial instability.

2. Note the patient's age:
• under age 18

• over age 35.

Rationales

1. A high-risk profile assists in prevention, early recognition, or reversal of problems and improvement of maternal condition and fetal outcome.

2. Age can affect fetal outcome.

• Increased adolescent fertility crosses all social, economic, and racial lines. Obstetric risks during early adolescence (ages 11 to 15) result from physiologic immaturity. Obstetric risks during late adolescence (ages 16 to 18) are associated with social factors and life-style choices, such as poor nutrition, smoking, alcohol and drug abuse, and sexually transmitted diseases. Teenage gravidas are at high risk for anemia, pre-eclampsia, and term or preterm low-birth-weight infants. Their offspring have an increased incidence of infections, accidents, cognitive defects, and behavioral problems. Failure of the adolescent patient to progress through psychosocial development tasks of adolescence commonly perpetuates the cycle—and consequences—of early pregnancy and childbirth.

• Changing women's roles, technological progress, more effective contraception, and economic imperatives have resulted in delayed childbearing for many women. The older pregnant patient is at increased risk for chronic hypertension, gestational or Type II (non-insulin-dependent) diabetes mellitus, placental accidents, and various medical and surgical conditions. These chronic, age-related conditions antedate the pregnancy and may affect it profoundly. Other risks for these women include ectopic pregnancy, spontaneous abortion, preterm labor, prolonged labor (especially in the nullipara), and preterm delivery. Implications for offspring include chromosomal anomalies, congenital malformations, low birth weight, and macrosomia. Also, perinatal mortality is increased. However, maternal and fetal outcomes are good if the older patient has no underlying chronic disease and receives prenatal care that includes genetic counseling, prenatal diagnosis, and tests for fetal well-being.

Interventions

3. Review immunization record, including rubella, measles, mumps, cholera, influenza, plague, typhoid, diphtheria, and tetanus.

4. Continue assessment of fundal height.

5. Assess fetal heart tones (FHT).

6. Assess fetal movement; query patient about frequency and intensity of fetal activity.

7. Review family pedigree, including ethnic, racial, and geographic factors. Correlate with maternal age. Assess need for maternal serum alpha-fetoprotein (MSAFP) screening.

8. Additional individualized interventions: _____

Rationales

3. Rubella vaccine is contraindicated in pregnancy because of its teratogenicity; lack of immunization necessitates immunization in immediate postpartum period; immunization for measles or mumps is also contraindicated. Diphtheria and tetanus toxoids may be given if no primary series was given or no booster was given within 10 years. Immunizations for cholera, influenza, plague, or typhoid are given to the patient at risk.

4. Increasing fundal height indicates uterine and fetal growth and may imply fetal well-being.

5. FHTs can be detected at 20 weeks' gestation with a fetoscope and as early as 12 weeks' gestation with a Doppler ultrasound device.

6. Fetal activity is perceived by patient at 20 weeks. Movements are sporadic and increase with maternal activity; they become significant when a marked change in frequency occurs (no fetal movement usually portends disappearance of FHT within 24 hours).

7. MSAFP determination is the most common initial prenatal screening test for inherited disorders. Ideally, it should be performed between weeks 15 and 18 of pregnancy. Elevated MSAFP levels are associated with neural tube defects and other anomalies typified by fetal edema or skin defects, underestimated gestational age, multiple gestation, decreased maternal weight, and fetal death. Low MSAFP levels are associated with chromosomal trisomies, increased maternal weight, overestimated gestational age, gestational trophoblastic disease, and fetal death.

8. Rationales: _____

Nursing diagnosis: *Altered nutrition: less than body requirements secondary to increased needs of pregnancy (2 goals)*

GOAL 1: Identify maternal nutritional status.

Interventions

1. Assess height, weight, and frame and compare with standardized charts for normal weight ranges. Note changes.

2. Perform a gross physical examination, including assessment of hair, nails, skin, eyes, and neuromuscular system.

Rationales

1. Assessment establishes baseline information and deviation from norm. Women whose weight is appropriate for height and frame should have a progressive gain of 25 to 35 lbs (11.5 to 16 kg) to support maternal changes and fetal growth. Underweight women may gain up to 40 lbs (18 kg); heavier or obese women should limit weight gain to 15 to 25 lbs (7 to 11.5 kg). Appropriate maternal weight gain is necessary for optimal fetal growth and development.

2. The well-nourished person exhibits shiny hair that is not easily plucked; firm, nonbrittle nails; smooth skin without lesions, rashes, or edema; bright, clear, shiny eyes with pink, moist membranes; and intact muscle innervation, tactile senses, and ability to perform activities of daily living without difficulty.

Interventions

3. Take a 24-hour diet recall, noting portion size, method of food preparation, ethnic preferences, food availability, food cravings, or unusual food habits (such as pica, a craving for dirt, starch, or other nonnutritive substances).

4. Additional individualized interventions: _____

Rationales

3. Recall identifies nutritional strengths and weaknesses. Teaching the patient about necessary changes and including her suggestions in menu changes facilitate compliance. Food cravings are usually benign and may be indulged if they do not interfere with or replace a well-balanced diet. Pica represents an aberration and requires treatment.

4. Rationales: _____

GOAL 2: Promote a well-balanced diet.

Interventions

1. Provide oral and written information on daily dietary requirements, using the food pyramid as a guide to food choices:
• bread, cereal, rice, and pasta group: 6 to 11 servings
• vegetable group: 3 to 5 servings
• fruit group: 2 to 4 servings
• milk, yogurt, and cheese group: 2 to 3 servings
• meat, poultry, fish, dry beans, egg, and nut group: 2 to 3 servings
• added sugars and naturally occurring and added fats and oils: use sparingly.

2. Advise against weight-reduction diets.

3. Advise patient to supplement diet with simple iron salts.

4. Advise patient to take vitamin-mineral supplements as indicated.

5. Advise patient to take folic acid supplements as indicated.

Rationales

1. Within ranges shown, gravida's diet should be increased to meet the additional dietary requirements of pregnancy. (See Appendix 2, Selected Daily Dietary Allowances—Maternal.) Increases should be based on caloric requirements. Generally, pregnant women require an additional 250 to 500 calories/day. Many of these calories should come from protein (preferably from animal sources). Increased servings from the milk, yogurt, and cheese group provide additional required amounts of vitamin D, calcium, and phosphorous as well as calories. Pregnant women should be encouraged to consume fresh fruits, vegetables, and other high-fiber foods.

2. Failure to gain 15 or more pounds is associated with catabolism of maternal tissue to provide for fetal growth and maternal accessory tissue. Weight gain is accounted for as follows:
• fetus: 7½ lb (3.4 kg)
• placenta: 1½ lb (0.7 kg)
• amniotic fluid: 1 lb (0.45 kg)
• uterine growth: 2½ lb (1.13 kg)
• increased blood volume: 3½ lb (1.6 kg)
• increased breast tissue: 2 lb (0.9 kg).

3. Even with a well-balanced diet, insufficient iron stores and the limited iron content of the typical diet necessitate supplementation to meet the increased needs of pregnancy. Pregnant women should take 30 to 60 mg of iron salts daily—preferably after the fourth month, when needs increase and the GI discomforts of early pregnancy have subsided.

4. Adolescents, vegetarians, women with multiple-gestation pregnancies, heavy smokers, and chemical substance abusers may have inadequate nutritional intake and may benefit from vitamin-mineral supplements.

5. Folic acid supplementation before conception is associated with reduced incidence of neural tube defects. Such supplementation is recommended for gravidas who have had offspring with spina bifida, anencephaly, or encephalocele. The Centers for Disease Control and Prevention (CDC) recommends that pregnant women take 4 mg of folic acid daily, starting 1 month before conception and continuing for the first 3 months of pregnancy. The CDC recommends 0.4 mg of folic acid daily for all fertile women.

Interventions

6. Assess patient's alcohol intake. Discourage alcohol consumption.

7. Additional individualized interventions: _____

_____

Rationales

6. Alcohol provides "empty" calories. No level of drinking during pregnancy is known to be safe; adverse fetal effects of maternal alcohol consumption may be profound.

7. Rationales: _____

_____

Nursing diagnosis: *Activity intolerance, possibly related to increasing hormone levels and to demands of pregnancy*

GOAL: Prevent or minimize activity intolerance and promote adequate rest.

Interventions

1. Assess sleep and rest patterns, home responsibilities, and employment status. Review hemoglobin and hematocrit values.

2. Offer advice about the need for adequate sleep and rest, including:
• 8 hours of uninterrupted sleep per day, plus one nap
• scheduled rest period at place of employment during each break
• napping at home while preschoolers are sleeping.

3. Advise that no restrictions on activity or travel are necessary.

4. Encourage exercise, including pelvic lifting or rocking, modified sit-ups, tailor-fashion sitting, and Kegel exercises.

5. As pregnancy progresses, advise changing position slowly and deliberately, and resting or sleeping on left side.

6. Additional individualized interventions: _____

_____

Rationales

1. Assessment provides baseline data and factors that may affect promotion of rest.

2. While the symptoms of fatigue cannot be prevented, its occurrence can be minimized.

3. Only activities of daily living that cause undue fatigue or possible risk to the fetus need to be altered.

4. These exercises promote muscle tone in preparation for delivery and more rapid return to prepregnant physical state.

5. Changing position slowly minimizes vertigo and risk of falls. Left-lying position reduces aortic compression and facilitates uteroplacental flow.

6. Rationales: _____

_____

Nursing diagnosis: *High risk for maternal urinary tract infection, possibly related to urinary stasis and silent bacteriuria*

GOAL: Prevent or minimize potential for infection.

Interventions

1. Assess for urinary frequency, urgency, dysuria, and hematuria. Perform urine examination by dipstick.

2. Offer the following advice about hygienic and prophylactic practices and about elimination:
• Maintain adequate hydration.

Rationales

1. Urinary frequency in the first and third trimesters is associated with the weight of the gravid uterus on the urinary bladder. The other symptoms are highly suggestive of infection and should be referred to physician.

2. These measures assist in prophylaxis:

• Adequate hydration keeps urine dilute and any possible colony count low.

Interventions

- Void when urge presents itself.
- Wipe from front to back after elimination.
- Wash hands after elimination.

3. Additional individualized interventions: _____

Rationales

- This minimizes stasis and possible colonization.
- This minimizes contamination by *Escherichia coli.*
- This minimizes contaminants and their spread.

3. Rationales: _____

Nursing diagnosis: *Altered sexuality patterns related to fatigue, genital changes, or fear of fetal injury*

GOAL: Provide information that will assist patient in maintaining normal sexual relations.

Interventions

1. Advise patient about sexual activity, including the following:
- Fatigue and breast tenderness in the first trimester, and abdominal bulk and fatigue in the third, may diminish sexual responsiveness.
- Intercourse need not be restricted unless membranes have ruptured or abortion, preterm labor, or bleeding threaten. (Note: Some practitioners advise against coitus during last month of pregnancy.)
- Sexual responsiveness is usually highest during the second trimester, when the discomforts of pregnancy are lowest.
- Changes in coital position may be necessary to accommodate the enlarged abdomen.

2. Assess for leukorrhea. Advise washing with mild soap and water after toileting. Douching is prohibited.

3. Additional individualized interventions: _____

Rationales

1. Physiologic response to pregnancy and perceptions concerning pregnancy may alter responsiveness and spontaneity. These feelings are normal and usually self-limiting; sexual activity is not associated with fetal injury.

2. Copious vaginal secretions are common and benign in pregnancy; their presence may inhibit sexual interest. Douching is associated with air embolism and ascending genital tract infection.

3. Rationales: _____

Nursing diagnosis: *Knowledge deficit related to normal pregnancy*

GOAL: Provide information to educate patient.

Interventions

1. Assess patient's knowledge of normal pregnancy, noting patient's age, previous experience, parity, marital status, and cultural expectations.

2. Present information on normal pregnancy sequentially with each visit. Provide pictures of fetal growth. Reinforce earlier teaching on health maintenance and allow time for questions.

3. Advise patient of danger signs that should be reported immediately, including vaginal bleeding, abdominal pain, edema of hands or fingers, persistent or severe headache, visual disturbances, persistent emesis, chills, pyrexia, dysuria, dyspnea, and significant change in fetal activity.

Rationales

1. This information provides a baseline for nursing action and teaching.

2. Sequential presentation allows patient time to internalize and synthesize information.

3. Each sign or symptom is highly suggestive of severe dysfunction.

Interventions

4. Demonstrate breast preparation for patients who plan to breast-feed.

5. Advise patient concerning birthing and anesthesia options.

6. Refer patient to childbirth preparation classes.

7. Teach patient signs of impending labor and criteria for going to hospital:
• rupture of membranes
• contractions in abdomen and back, regular, 5 to 10 minutes apart, and increasing in intensity and duration.

8. Additional individualized interventions: _____

_____

Rationales

4. Teaching the patient these techniques facilitates breast-feeding without discomfort or anxiety.

5. This incorporates the patient into the health care team, allows time for informed decision-making, and gives the patient a sense of control.

6. These classes involve the parents in the birthing and parenting processes (see Appendix 13: Parent Teaching Guides).
7. This information enables the patient to recognize the signs of labor and make an informed decision before taking action.

8. Rationales: _____

_____

ASSOCIATED APPENDICES
• Selected Daily Dietary Allowances—Maternal (Appendix 2)
• Selected Substances and Fetal Abnormalities (Appendix 3)
• Aspects of Psychological Care—Maternal (Appendix 4)
• The Family and Home Assessment (Appendix 7)

ADDITIONAL NURSING DIAGNOSES
• Constipation related to decreased peristalsis and increased water and electrolyte absorption
• High risk for fetal poisoning or trauma related to maternal use of nicotine or intoxicants
• Sleep pattern disturbance related to change in body size and contour

Abortion

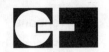

DEFINITION
Abortion is the spontaneous or induced loss of the products of conception before the occurrence of fetal viability, measured as a gestational age of less than 20 weeks or a fetal weight of 500 grams or less. Abortions occurring before the 12th week of gestation are termed early; those between the 12th and 20th week, late. This distinction is necessary because anatomic and physiologic changes in the latter weeks of gestation make treatment more difficult. Spontaneous abortions are classified as threatened, inevitable, missed, incomplete, complete, habitual, and septic. Septic abortion is more commonly—though not exclusively—associated with self-induced instrumentation. Complications include hemorrhage, septic or endotoxic shock, acute renal failure, and death.

ETIOLOGY AND PRECIPITATING FACTORS
• First-trimester abortions are associated with embryonic, fetal, or placental abnormalities caused by congenital or genetic defects and by alterations in the intrauterine environment caused by endocrine imbalance or exposure to teratogens.
• Second-trimester abortions are associated more with maternal problems, such as infection, endocrine dysfunction, severe malnutrition, drug ingestion (including alcohol or tobacco), manipulation of or abnormalities of the reproductive viscera, and possibly Rh isoimmunization and blood group incompatibility between mates. The role of physical and emotional trauma is suspect.

PHYSICAL FINDINGS
Cardiovascular
• tachycardia
• tachypnea
• hypotension
• restlessness
• pyrexia

Genitourinary
• Threatened
  □ protracted vaginal spotting or slight bleeding for days or weeks
  □ mild, menstrual-like cramps or low backache
  □ closed cervix
  □ no passage of tissue
  □ uterine size congruent with length of pregnancy
• Inevitable
  □ moderate vaginal bleeding; passage of clots
  □ uterine contractions, pain
  □ dilated cervix
  □ ruptured membranes
  □ uterine size congruent with length of pregnancy

• Incomplete
  □ profuse, bright red vaginal bleeding
  □ severe uterine cramping
  □ dilated cervix
  □ partial or full placental retention in utero; passage of some placental tissue
  □ uterine size smaller than warranted by length of pregnancy
• Complete
  □ possible scant vaginal bleeding
  □ possible mild menstrual-like cramps
  □ passage of fetus, membranes, and placenta
  □ closed cervix after passage
  □ uterine size smaller than warranted by length of pregnancy
• Septic
  □ possible vaginal or cervical lacerations or puncture wounds; gross trauma
  □ possible bleeding; foul-smelling, purulent vaginal discharge
  □ possible uterine cramping or tenderness
  □ cervical pain on palpation
  □ possible dilated cervix
  □ uterine size smaller than warranted by length of pregnancy; possibly larger in cases of pronounced infectious process

DIAGNOSTIC STUDIES
• Accurate and complete history and physical examination, including pelvic examination, may furnish enough data for a definitive diagnosis.
• Sonography identifies poorly formed or absent gestational sac in impending abortion, uterine abnormalities, and placental location and abnormalities; it also confirms presence or absence of fetal viability.

Laboratory data
• Urine pregnancy test—negative or weakly positive.
• Hemoglobin (Hb) and hematocrit (HCT) values—generally decrease.
• White blood cell (WBC) count—increases, most often in complete and septic abortions.
• Blood and urine cultures—positive anaerobic or aerobic in septic abortion.
• Tissue cytology—may confirm fetal or placental tissue.

Nursing diagnosis: *High risk for injury related to pregnancy termination caused by maternal or fetal abnormality (3 goals)*

GOAL 1: Recognize signs of threatened abortion.

Interventions

1. Monitor for signs of threatened abortion. Begin by determining date of last menstrual period (LMP), estimation of gestational age, and pregnancy test results. Then assess for the following:
• vaginal bleeding or spotting
• menstrual-like cramping or low backache, notably after onset of bleeding.

2. Prepare patient for ultrasonography, as ordered. Tell the patient the following:

• Do not void before examination.

• Withhold fluids before examination.

3. Additional individualized interventions: _____

Rationales

1. Identifying LMP assists in confirming and dating pregnancy. Positive pregnancy test may assist in confirmation of diagnosis. Painless vaginal spotting or bleeding in early pregnancy is common. Fewer than half these patients abort. Pain accompanying bleeding has a poorer prognosis.

2. Ultrasonography assists in determining placental site and integrity, stage of abortion, and possible fetal viability.
• The distended bladder pushes the uterus out of the pelvis and facilitates imaging.
• Although fluids assist in urine production, food and fluids are usually withheld from patient in anticipation of possible surgery.

3. Rationales: _____

GOAL 2: Recognize early signs of cervical incompetence and minimize its sequelae.

Interventions

1. Monitor for early cervical incompetence, including:
• history of cervical trauma
• dilatation of cervical os in second, possibly early third, trimester
• absence of pain
• in utero exposure to diethylstilbestrol
• repeated, unexplained late-term abortions or preterm deliveries.

2. Additional individualized interventions: _____

Rationales

1. Should cervical incompetence be identified, surgical reinforcement of the weakened cervix can be performed if dilation is less than 4 cm.

2. Rationales: _____

GOAL 3: Prevent or minimize the risk of progression of abortion.

Interventions

1. Assess for current use of intrauterine device (IUD); assist physician in its removal.

2. Instruct the patient about at-home medical regimen, including:
• bed rest
• no sexual intercourse, douching, or cathartics
• need to communicate persistent or increased bleeding or cramping to appropriate health care personnel.

3. Additional individualized interventions: _____

Rationales

1. If tail of the IUD is visible, removal may be medically indicated to lessen the risk of late abortion, infection, and prematurity.

2. Bed rest, associated with decreased bleeding and cramping, and abstinence are the only effective measures to minimize or prevent progression of abortion. Increasingly severe symptoms warrant hospitalization and medical intervention.

3. Rationales: _____

Collaborative problem: *High risk for fluid volume deficit related to hemorrhage (2 goals)*

GOAL 1: Identify signs of increased bleeding.

Interventions

1. Assess patient for bleeding—every hour, or as patient's condition warrants:

• Note vaginal bleeding: color, number of perineal pads used, degree of saturation, and weight; bleeding accompanied by gushes of fluid.

• Note passage of large or numerous clots, tissue; save all tissue passed.

• Watch patient for signs of restlessness, tachycardia, hypotension, diaphoresis, or pallor.

2. Monitor Hb and hematocrit (HCT) values.

3. Additional individualized interventions: _____

Rationales

1. In an incomplete abortion, partially retained placental tissue impedes uterine contraction and results in profuse bleeding. Severe hypovolemia may develop quickly.

• Accurate assessment helps evaluate blood loss. (*Note:* one saturated pad represents 100 ml blood loss.)

• Examination of tissue assists in staging abortion. In complete abortion, abortus and full placenta have been passed.

• Deterioration into hemorrhagic shock warrants rapid intervention to reverse the process.

2. Decreasing Hb and HCT values are consistent with blood loss and provide a data base for blood replacement needs.

3. Rationales: _____

GOAL 2: Restore and maintain normovolemia.

Interventions

1. Monitor patient's vital signs as condition warrants.

2. Monitor blood study trends, including Hb and HCT values, and coagulation profile.

3. Type and crossmatch for two units of blood, as ordered.

4. Administer whole blood, packed red blood cells, or clotting factors, as ordered.

5. Monitor fluid intake and output.

6. Administer oxytocin drip, as ordered. Monitor vital signs, fluid intake and output, and uterine contractions. Administer analgesics.

7. Prepare the patient for surgery.

8. Additional individualized interventions: _____

Rationales

1. Increasing pulse and falling blood pressure indicate continuing blood loss.

2. Clinical and laboratory profiles assist in evaluating patient need, status, and effectiveness of treatment.

3. Procedure ensures blood supply for immediate use.

4. Replacement of blood or blood products may be necessary to restore adequate volume.

5. Output reflects renal perfusion.

6. Oxytocin is indicated in inevitable, incomplete, or missed abortions; the drug stimulates uterine contraction and facilitates complete expulsion of the products of conception. *Note:* Discontinue drug if tetanic uterine contractions occur.

7. Surgical dilatation and curettage are indicated if complete passage of abortus and placenta have not been ascertained. Inevitable or incomplete abortions warrant complete evacuation of products of conception.

8. Rationales: _____

Collaborative problem: *High risk for infection related to incomplete or self-induced abortion*

GOAL: Recognize signs of infection.

Interventions	Rationales
1. Monitor for signs of infection, including: • fever more than 100.4° F (38° C) and chills; foul, purulent vaginal discharge • constant low back, pelvic, or abdominal pain and elevated WBC count.	1. Instrumentation, in self-induced abortions, or the retained products of conception may cause metritis, parametritis, or peritonitis. Profound sepsis, bacterial shock, acute renal failure, and death may occur if the condition goes unchecked.
2. Administer tetanus toxoid if patient has been previously immunized or tetanus immune globulin (human) to inadequately immunized patient.	2. Protection against the *Clostridium tetani* anaerobe is indicated in suspected or confirmed self-induced abortion.
3. Obtain anaerobic and aerobic blood cultures, including smear for Gram stain from cervix or products of conception, if feasible.	3. Laboratory data identifies causative organisms.
4. Screen patient for drug allergies. Administer broad-spectrum antibiotics after cultures are obtained.	4. Antibiotics may be given prophylactically if suspicion of self-induction exists. In confirmed septic abortion, drug therapy is initiated to combat infection.
5. Prepare the patient for surgery.	5. Complete evacuation of uterine contents is necessary to rid the infection source.
6. Additional individualized interventions: _____	6. Rationales: _____

Collaborative problem: *High risk for maternal injury related to fetal autolysis or Rh isoimmunization (2 goals)*

GOAL 1: Prevent Rh isoimmunization.

Interventions	Rationales
1. Note blood Rh factor of patient and mate.	1. Rh-negative, nonsensitized patients with Rh-positive mates are candidates for treatment.
2. Administer $Rh_o(D)$ immune globulin (RhoGAM) within 72 hours of abortion.	2. If the Rh of the products of conception is positive or unknown, RhoGAM must be given to prevent maternal isoimmunization.
3. Additional individualized interventions: _____	3. Rationales: _____

GOAL 2: Recognize the signs of coagulopathy.

Interventions	Rationales
1. Monitor for signs of fetal death in first half of pregnancy, including: • history of normal early pregnancy: amenorrhea, possible nausea and vomiting, breast changes, and uterine enlargement • possible subsequent vaginal bleeding • lack of change or decrease in uterine size • mammary regression to prepregnant state; weight loss.	1. The majority of missed abortions terminate spontaneously and follow the sequence of any other spontaneous abortion.

Interventions	Rationales
2. Monitor for coagulopathy, including: • multisite bleeding, including frank bleeding from slight trauma, ecchymoses, petechiae, hematomas, or bleeding from mucous membranes • prothrombin time greater than 15 seconds (may vary widely) • partial thromboplastin time greater than 60 seconds (may vary widely) • fibrinogen levels less than 150 mg/dl • platelet count less than 100,000/mm³ • fibrin degradation products greater than 100 mcg/ml.	2. Prolonged retention of a dead fetus results in the release of thromboplastins, which may cause disseminated intravascular coagulation. Correction is directed at control of the defect by possible heparin infusion, followed by surgical intervention.
3. Prepare the patient for surgery.	3. Uterine evacuation of the retained dead products of conception is necessary.
4. Additional individualized interventions: _____	4. Rationales: _____

Nursing diagnosis: *Pain related to uterine contractions*

GOAL: Decrease or minimize pain.

Interventions	Rationales
1. Establish rapport with patient and significant others. Call patient by preferred name. Do not leave patient unattended for long periods of time.	1. A positive relationship facilitates trust and decreases anxiety. Regressive behaviors, anger, resistance, or noncompliance may thereby decrease.
2. Assess for pain and its characteristics, including quality, frequency, location, and intensity.	2. Pain profile may indicate late staging of incomplete or inevitable abortion.
3. Minimize distracting environmental stimuli.	3. External stimuli may increase pain perception.
4. Perform comfort measures, including position changes, relaxation techniques, rubdowns, and pharmacologic analgesia.	4. Increased tissue perfusion plus stimulation of large afferent, sensory fibers decrease sensation or perception of pain.
5. Additional individualized interventions: _____	5. Rationales: _____

Nursing diagnosis: *Anxiety related to pregnancy outcome and to uncertainty of future pregnancies*

GOAL: Reduce or minimize anxiety.

Interventions	Rationales
1. Accept the patient's reaction to the loss.	1. Silence, anger, bewilderment, denial, and regressive behaviors are possible reactions. Allowing the patient to act out facilitates her coping mechanisms and grief resolution.
2. Provide information in a clear, forthright manner. Include, as appropriate in spontaneous abortions, the implications of the following information: Incompetent cervix is characterized by repeated spontaneous abortion. Habitual abortion is defined as three or more successive abortions.	2. Providing understandable information will help reduce patient's anxiety about her condition.

Interventions

- Surgical repair of an incompetent cervix has a very high success rate (85% to 90%).

- Death of the embryo in very early pregnancy occurs before spontaneous abortion.
- Early abortions are commonly associated with chromosomal abnormalities.
- Risk of future abortions is only slightly higher than for the population as a whole.

- Late abortions are associated with maternal abnormalities.

- Resumption of ovulation occurs from as early as 2 weeks postabortion.

3. Additional individualized interventions: _____

_____

Rationales

- The high success of this treatment option may decrease anxiety.

- Anxiety and guilt feelings associated with surgical uterine evacuation may be reduced or eliminated.
- This assures the patient that she is not at fault for having "caused" the abortion.
- The likelihood of a positive pregnancy outcome may offer hope and decrease anxiety during an emotionally devastating period.
- Extensive history, hormonal assessment, endometrial biopsy, and hysterosalpingography of the woman and karyotyping of both parents may identify the cause of habitual abortions.
- Many physicians recommend delaying future pregnancies until two or three normal menstrual cycles have occurred. Contraceptive information is critical in cases of self-induced or selected therapeutic abortions.

3. Rationales: _____

_____

Nursing diagnosis: *Spiritual distress related to pregnancy outcome*

GOAL: Reduce or minimize distress.

Interventions

1. Accept patient's response to loss in a calm, nonjudgmental manner.

2. Arrange for baptism of the dead fetus, if requested.

3. Provide patient and partner with referral to religious or counseling services.

4. Additional individualized interventions: _____

_____

Rationales

1. Self-blame is frequently associated with abortion, whether spontaneous or induced.

2. Acknowledging religious beliefs and facilitating religious rites may offer consolation.

3. Dysfunctional grieving, impaired family relationships, and severe depression may require professional counseling.

4. Rationales: _____

_____

ASSOCIATED PLANS AND APPENDICES
- Normal Antepartum
- Preparing for Nonemergency Surgery (Appendix 5)
- Selected Methods of Family Planning (Appendix 6)

ADDITIONAL NURSING DIAGNOSES
- Altered sexuality patterns related to required pregnancy postponement
- Ineffective individual coping related to repeated loss of a desired pregnancy
- Powerlessness related to undiagnosed cause of habitual loss of a desired pregnancy

Abruptio Placentae

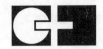

DEFINITION
Abruptio placentae is the premature separation of the placenta from the uterus before fetus delivery. Premature separation of the normally implanted placenta usually occurs in the third trimester, with possible occurrence ranging from 20 to 28 weeks' gestation to second-stage labor. Severity ranges from marginal separation to life-threatening, complete detachment. Presenting symptoms are in proportion to the degree of separation and to the amount of maternal blood lost. Minimal vaginal bleeding, associated with mild separation, accompanied by strong fetal heart tones (FHT) of normal rate and rhythm may be treated conservatively with bed rest. Marked detachment may result in fetal distress, irreversible neurologic damage, or fetal death. Maternal complications include hemorrhage and shock, hypofibrinogenemia, disseminated intravascular coagulation (DIC), renal failure, Couvelaire uterus (uteroplacental apoplexy), and death.

ETIOLOGY AND PRECIPITATING FACTORS
• Etiology unknown
• Patient at risk: maternal age greater than 35, parity of 5 or greater, history of chronic or pregnancy-induced hypertension, previous abruptio placentae, diabetes, vascular or renal disease, inferior vena cava compression, abdominal trauma, uterine anomaly or tumor, sudden decompression of uterus (after amniotomy in hydramnios or delivery of first twin), history of smoking, or shortened umbilical cord.

PHYSICAL FINDINGS
Cardiovascular
• tachycardia
• hypotension
• vertigo
• syncope
• diaphoresis
• pallor
• cyanosis

Genitourinary
• uterine tenderness or tension ranging from absent to minimal to boardlike (dependent on degree of separation)
• vaginal bleeding ranging from none to scant to profuse, dark red in color
• increased uterine size
• increased uterine tone
• proteinuria (in severe abruptio placentae)
• oliguria or anuria
• high to engaged presenting part

Integumentary
• cold, moist skin
• dry mucous membranes

Neurologic
• lethargy
• confusion
• somnolence

Respiratory
• tachypnea
• increasing shallow respirations

Subjective
• feelings of thirst, cold, apprehension
• marked pain in moderate to severe abruptio placentae
• uterine pain that is localized or diffused, unrelenting, and excruciating

DIAGNOSTIC STUDIES
• Accurate and complete history and physical examination may furnish data for a definitive diagnosis.
• Vaginal examination, which may be performed by the physician to rule out placenta previa, is done only if delivery is imminent and if setups for both vaginal and cesarean section deliveries are immediately available.
• Ultrasonography reveals placental implantation site, fetal viability, gestational age, position and station, and possibly hemorrhage site and retroplacental blood clot; rules out placenta previa.
• Internal fetal monitoring may reveal late deceleration related to uteroplacental insufficiency, fetal hypoxia, or the absence of FHT.
• Apt test of amniotic fluid may reveal maternal blood that turns amniotic fluid port wine in color.

Laboratory data
• Hemoglobin (Hb) and hematocrit (HCT) values—decreases
• Coagulation factors—may decrease
• Fibrinogen degradation products—may increase
• Folic acid levels—may decrease

Collaborative problem: *Fluid volume deficit related to bleeding (3 goals)*

GOAL 1: Identify signs of bleeding.

Interventions

1. Assess bleeding every 30 minutes, or as patient's condition warrants:

• Record onset and amount of vaginal bleeding before admission.

• Monitor vital signs and compare with baseline; note capillary blanch test and pulse pressure.

• Note vaginal bleeding: color, number of perineal pads used, degree of saturation, and weight.

• Measure fundal height from superior aspect of symphysis pubis to top of uterine fundus.

2. Monitor Hb and HCT values.

3. Monitor coagulation factors, noting:
• prothrombin time longer than 15 seconds (may be normal, prolonged, or shortened)
• partial thromboplastin time longer than 60 to 80 seconds (may be normal, prolonged, or shortened)
• fibrinogen levels less than 150 mg/dl
• platelet count less than 100,000/mm³
• fibrinogen degradation products greater than 100 mcg/ml
• multisite bleeding, including frank bleeding, ecchymoses, petechiae, hematomas, or bleeding from mucous membranes or sites of invasive procedures.

4. Additional individualized interventions: '_____

Rationales

1. Overt, retroplacental bleeding may occur. Blood passes behind the membranes and exits externally through the cervix and vagina. Covert, internal bleeding occurs when blood is trapped behind the placenta.

• Blood loss may be as much as half the pregnant blood volume.

• A decreased refill time in the capillary blanch test indicates decreased peripheral circulation; a narrowing pulse pressure indicates early shock. Patient may lose 500 to 600 ml of blood before arterial blood pressure or cardiac output are significantly affected. Maternal hypervolemia, hypertension, and initial compensatory mechanisms may mask signs of shock: restlessness, tachycardia, hypotension, and tachypnea.

• Accurate assessment helps estimate blood loss and replacement needs. (*Note:* 1 gram of blood by weight equals 1 ml; a saturated pad equals approximately 100 ml.)

• Fundal height reflects gestational age. Increases may indicate covert bleeding.

2. Decreasing Hb and HCT values are consistent with blood loss.

3. These signs and symptoms suggest DIC. DIC requires prompt treatment with blood replacement and correction of underlying pathology.

4. Rationales: _____

GOAL 2: Restore and maintain normovolemia.

Interventions

1. Maintain hydration.

• Start I.V. infusion of crystalloid or balanced saline solution using a large-bore needle.

• Monitor fluid intake and output and specific gravity every hour.

Rationales

1. Rapid fluid replacement is necessary to correct hypovolemia.

• Fluids are provided while awaiting typing and crossmatching of blood products. Patient is not given food or fluids in anticipation of possible surgery.

• Fluid intake and output measurement helps to assess kidney function. Minimum physiologically acceptable urine output is 30 ml/hour. Premature labor is associated with dehydration. Decreased kidney perfusion may result in renal failure. Decreased urine output and specific gravity, decreased creatinine clearance, and increased blood urea nitrogen and creatinine levels indicate impending or actual kidney failure.

Interventions

• Monitor central venous pressure (CVP) line.

2. Administer fresh whole blood, cryoprecipitate, plasma, or platelets, as ordered.

3. At postpartum, perform uterine massage; note uterine contractility.

4. Additional individualized interventions:_____

Rationales

• Normal CVP readings during pregnancy are between 8 and 10 cm H_2O. Readings of 15 to 20 cm H_2O indicate circulatory overload.

2. Large volumes of blood may be required to replace loss. Plasma or cryoprecipitate may be given to correct decreasing fibrinogen levels.

3. Massage stimulates contraction. Decreased uterine contractility, coupled with blood between the myometrial fibers, is characteristic of Couvelaire uterus. Trapped blood makes the uterus feel deceptively firm.

4. Rationales: _____

GOAL 3: Optimize tissue perfusion.

Interventions

1. Maintain bed rest, left lateral position preferred. Elevate feet 30 degrees.

2. Administer oxygen by mask at 7 to 10 liters/minute, as patient condition warrants.

3. Additional individualized interventions: _____

Rationales

1. Bed rest decreases physiologic and metabolic demands. Left lateral position decreases pressure on the vena cava, facilitating venous return and cardiac output. Elevation of feet facilitates blood flow to vital organs.

2. Supplemental oxygen enhances tissue perfusion at the alveolocapillary membrane.

3. Rationales: _____

Nursing diagnosis: *Pain related to uterine tonicity, fundal tenderness, and unrelenting, uncharacteristic uterine contractions*

GOAL: Decrease or minimize pain.

Interventions

1. Establish rapport with patient and significant others. Call patient by preferred name. Check patient frequently.

2. Assess for pain and its characteristics, including quality, frequency, location, and intensity.

3. Minimize distracting environmental stimuli.

4. Perform comfort measures, including position changes, relaxation techniques, rubdowns, effleurage, and pharmacologic analgesia.

5. Additional individualized interventions: _____

Rationales

1. A positive relationship facilitates trust and decreases anxiety. Regressive behaviors, anger, resistance, or noncompliance may thereby decrease.

2. Pain profile may indicate degree and severity of the separation.

3. External stimuli may tend to increase perception of pain. Unwarranted interruptions of rest periods sap patient's emotional reserve.

4. Increased tissue perfusion plus stimulation of large afferent, sensory fibers decrease sensation and perception of pain. Analgesics are given cautiously because they may compromise fetal status.

5. Rationales: _____

Nursing diagnosis: *Fear related to fetal distress or death*

GOAL: Minimize fear.

Interventions	**Rationales**
1. Provide information in a clear, forthright manner. Ascertain patient's understanding of information given.	1. Open communication gives patient a sense of control and helps decrease fear. Infant survival depends on gestational age and maturity and extent or severity of abruption. A realistic appraisal of deteriorating stability of undeveloped fetus permits for early grieving.
2. Additional individualized interventions: _____	2. Rationales: _____

Collaborative problem: *High risk for fetal injury related to uteroplacental hemorrhage and compromised gas exchange (2 goals)*

GOAL 1: Detect early signs of fetal distress.

Interventions	**Rationales**
1. Assess fetal status with each maternal assessment, including fetal heart rate (FHR) patterns and variability, fetal activity, and uterine contractility. Compare with baseline.	1. Indicators of fetal distress include hyperactivity; FHT that are slow, irregular, or clinically difficult to hear; late decelerations; and increased FHR with decreased variability.
2. Additional individualized interventions: _____	2. Rationales: _____

GOAL 2: Promote safe delivery of the preterm infant.

Interventions	**Rationales**
1. Facilitate labor and monitor its progress.	1. Fetal distress, loss of fetal viability, or uncontrolled vaginal bleeding with a ripe cervix warrant delivery. Oxytocin infusion or amniotomy may be performed to facilitate a vaginal delivery. Vaginal delivery is preferable if the fetus has died and DIC is probable. If the cervix is not ripe or if fetal distress occurs, delivery by cesarean section is appropriate. Prompt delivery of a compromised fetus is critical to its survival.
2. Notify pediatric and neonatal staff of impending delivery. Obtain necessary resuscitative equipment.	2. Ability of the fetus to survive outside the uterus depends on its gestational age and respiratory, neurologic, thermoregulatory, and gastrointestinal maturity. Survival of the preterm infant depends on aggressive resuscitation and sustained intensive care.
3. Additional individualized interventions: _____	3. Rationales: _____

ASSOCIATED PLANS AND APPENDICES
• Inappropriate Size or Weight for Gestational Age, Small
• Normal Antepartum
• Pregnancy Complicated by Diabetes Mellitus
• Pregnancy-Induced Hypertension
• Preterm Infant, Less Than 37 Weeks
• Aspects of Psychological Care—Maternal (Appendix 4)

ADDITIONAL NURSING DIAGNOSES
• Knowledge deficit related to risk profile and recurrence ratio

Acquired Immunodeficiency Syndrome (AIDS) — Maternal

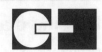

DEFINITION

Acquired immunodeficiency syndrome (AIDS) represents end-stage infection with the human immunodeficiency virus (HIV). AIDS begins with acquisition of HIV and generally progresses from an antibody-negative, asymptomatic carrier state through seroconversion and possible acute seroconversion syndrome to an antibody-positive, asymptomatic carrier state, and then to opportunistic infections or malignancies.

AIDS is characterized by profound, irreversible immunosuppression that cannot be explained by congenital conditions or by immunosuppressive or cytotoxic drug therapy. The disease affects both cell-mediated immunity and, to a lesser extent, humoral (antibody-mediated) immunity. Helper T lymphocytes or CD4 lymphocytes are the primary targets of HIV. Loss of these cells accounts for much of the immunologic dysfunction in persons with AIDS, and leads to opportunistic infections caused by bacteria, fungi, protozoa, and viruses. *Pneumocystis carinii* pneumonia (PCP) is the most common and serious of these infections.

Various cancers also occur in persons with AIDS, such as Kaposi's sarcoma and invasive cervical carcinoma. A broad range of AIDS indicator diseases are included in the surveillance definition for AIDS established by the Centers for Disease Control and Prevention (CDC). (See Appendix 13: 1993 CDC Revised Classification System for HIV Infection/AIDS Surveillance Case Definition.

Because the number of women diagnosed with AIDS has risen sharply and because AIDS carries a grim prognosis, preventing HIV transmission is crucial. Management is directed at counseling about disease prevention and the benefits of delaying pregnancy in HIV-infected women until more is known about perinatal transmission and control. Virus transmission from mother to fetus may occur during pregnancy or during labor and delivery. Breast-feeding has been implicated in HIV transmission after delivery. This plan focuses solely on women who are at high risk for acquiring HIV and who are or may become pregnant.

ETIOLOGY AND PRECIPITATING FACTORS

• Etiology: The causative agent of HIV-1 is a spherical, enveloped, single-stranded ribonucleic acid (RNA) retrovirus. Viral RNA is converted to deoxyribonucleic acid by the enzyme reverse transcriptase and is incorporated into the host cell.
• Patients at risk in heterosexual population: I.V. drug users; heterosexual, homosexual, or bisexual women with current or previous multiple sex partners; prostitutes; recipients of blood or blood products; women with a history of or current sexually transmitted diseases (STDs) or HIV-related illnesses; and women with partners who:
 □ are I.V. drug abusers
 □ are hemophiliacs and received blood or blood products before 1985
 □ are seropositive and asymptomatic
 □ have AIDS
 □ are bisexual
 □ have multiple sex partners
 □ engage in high-risk homosexual or heterosexual activity, including unprotected vaginal or anal intercourse, fellatio, cunnilingus, fisting (insertion of hand or fist into rectum), or rimming (rectal-oral contact).

PHYSICAL FINDINGS

• Acute seroconversion syndrome: fever, malaise, raised red rash on trunk, sore throat, arthralgia, lymphadenopathy
• AIDS-related complex: malaise, fatigue, weight loss, intermittent fever, chronic diarrhea, and generalized lymphadenopathy
• Early manifestations of HIV infection: persistent generalized lymphadenopathy (PGL) lasting more than 3 months; painless nodules measuring ¾" (2 cm) or more in diameter found at two or more sites outside the groin; thrush and candidiasis; herpes simplex
• Later manifestations of AIDS: findings vary greatly and depend on the opportunistic infection, cancer, or neurologic dysfunction manifested

DIAGNOSTIC STUDIES
HIV antibody detection

• Enzyme-linked immunosorbent assay (ELISA) to detect HIV antibodies. This sensitive and specific test usually becomes reactive within 6 to 12 weeks of HIV infection. However, seroconversion may be delayed 6 to 18 months. Usually, a repeat test is performed if initial results are positive.
• Western blot test: a positive result confirms a repeatedly reactive ELISA result.

HIV antigen detection

• Direct identification of HIV in host tissue by viral culture (used mainly in research)
• Positive results of any other highly specific licensed test for HIV
• Detection of p24 antigen (aids diagnosis in patients with indeterminate Western blot tests)

Other laboratory data

• CD4 count: decreased absolute number per microliter of blood (normal count is 1,000 to 1,300/microliter) or decreased percentage. (See Appendix 13.)
• CD4-CD8 ratio: decreased (normal ratio is 2:1)
• Beta-2 microglobulin: increases during acute phase of infection, decreases during antibody production, and then rises again with clinical diagnosis

• Neopterin: increases at a rate inversely proportional to CD4 count
• Soluble interleukin-2 receptors, immunoglobulin A, and delayed hypersensitivity skin test reactions may be useful, although they are less specific and predictive.

Collaborative problem: *High risk for maternal HIV infection related to sexual practices, illicit drug use, or exposure to infected blood products or carrier (3 goals)*

GOAL 1: Identify high-risk female population.

Interventions

1. Obtain gynecologic history. Include menstrual and obstetric histories and status of offspring, use of contraceptives and STD prophylaxis, history of STDs and vaginal and pelvic infections, sexual activities (including multiple sex partners), health and life-style of sex partners, and drug use. Review previous Papanicolaou test results.

2. Perform gynecologic examination. Examine vaginal and rectal areas, noting any lesions or signs of infection. Obtain Papanicolaou smear and laboratory screen for STDs.

3. Counsel and refer patient for HIV testing.

4. Additional individualized interventions: _____

Rationales

1. A lag exists between the time of HIV infection and the appearance of HIV antibodies. During this interim, the patient is a seronegative, asymptomatic HIV carrier. (However, asymptomatic women may be seropositive.) Comprehensive evaluation of all women promotes identification of high-risk patients and determines potential for exposure to HIV.

2. Examination may reveal gynecologic manifestations of HIV. Cervical dysplasia or neoplasia, human papillomavirus infection, ulcerative genital disease, recurrent *Candida* vaginitis, and pelvic inflammatory disease (PID) have been associated with HIV infection.

3. Counseling should relate test results to behavioral risk factors, disease control, and pregnancy prevention or management. Seronegative patients should be counseled because high-risk behaviors that required referral for testing may keep them at risk for HIV infection. Seropositive patients should be counseled to develop an individualized plan to prevent HIV transmission and to receive preventive health and social services.

4. Rationales: _____

GOAL 2: Minimize risk of infection in high-risk women.

Interventions

1. Review results of ELISA and Western blot tests; integrate results with history of high-risk life-style. (Voluntary HIV testing of women in prenatal clinics or high-prevalence areas, exclusive of self-described histories and risk behaviors, may be recommended.)

2. If pregnancy test is negative, advise patient about family planning methods.

Rationales

1. Seronegativity may indicate that antibodies have not yet developed. Women whose sex partners are HIV-positive (whether symptomatic or not) or whose life-styles put them at risk for HIV are at high risk for acquiring the disease.

2. The overwhelming majority of women with HIV are in their childbearing years (ages 15 to 44). Pregnancy should be delayed as long as patient remains at high risk. *Note:* Except for condoms, family planning methods do not prevent transmission of HIV and other STDs. Oral contraceptives do not prevent STDs and may have multiple drug interactions. The intrauterine device (IUD) may increase the risk of disease transmission by the HIV-positive woman and may promote susceptibility to ascending genital infection.

CDC RECOMMENDATIONS FOR LATEX CONDOM USE

The Centers for Disease Control and Prevention has published the following guidelines for correct use of latex condoms.
• Store condoms in a cool, dry place out of direct sunlight.
• Do not use condoms after the expiration date printed on the package.
• Do not use condoms in damaged packages or that show obvious signs of deterioration, such as brittleness, stickiness, or discoloration—regardless of the expiration date.
• Use a new condom for each new act of sexual intercourse.
• Handle condoms carefully to avoid damaging them with fingernails, teeth, and other sharp objects.

• Put the condom on after the penis is erect and before any genital contact with the partner.
• Leave space in the tip of the condom, but make sure no air is trapped in the tip.
• Ensure adequate lubrication during intercourse. If necessary, use an exogenous lubricant—but only one that is water-based, such as K-Y Jelly or glycerin. Do not use oil-based lubricants (for example, petroleum jelly, mineral oil, massage oils, body lotions, cooking oils, or shortening) because these may weaken latex.
• To prevent spillage, withdraw while the penis is still erect. During withdrawal, hold the condom firmly against the base of the penis.

Adapted from Centers for Disease Control. "Update: Barrier Protection Against HIV Infection and Other Sexually Transmitted Diseases," *Morbidity and Mortality Weekly Report* 42(30): August 6, 1993.

Interventions

3. Advise patient to use "safer sex" practices (see "Knowledge deficit related to modes of HIV transmission," page 28) to minimize risk of infection.

4. Advise patient not to share personal items that may be soiled with blood or body fluids, such as razors and toothbrushes.

5. Refer I.V. drug user to professional counselors and detoxification center. Strongly discourage sharing of needles and syringes. If patient continues to inject I.V. drugs, instruct patient to clean "works" with bleach and to use only clean, unused paraphernalia.

6. Follow universal precautions as well as institutionally prescribed infection control measures. (See Appendix 14: CDC Guidelines for Preventing HIV Transmission in Health Care Settings, page 337.)

7. Limit the practice of HIV-positive caregivers during exposure-prone invasive gynecologic and obstetric procedures. CDC recommends that such persons:
• use universal precautions when using and disposing of needles and other sharp instruments. These workers also should comply with guidelines for disinfection and sterilization of reusable devices used in invasive procedures.
• refrain from all direct patient care and from handling patient care equipment and devices used in invasive procedures when exudative lesions or weeping dermatitis are present
• refrain from performing exposure-prone procedures until they have been advised by an expert review panel. (Practitioners who perform invasive procedures should know their HIV antibody status.)

8. Additional individualized interventions: _____

Rationales

3. HIV has been isolated from blood, semen, vaginal secretions, saliva, tears, urine, cerebrospinal fluid, amniotic fluid, and breast milk. However, only blood, semen, vaginal secretions and possibly breast milk have been associated with disease transmission.

4. Blood and body fluids are sources of infection. Contact with infected body fluids is required for disease transmission. HIV is not transmitted through casual contact or close, nonsexual contact.

5. Sharing of drug paraphernalia, the practice of aspirating and reinjecting venous blood during I.V. drug use, and the high incidence of exchanging sex for drugs increase the chances for HIV transmission in I.V. drug users. Destructive drug-abusing behaviors and the effects of mind-altering drugs foster noncompliance and make HIV transmission likely.

6. Health care workers should consider AIDS prophylaxis when caring for all patients, not just those who are HIV-positive, diagnosed, or symptomatic.

7. The risk of HIV transmission by an HIV-infected health care provider is small. HIV-infected caregivers who do not perform invasive procedures and who adhere to universal precautions pose no transmission risk.

8. Rationales: _____

GOAL 3: Identify AIDS-associated manifestations in high-risk pregnant patients.

Interventions

1. Determine estimated date of confinement; correlate with history and clinical profile. Perform routine prenatal testing as well as hepatitis B, cytomegalovirus, and toxoplasmosis tests.

2. Evaluate CD4 counts.

3. Assess for fatigue, malaise, heartburn, anorexia, weight loss, increased temperature, night sweats, bleeding and swollen gums, nasal congestion, shortness of breath, and emotional lability. Relate to CD4 count.

4. Assess patient history for the following, then correlate with physical findings: 1- to 2-week episode of fever, malaise, rash, arthralgia, and generalized lymphadenopathy.

5. Review dates and results of Papanicolaou smears, colposcopic examinations, and colposcopically directed biopsy.

6. Perform review of symptoms and complete physical examination. Include EENT, respiratory, integumentary, neurologic, GI, and gynecologic systems.

7. Assess for pyrexia, chest tightness, shortness of breath, cough, and dyspnea on exertion.

Rationales

1. Cell-mediated immunity is somewhat suppressed during normal pregnancy. HIV-infected patients may become symptomatic at any point. The benefits of HIV treatment must be balanced against possible health risks to the fetus. Except during advanced stages of HIV disease, pregnancy does not appear to influence the course of HIV infection or hasten its progression. HIV infection in asymptomatic, seropositive women does not seem to increase the risk of complications during pregnancy or result in preterm or low-birth-weight infants. Little data exists on the risks of fetal HIV infection. Rates of vertical perinatal transmission of HIV from mother to infant range from 13% to 30%. Infants of HIV-positive women may test positive for HIV antibodies for up to 18 months.

2. CD4 counts drop dramatically (by up to 50%) within months of initial HIV infection, although great variation exists among patients. As the CD4 count decreases, the risk and severity of opportunistic infection increase.

3. These signs and symptoms are associated both with normal pregnancy and with HIV-associated illnesses, possibly complicating assessment and diagnosis. CD4 counts are indicators of immune dysfunction and HIV progression. Clinical manifestations and CD4 counts serve as guides to management.

4. These signs and symptoms may indicate acute retroviral seroconversion syndrome. After the syndrome resolves, patient typically becomes an asymptomatic, seropositive HIV carrier. Generalized lymphadenopathy persists and CD4 count continues to fall. Patients with CD4 counts below 500/microliter are candidates for PCP prophylaxis. CD4 counts below 200/microliter or CD4 percentages below 14% represent severe immunosuppression; PCP prophylaxis is recommended. Aerosolized pentamidine (Nebupent) generally is effective and its low therapeutic serum levels make it relatively safe for the fetus. Oral trimethoprim-sulfamethoxazole (Bactrim) may be given, although fetal malformations have occurred. No antiviral drug is safe during pregnancy.

5. False-negative cytologic findings are more common in HIV-infected women. Colposcopic testing is indicated if Papanicolaou test results are abnormal or inconclusive. The prevalence of cervical dysplasia is higher and the course of cervical neoplasia more aggressive in HIV-infected women. Invasive cervical carcinoma is an AIDS indicator disease.

6. HIV infection leads to a wide range of pathologic conditions, as indicated by the conditions listed in the CDC case definition. (See Appendix 14.)

7. Recurrent acute pneumonia or pulmonary tuberculosis may be presumptive of AIDS indicator diseases. PCP is the most common serious opportunistic infection in HIV-positive women.

Interventions

8. Assess for genital discomfort, lesions, discharge, erythema, edema, excoriation, fissures, and abdominal or pelvic pain. Obtain cultures for gonorrhea and *Chlamydia*. Perform Venereal Disease Research Laboratory (VDRL) test for syphilis.

9. Assess cognition, emotional condition, and motor and sensory function. Note complaints of headache, lethargy, confusion, weakness, or paresthesias and any motor or sensory deficits.

10. Perform tuberculin skin test (purified protein derivative) and obtain smears and cultures, as indicated. Relate response time to anergy and HIV status.

11. Refer HIV-infected pregnant patient to a facility with staff expertise in HIV disease management.

12. Additional individualized interventions: _____

Rationales

8. Herpes, syphilis, and other STDs may promote sexual transmission of HIV. Manifestations of PID may be atypical. Recurrent candidiasis is common and highly resistant to treatment; its presence portends severe opportunistic infection. HIV-related thrush and unexplained fever may increase the risk of PCP.

9. Neurologic manifestations may indicate HIV infection or may be associated with late-stage syphilis. Altered sensorium or emotional lability also may indicate drug use.

10. Tuberculosis (TB) is an AIDS indicator disease. The risk of developing active TB increases when TB and HIV coexist.

11. Health care management for HIV disease is highly specialized and requires a focused multidisciplinary team to address a broad range of physical and psychosocial problems.

12. Rationales: _____

Nursing diagnosis: *Knowledge deficit related to modes of HIV transmission*

GOAL: Provide information about HIV transmission.

Interventions

1. Review patient's medical history, sexual orientation and practices, drug use, educational background, and cultural influences.

2. Assist patient in developing a personalized risk assessment.

3. Provide information in a clear, nonjudgmental manner. Use language with which patient is comfortable and familiar. Allow time for questions. Clarify written materials and repeat instructions as often as necessary.

4. Provide the following information on sexual options:
• Sexual abstinence or a long-term monogamous relationship with a faithful, uninfected partner is the best protection against AIDS. Emphasize that neither partner can have a history of I.V. drug abuse and that both must refrain from subsequent I.V. drug abuse.
• Safer sexual practices include dry kissing and nongenital touching and masturbation.
• Possibly safer sex practices include consistent and correct use of a latex condom throughout vaginal or anal intercourse or during oral sex. (See *CDC recommendations for latex condom use,* page 26.)
• Risky sexual practices include wet (open-mouth) kissing, oral sex on females, oral sex on males without a condom, and use of alcohol, marijuana, amyl nitrate, amphetamines, and other mind-altering substances during sexual relations.

Rationales

1. These data help create a physiologic profile and database for patient teaching. A patient-centered approach promotes receptivity to learning.

2. Compliance with risk reduction is enhanced when the patient is an active participant.

3. The devastating implications of an AIDS diagnosis may impede the patient's receptivity to health teaching. The practitioner who is well versed in HIV disease progression and control, behavior modification, human sexuality, cultural influences, and local mores can best serve as a patient advocate and change agent.

4. This information clearly defines various sexual practices and their consequences. Modification of sexual behavior is critical to reducing the risk of HIV transmission.

Interventions	Rationales
• High-risk practices include vaginal or anal intercourse without a condom; recipient role in anal sex; rimming; fisting; sharing of sex toys; any practice that puts body fluids in contact with the partner or with open or abraded skin; and sharing of I.V. needles and syringes.	
5. Discourage breast-feeding in high-risk or HIV-positive women.	5. HIV has been isolated in breast milk and has been implicated in disease transmission.
6. Discourage high-risk women from donating blood or organs for transplantation.	6. Blood and tissues may harbor HIV. Blood and blood products are the most efficient agents of viral transmission.
7. Additional individualized interventions: _____	7. Rationales: _____

Nursing diagnosis: *Ineffective individual coping related to AIDS diagnosis and its implications*

GOAL: Support and bolster patient's established coping mechanisms.

Interventions	Rationales
1. Assess patient's coping abilities, integrating verbal and nonverbal responses and patient's interaction with family, friends, and health care workers.	1. Assessment identifies sources of strength and possible avenues of reinforcement.
2. Explore patient's understanding of condition and (if applicable) of pregnancy.	2. Rates of pregnancy termination and repeat pregnancies are similar in HIV-infected and noninfected women. The meaning of pregnancy, patient's health status, drug use, cultural and religious influences, perception of risk, and access to health care are factors in decisions about health care.
3. Maintain nonjudgmental approach. Accept patient's response to illness. Ensure confidentiality.	3. Fear of abandonment, violence from partner, family disruption, debilitation, disfigurement, and death may trigger various emotional reactions.
4. Provide and assist patient with options for care. Make referrals, as appropriate.	4. Confusion, denial, passivity, dependency, powerlessness, and low frustration tolerance — when coupled with great anxiety — may signal limited coping ability. Support groups, family counselors, and financial and religious or pastoral counselors may provide significant support.
5. Additional individualized interventions: _____	5. Rationales: _____

ASSOCIATED PLANS AND APPENDICES
• Acquired Immunodeficiency Syndrome — Infant
• Aspects of Psychological Care — Maternal (Appendix 4)
• Selected Methods of Family Planning (Appendix 6)
• 1993 CDC Revised Classification System for HIV Infection/AIDS Surveillance Case Definition (Appendix 13)
• CDC Guidelines for Preventing HIV Transmission in Health Care Settings (Appendix 14)

ADDITIONAL NURSING DIAGNOSES
• Hopelessness related to projected mortality associated with AIDS diagnosis
• Noncompliance with sexual prophylaxis related to denial of condition, fear of abandonment, or altered sensorium secondary to illicit drug use
• Spiritual distress related to perceived guilt associated with sexual practices

Ectopic Pregnancy

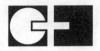

DEFINITION

Ectopic pregnancy is the implantation of the fertilized ovum outside the uterine cavity. The most common site of implantation is the fallopian tube, generally the right one. Other possible sites include the interstitium, the tubo-ovarian ligament, ovary, abdominal cavity, and external cervical os.

Ectopic pregnancy is second only to spontaneous abortion as a primary cause of bleeding in the first trimester, and presenting symptoms and diagnosis generally occur within that period. After implantation, amenorrhea and the nausea and vomiting associated with pregnancy may occur. Slight vaginal bleeding ("spotting"), adnexal fullness, and unilateral or bilateral cramping and tenderness associated with an unruptured ectopic pregnancy may occur. When the thin, relatively inelastic fallopian tube can no longer accommodate the growing fetus, rupture becomes inevitable. The extent of bleeding is dependent on the size and number of ruptured vessels. Blood from eroded vessels and the products of conception spill into the pelvic or peritoneal cavities. Complications include hemorrhage, shock, and peritonitis. Ectopic pregnancy requires surgical intervention.

Rarely, an abdominal pregnancy may be carried to term. Delivery is accomplished through a laparotomy; the umbilical cord is cut and the placenta left in place where it will be absorbed by the viscera to which it is attached.

ETIOLOGY AND PRECIPITATING FACTORS

• Any condition that impedes or prevents the predesigned passage of the fertilized ovum from the ovary through the fallopian tube to the uterus may result in an ectopic pregnancy: endosalpingitis, pelvic inflammatory disease (PID), diverticula, adhesions (especially from endometriosis or puerperal infection), tumors, tubal surgery, hormonal factors, tubal infection, and scarring resulting from intrauterine devices (IUDs), sexually transmitted disease (STD), or induced abortion.

PHYSICAL FINDINGS
Cardiovascular
• occasional tachycardia
• hypotension
• vertigo
• syncope
• diaphoresis
• pallor

Gastrointestinal
• diarrhea
• possible nausea and vomiting
• Cullen's sign (periumbilical ecchymoses)

Genitourinary
• amenorrhea or abnormal menses followed by spotting or cramping; bleeding may be mistaken for menses
• scant, dark brown vaginal bleeding
• increased uterine size: nearly the same size as gestational age would warrant during first 3 months
• unilateral or bilateral pelvic tenderness or pain, notably on movement of cervix during pelvic examination (chandelier effect)
• palpable mass on the fallopian tube or in the cul-de-sac on pelvic examination
• asymmetric uterus in interstitial pregnancies
• pelvic distention or feeling of fullness
• sudden and acute abdominal or pelvic pain; referred shoulder or neck pain; rebound tenderness and guarding

DIAGNOSTIC STUDIES
• Accurate and complete history and physical examination furnish enough data for a tentative diagnosis.

Laboratory data
• Beta-subunit assay for human chorionic gonadotropin — low or falling levels.
• White blood cell (WBC) count — may increase.
• Red blood cell (RBC) count — decreases.
• Hemoglobin (Hb) and hematocrit (HCT) values — decrease.
• Erythrocyte sedimentation rate (ESR) — may increase.
• Ultrasonography — may reveal extrauterine pregnancy or absence of intrauterine pregnancy.
• Culdocentesis (fluid aspirate from the vaginal cul-de-sac) — reveals nonclotting blood.
• Laparoscopy — visualizes extrauterine pregnancy and enlarged or ruptured fallopian tube.

Collaborative problem: *Fluid volume deficit related to bleeding (2 goals)*

GOAL 1: Identify signs of bleeding.

Interventions	Rationales
1. Assess bleeding every 30 minutes or as patient condition warrants: • Monitor vital signs.	1. Blood loss affects fluid volume balance. • Vital signs may remain within normal limits initially. Careful evaluation of vital signs and cardiopulmonary status is critical because bleeding is internal and extent of actual blood loss is not evident. Tachycardia, hypotension, tachypnea, and restlessness are consistent with intense blood loss and resulting shock.
• Assess vaginal bleeding: color, number of perineal pads used, degree of saturation, and odor; confirm date of last menstrual period.	• Scant, dark red vaginal blood in suspected or confirmed early pregnancy, accompanied by abdominal or pelvic pain and a palpable mass on the fallopian tube or in the cul-de-sac, is consistent with a diagnosis of ectopic pregnancy. (*Note:* Saturated pad represents approximately 100 ml blood loss.)
2. Monitor blood studies.	2. Falling RBC count and Hb and HCT values are consistent with blood loss. Accurate assessment assists in calculating replacement needs.
3. Additional individualized interventions: _____	3. Rationales: _____

GOAL 2: Restore and maintain normovolemia.

Interventions	Rationales
1. Administer I.V. infusion of prescribed solution using large-bore needle; withdraw blood for typing and cross-matching that will include Rh determination.	1. Fluids are provided while awaiting typing and cross-matching of blood products. Food and fluids are withheld from patient before surgery. An Rh-negative nonsensitized mother with conceptus of unknown or positive Rh will require an injection of Rh_o (D) immune globulin (RhoGAM) within 72 hours of abortion to prevent isoimmunization.
2. Administer whole blood, as ordered.	2. Large volumes of blood may be required to replace loss.
3. Prepare patient for surgery: • Monitor trends of vital signs and results of laboratory testing and refer to physician as necessary. • Assist in obtaining informed consents. • Assist with physical preparation.	3. Continual monitoring is necessary to screen for and rule out other disorders that share similar signs and symptoms: appendicitis, salpingitis, ovarian torsion, ruptured corpus luteum, ovarian cyst, and uterine abortion. Laparotomy may be necessary to confirm the diagnosis of ectopic pregnancy. Surgical intervention varies with the location of the gestational sac; a salpingectomy—removal of the affected tube—may be performed as part of laparotomy. Every attempt is made to conserve the ovaries. The products of conception are removed and the bleeding controlled.
4. Additional individualized interventions: _____	4. Rationales: _____

Nursing diagnosis: *High risk for infection related to the trauma of rupture and peritoneal inflammation*

GOAL: Recognize early signs of infection.

Interventions	Rationales
1. Monitor vital signs, including temperature.	1. Temperature may be low, normal, or up to 100.4° F (38° C). Pyrexia is consistent with generalized infection and a temperature greater than 100.4° F may distinguish salpingitis from ruptured tubal pregnancy; antibiotic therapy is initiated before surgery and continues after surgery prophylactically as well as with actual infections.
2. Monitor WBC count and ESR.	2. An ESR within normal limits is consistent with early or unruptured ectopic pregnancy. Increases are seen in ruptured ectopic pregnancy. A transient, moderately elevated WBC count is associated with the trauma of rupture. Levels usually return to normal within 24 hours. Persistent, elevated WBC count is associated with infection, as well as PID.
3. Assess for pain trends and their characteristics. Administer analgesics cautiously, but do not withhold.	3. Analgesics may mask as well as alleviate the pain of intraperitoneal rupture and subsequent peritonitis. Scrupulous attention should be paid to abdominal size and tension and guarding. Cullen's sign may be visible.
4. Additional individualized interventions: _____	4. Rationales: _____

Nursing diagnosis: *Pain related to disruption of pelvic tissue*

GOAL: Minimize pain.

Interventions	Rationales
1. Assess for pain and its characteristics, including quality, frequency, location, and intensity.	1. Pain profile may assist in formulating the medical diagnosis.
2. Establish rapport with patient and significant others. Call patient by preferred name. Do not leave patient unattended for long periods.	2. A positive relationship facilitates trust and decreases anxiety. Regressive behaviors, anger, resistance, and noncompliance may thereby decrease.
3. Minimize distracting environmental stimuli.	3. External stimuli may tend to increase perception of pain. Unwarranted interruptions of rest periods sap patient's emotional reserve.
4. Perform comfort measures, including position changes, relaxation techniques, rubdowns, effleurage, and pharmacologic analgesia.	4. Increased tissue perfusion plus stimulation of large afferent, sensory fibers decrease sensation or perception of pain.
5. Additional individualized interventions: _____	5. Rationales: _____

Nursing diagnosis: *Fear related to loss of pregnancy and threat to fertility*

GOAL: Minimize fear.

Interventions

1. Provide information in a clear, forthright manner. Ascertain patient's understanding of information given.

2. Be supportive and nonjudgmental. Accept patient's emotional response and allow her to cope in the manner she has established for herself.

3. Teach patient these measures to minimize the risk of ectopic pregnancies:
• Treat genital infections and PID promptly (the risk of ectopic pregnancy is increased in confirmed PID or a history of surgery to the fallopian tubes).
• Avoid IUD use (IUDs may contribute to ectopic pregnancies).

4. Additional individualized interventions: _____

Rationales

1. Open communication gives patient a sense of control and helps decrease fear. Fetal death accompanies rupture of the ectopic pregnancy.

2. Because ectopic pregnancy may result from STD and resulting PID, patient may perceive disorder as a punishment for dysfunctional relationships or sexual indiscretions.

3. Discussion of measures to reduce (not prevent) incidence of ectopic pregnancy should be deferred until patient's condition is stabilized, pain controlled, and receptivity to teaching demonstrated.

4. Rationales: _____

ASSOCIATED PLANS AND APPENDICES
• Normal Antepartum
• Sepsis Neonatorum and Infectious Disorders
• Aspects of Psychological Care—Maternal (Appendix 4)
• Preparing for Nonemergency Surgery (Appendix 5)

ADDITIONAL NURSING DIAGNOSES
• Ineffective breathing pattern related to abdominal incision
• Powerlessness related to loss of fetus and possible infertility
• Sexual dysfunction related to pelvic tenderness

Hydatidiform Mole (Molar Pregnancy)

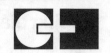

DEFINITION
Hydatidiform moles are neoplastic anomalies of trophoblastic tissue usually located in the uterus. They are characterized by proliferation of trophoblastic cells and edema of villous stroma. They may invade local structures or metastasize. In most cases, no fetal growth occurs, although fetal blood may be present in the villi. Trophoblastic tissue proliferates rapidly and warrants surgical evacuation from the uterus. Complications of a local mole include invasion, uterine hemorrhage, intrauterine infection, pregnancy-induced hypertension, and sepsis. The molar pregnancy may precede choriocarcinoma, a malignant, widely metastatic tumor.

ETIOLOGY AND PRECIPITATING FACTORS
• etiology unknown
• patient at risk: maternal age greater than 45; maternal place of origin may be Asia, Mexico, or native Alaska; use of the ovarian stimulant clomiphene citrate (Clomid); low socioeconomic status coupled with a low-protein diet

PHYSICAL FINDINGS
Cardiovascular
• possible hypertension*
• possible edema*

Gastrointestinal
• severe nausea
• vomiting

Genitourinary
• increased uterine size, larger than estimated gestational age would warrant

• persistent vaginal bleeding: dark brown spotting or profuse bleeding with concurrent discharge of hydatid vesicles
• ovarian enlargement, tenderness on palpation
• soft, thin cervix on pelvic examination
• no palpation of fetal parts; no fetal heart tones
• proteinuria

DIAGNOSTIC STUDIES
• Accurate and complete history and physical examination may furnish sufficient data for a tentative diagnosis.
• Ultrasonography fails to reveal amniotic sac or a fetus within; may reveal a characteristic molar pattern.
• Contrast medium injected into the amniotic cavity reveals a moth-eaten pattern on X-ray (seldom used since availability of sonography).
• Fetal indirect (external) electronic monitor or Doppler stethoscope reveals no fetal heart tones.

Laboratory data
• serum and urine human chorionic gonadotropin (HCG) — strongly positive, especially after first trimester
• hemoglobin and hematocrit values and red blood cell count — decrease
• urinalysis — reveals proteinuria
• histologic examination — grapelike, vesicular tissue confirms the diagnosis

---

Nursing diagnosis *High risk for fluid volume deficit related to bleeding*

GOAL: Identify signs of bleeding.

Interventions

1. Assess vaginal bleeding every 30 minutes, or as patient condition warrants:

• Note onset and amount of vaginal bleeding before hospitalization, noting any tissue passed. Upon hospitalization save all clots and tissue passed.
• Monitor vaginal bleeding: color, number of perineal pads used, and degree of saturation.

• Monitor vital signs.

Rationales

1. Accurate assessment assists in differentiation of hydatidiform mole from spontaneous abortion.

• A definite diagnosis is made by histologic examination of the hydatid tissue passed vaginally.

• Accurate assessment helps estimate blood loss and replacement needs; spotting may result in anemia, which is treated with iron replacement therapy. More profuse blood loss may necessitate transfusion of blood products.

• Hypotension, tachycardia, tachypnea, and restlessness may indicate shock associated with blood loss.

Interventions

2. Additional individualized interventions: _____

_____

Rationales

2. Rationales: _____

_____

Collaborative problem: *High risk for infection related to uterine bleeding, inflammation, irritation, or invasion*

GOAL: Recognize early signs of infection.

Interventions

1. Assess patient for signs of infection, including:
• chills, pyrexia (note temperature trends)
• headache
• anorexia
• foul-smelling, purulent vaginal discharge
• low back or abdominal pain
• malaise, lethargy
• elevated white blood cell count.

2. Administer antibiotics, as ordered. Note drug allergies.

3. Additional individualized interventions: _____

_____

Rationales

1. Trend analysis assists in the detection and diagnosis of infection. Intrauterine infection may progress to septicemia.

2. Broad-spectrum antibiotic therapy is initiated either prophylactically or in the presence of actual infection. Vaginal cultures should be performed before therapy begins, and the drug regimen should be modified upon evaluation of culture and sensitivity reports.

3. Rationales: _____

_____

Nursing diagnosis: *High risk for maternal injury related to rapidly expanding uterine size and blood loss*

GOAL: Minimize injury.

Interventions

1. Prepare the patient for surgery.

2. Additional individualized interventions: _____

_____

Rationales

1. Surgical evacuation of the mole is essential. Induced abortion by suction curettage is the treatment of choice and may be followed by oxytocin stimulation to control postpartum bleeding if there is no predisposition to ruptured uterus from overdistention. Firming of the uterine wall precedes uterine dilatation and curettage.

2. Rationales: _____

_____

Nursing diagnosis: *Altered health maintenance related to potential metastatic disease*

GOAL: Monitor for malignant conversion.

Interventions

1. Assess HCG titers for 1 year or more on schedule prescribed.

Rationales

1. HCG levels should progressively decrease. Measurable amounts should not be in the urine after 8 weeks.

Interventions

Rationales

Failure to decrease or actual increases may indicate malignant growth from converted trophoblastic tissue. Chemotherapy with dactinomycin (Cosmegen) or methotrexate (Folex) is the treatment of choice.

2. Counsel patient on reliable family planning methods.

2. Pregnancy should be avoided for 1 year because the increased HCG resulting from pregnancy may confuse diagnosis of malignant disease.

3. Assess concurrently with HCG titer readings:
• cachexia, weight loss, weakness, pyrexia
• hemorrhagic nodules on vulva or vagina
• cough, hemoptysis
• abdominal masses or tenderness
• jaundice, ascites, dependent edema
• bony mass, bone pain, immobility
• skin changes.

3. Presence of any or all of these signs and symptoms suggests metastatic choriocarcinoma (chorioepithelioma).

4. Additional individualized interventions: _____

4. Rationales: _____

Nursing diagnosis: *Dysfunctional grieving related to fetal loss and protracted postoperative treatment course*

GOAL: Minimize grief.

Interventions

Rationales

1. Accept the patient's verbal and nonverbal response to fetal loss.

1. The loss and perceived impaired childbearing capability may devastate the patient. She may need to grieve over the loss at any period of gestation.

2. Counsel the patient about future pregnancies.

2. If HCG levels have been normal for 1 year, probability for recurrence of a mole is low (about 2%).

3. Additional individualized interventions: _____

3. Rationales: _____

ASSOCIATED PLANS AND APPENDICES
• Pregnancy-Induced Hypertension
• Aspects of Psychological Care—Maternal (Appendix 4)
• Preparing for Nonemergency Surgery (Appendix 5)

ADDITIONAL NURSING DIAGNOSES
• Altered nutrition: less than body requirements related to low socioeconomic status and resulting low-protein diet
• Fear related to potential metastases
• Knowledge deficit related to types and use of contraceptives
• Sexual dysfunction related to need for family planning

---

*One of the triad of symptoms of preeclampsia, the only true pregnancy-induced hypertension seen before the 24th week of gestation.

ANTEPARTUM
Hyperemesis Gravidarum

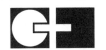

DEFINITION
Hyperemesis gravidarum is pernicious or malignant nausea or vomiting associated with pregnancy; it progresses to dehydration, starvation, and an acid-base imbalance. It is unlike morning sickness, the transient nausea and vomiting that occur during the first trimester possibly in response to increasing human chorionic gonadotropin (HCG) and estrogen levels. Instead, it is severe and unremitting and may persist past the first trimester. It must be treated before fetal damage results. Untreated, it may be associated with electrolyte and acid-base imbalances and liver damage; hemorrhagic retinitis is a grave maternal complication associated with high mortality. Usually, prognosis is good with appropriate treatment.

ETIOLOGY AND PRECIPITATING FACTORS
• coincident with elevated HCG levels of pregnancy as well as even higher levels associated with multiple pregnancy or hydatidiform mole
• hypoglycemia resulting from altered carbohydrate metabolism in early pregnancy
• psychological factors

PHYSICAL FINDINGS
Cardiovascular
• tachycardia
• hypotension
• vertigo
• syncope

Gastrointestinal
• severe nausea
• marked emesis
• mucosal bleeding
• ptyalism

Genitourinary
• oliguria
• ketonuria

Integumentary
• pale, dry skin; decreased turgor
• dry mucous membranes and lips
• sunken eyeballs
• jaundice

Metabolic
• low-grade fever
• weight aberration (failure to gain weight or actual weight loss)
• fruity breath

Neurologic
• lethargy
• confusion
• somnolence
• polyneuritis or peripheral neuropathy

Subjective
• sour taste in mouth
• feelings of thirst

DIAGNOSTIC STUDIES
• Accurate and complete history and complete physical examination are necessary to differentiate from the transient discomfort of early pregnancy and to rule out other conditions that may cause vomiting.

Laboratory data
• potassium, sodium, chloride, protein levels—decrease
• blood urea nitrogen, nonprotein nitrogen, uric acid levels—increase
• hemoglobin and hematocrit values—increase
• urinalysis—reveals ketones and possibly protein; specific gravity increases
• vitamin levels—decrease

Nursing diagnosis: *Altered nutrition: less than body requirements related to nausea, emesis, and subsequent inconsistent or insufficient food intake (3 goals)*

GOAL 1: Recognize early signs of nutritional alteration.

Interventions

1. Weigh at each prenatal clinic visit and, if hospitalized, daily on same scale, at same time of day, wearing same type of clothing. Note pattern of weight gain.

Rationales

1. Consistency ensures accuracy of measurement and minimizes diurnal variation. A total gain of 22 to 28 lb (10 to 13 kg) is optimal for fetal growth and maternal changes. Weight gain expectations include 2 to 4 lb (1 to 2 kg) for the first trimester and 0.9 lb (0.4 kg) per week for remainder of pregnancy.

Interventions

2. Monitor intake by 24-hour patient dietary recall.

3. Assess for edema, noting tight or constrictive shoes, feelings of being bloated, and benign, dependent leg edema.

4. Assess for ketones in urine.

5. Additional individualized interventions: _____

Rationales

2. Recall provides a data base for assessment.

3. The clinical presentation of edema may mask true failure to gain weight. Weight gain should reflect maternal and fetal growth and not retained excess fluid.

4. Ketonuria is a sign that stored reserves are being used for all growth; it is associated with fetal brain damage.

5. Rationales: _____

GOAL 2: Recognize morning sickness and minimize discomfort of nausea and vomiting.

Interventions

1. Monitor patient for signs of morning sickness:
• Nausea is experienced from first missed period to end of 3rd month of gestation and usually resolves spontaneously at beginning of 4th month.
• Condition may or may not be accompanied by emesis.
• Condition may be more intense upon arising.
• Condition may be aggravated by fatigue.

2. Provide nonmedical methods to minimize symptoms, including:
• high-protein bedtime snack
• dry carbohydrates 30 minutes before rising
• delay in mealtime until nausea has subsided, but no skipping of meals
• no fluids with meals
• frequent small meals rather than three large ones
• no foods that are greasy, spicy, gas-forming, or have a pronounced aroma
• no periods of more than 12 hours without eating.

3. Use all prescription and over-the-counter antiemetic drugs with caution.

4. Additional individualized interventions: _____

Rationales

1. Symptomatology may be a result of hormonal changes, maternal hypoglycemia, and decreased gastric motility as well as fatigue, emotional factors, and cultural expectations.

2. Treatment is palliative and focuses on minimizing both stressors and maternal hypoglycemia.

3. Many drugs have teratogenic effects in pregnancy, notably in early pregnancy.

4. Rationales: _____

GOAL 3: Recognize pronounced or protracted emesis.

Interventions

1. Assess emesis, noting its onset, frequency, duration, time of day, relationship to intake, and precipitating and alleviating factors; also note this information for each episode: color, amount, consistency, and the presence of undigested food, mucus, blood, or bile.

2. Assess abdomen every 2 hours or as patient condition warrants, including size, contour, bowel sounds, pain, tenderness, or guarding; also note vital signs.

3. Additional individualized interventions: _____

Rationales

1. Vomitus may represent loss of acidic gastric contents or lower gastrointestinal alkaline products; proper assessment is essential to reverse developing acid-base and electrolyte imbalances.

2. Accurate assessment can assist in the diagnosis of various disorders that cause vomiting: liver disease, kidney infection, pancreatitis, gastrointestinal obstruction or lesions, drug toxicity, or intracranial lesions.

3. Rationales: _____

Collaborative problem: *Fluid volume deficit related to protracted emesis (2 goals)*

GOAL 1: Recognize signs of fluid volume deficit.

Interventions

1. Monitor the patient for signs and symptoms of fluid volume deficit:
• dry skin with poor turgor and dry mucous membranes
• sunken eyeballs
• concentrated urine and oliguria
• malaise
• hypotension, vertigo, and syncope.

2. Assess hemoglobin and hematocrit values.

3. Additional individualized interventions: _____

Rationales

1. Restoration of fluid balance is essential to maintain homeostatic mechanisms and for maternal and fetal well-being.

2. Increased hemoglobin and hematocrit values may indicate hemoconcentration.

3. Rationales: _____

GOAL 2: Restore and maintain normovolemic state; minimize emesis and promote optimal nutrition.

Interventions

1. Restrict all oral intake for 24 to 48 hours.

2. Administer balanced I.V. solution with electrolytes, glucose, and vitamins added.

3. Permit oral intake after all vomiting has ceased for 24 hours. If vomiting occurs after foods have been initiated, revert to previous menu.
• Begin with clear fluids, not to exceed 100 ml, alternated every 1 to 1½ hours with dry toast or crackers.
• Progress to soft diet.
• Progress to regular diet; all portions should be small (six to seven meals per day) and well-prepared.

4. Additional individualized interventions: _____

Rationales

1. Restriction allows stomach to rest and irritated gastric mucosa to heal.

2. This solution provides fluids to reverse deficit and corrects acid-base imbalances, altered electrolyte levels, and hypovitaminosis.

3. Careful and slow introduction of food is usually effective.

4. Rationales: _____

Nursing diagnosis: *Fear related to hospitalization and pregnancy outcome*

GOAL: Minimize patient's fear.

Interventions

1. Accept the patient's verbal and nonverbal responses to illness.

2. Provide information in a clear, forthright manner.

3. Be supportive and nonjudgmental. Accept patient's emotional response and allow her to cope in the manner she has established for herself.

Rationales

1. Acceptance facilitates good rapport and trust.

2. Pregnancy outcome is determined by severity and duration of disorder; the disorder, once controlled, usually does not recur. Open communication gives patient a sense of control and helps decrease fear.

3. Patient may need to initiate anticipatory grieving over the pregnancy, which may result in a low-birth-weight infant.

Interventions	Rationales
4. Provide information on counseling; refer to appropriate health care professional, if necessary.	4. Ambivalence toward pregnancy and reactions to stress may play a significant role in disorder etiology.
5. Inform family and significant others of patient's condition, especially because visitors are limited in early hospitalization.	5. Family interaction bolsters patient's established support system.
6. Additional individualized interventions: _____	6. Rationales: _____

Nursing diagnosis: *Pain related to repeated episodes of vomiting*

GOAL: Minimize discomfort.

Interventions	Rationales
1. Provide a clean, odor-free environment. Keep emesis basin and bedpan out of sight, but within reach. Keep dietary food cart away from patient's room. Remove patient's tray as soon as possible after meal completion.	1. Some odors may trigger vomiting.
2. Provide mouth care before each meal and snack and after each episode of vomiting.	2. Good oral hygiene contributes to patient comfort and sense of well-being.
3. Place the patient in high Fowler's position or seated upright for 30 minutes after each feeding.	3. This position minimizes gastric reflux.
4. Additional individualized interventions: _____	4. Rationales: _____

ASSOCIATED PLANS AND APPENDICES
• Normal Antepartum
• Selected Daily Dietary Allowances—Maternal (Appendix 2)
• Aspects of Psychological Care—Maternal (Appendix 4)

ADDITIONAL NURSING DIAGNOSES
• Constipation related to inadequate food intake
• Impaired home maintenance management related to debilitating emesis and subsequent generalized paresis
• Sensory-perceptual alteration (gustatory) related to persistent emesis

ANTEPARTUM
Multiple Gestation

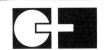

DEFINITION
Multiple gestation is the concurrent development of two or more embryos in utero. The fertilization of two separate ova results in dizygotic, or fraternal, twins; twins arising from a single fertilized ovum result in monozygotic, or identical, twins. Concurrent development of more than two fetuses involves either or both of the fertilization processes. Zygosity is usually established by postpartum examination of the placenta and membranes. Management—primarily bed rest—is directed at delaying the onset of labor and the delivery of preterm infants, at least until fetal lungs have sufficiently matured. Atraumatic delivery of viable infants is of prime concern. Maternal complications include exaggerated discomforts of pregnancy, anemia, hydramnios, pregnancy-induced or pregnancy-aggravated hypertension, placenta previa, abruptio placentae, umbilical cord accidents, preterm delivery with a complicated labor, postpartum hemorrhage, possible coagulopathy, or spontaneous abortion and prenatal death. Implications for the fetus include congenital malformation (more common in monozygotic twins), death in utero of one fetus, shunting of blood between placentas, retarded intrauterine growth or discordant growth, premature birth and subsequent low birth weight, and respiratory impairment.

ETIOLOGY AND PRECIPITATING FACTORS
• Monozygotic twinning is a random occurrence essentially unrelated to heredity, age, race, parity, or treatment for infertility.
• Dizygotic twinning is affected by these factors, revealed by a frequency profile:
  □ race—higher rates in blacks; lower rates in Asians
  □ women who were dizygotic twins carry an autosomal recessive genotype
  □ increased maternal age and parity—age 35 or more; parity more than 4
  □ elevated endogenous follicle-stimulating hormone implicated
  □ use of agents to treat infertility, such as gonadotropin or clomiphene citrate (Clomid), commonly results in ovulation of multiple ova.

PHYSICAL FINDINGS
Genitourinary
• uterine size greater than gestational age would warrant
• palpation of a large number of fetal parts on all sides of the abdomen
• distinct, asynchronous fetal heart tones at or after 20 weeks' gestation

DIAGNOSTIC STUDIES
• Ultrasonography reveals separate gestational sacs.

Nursing diagnosis: *High risk for maternal and fetal injury related to physiologic demands of a multifetal pregnancy (2 goals)*

GOAL 1: Recognize signs of multifetal pregnancy.

Interventions
1. Note date of last menstrual period and maternal history. Monitor weight, fundal height, fetal heart tones, and multiple areas of fetal activity at each clinic visit.

2. Additional individualized interventions: _____

Rationales
1. Early management of a multifetal pregnancy can decrease perinatal mortality and morbidity.

2. Rationales: _____

GOAL 2: Minimize the physiologic stressors associated with multifetal pregnancies.

Interventions
1. Counsel patient about increased dietary requirements, including:
• intake of additional 300 kcal/day
• increased protein intake up to 1.5 grams/kg of body weight
• iron supplementation of 60 to 100 mg/day
• vitamin and mineral supplementation.

Rationales
1. Increased resting metabolic rate, fetal mass, and maternal changes require additional calories to support growth and activity. Extra protein is required to provide for fetal growth and accessory maternal tissue, especially uterine and placental tissue. Maternal blood volume is approximately 500 ml greater with twins than with single-fetus pregnancies.

Interventions	**Rationales**
2. Encourage multiple small meals.	2. Pressure of the expanding uterus on the stomach may decrease appetite. Small, frequent meals may facilitate intake of required foods.
3. Weigh patient at each clinic visit.	3. Progressive weight gain, uncomplicated by edema, usually indicates diet adequacy. Failure to gain has a poor prognosis.
4. Counsel the patient about increased rest needs, suggesting that she get 10 hours of sleep per night and 2 hours per afternoon. Patient may be hospitalized as early as beginning of third trimester.	4. Bed rest has been associated with facilitation of fetal growth, increased birth weight, and prevention of prematurity.
5. Additional individualized interventions: _____ _____	5. Rationales: _____ _____

Collaborative problem: *Discomfort related to increased uterine size (2 goals)*

GOAL 1: Minimize discomfort.

Interventions	**Rationales**
1. Counsel patient on ways to minimize discomfort, such as bed rest in left lateral position, use of maternity girdle, and use of thromboembolic stockings.	1. Bed rest minimizes mechanical pressure on the lower back. The left lateral position facilitates uterine and kidney perfusion, reducing maternal hypertension to which these patients are prone. The maternity girdle provides muscle support. Pressure of the enlarged uterus on pelvic vessels impedes blood flow to and from the legs. Stockings compress superficial leg veins and facilitate venous return from deep leg veins.
2. Additional individualized interventions: _____ _____	2. Rationales: _____ _____

GOAL 2: Recognize excessive accumulation of amniotic fluid.

Interventions	**Rationales**
1. Monitor fundal height, weight gain unrelated to intake or edema, onset of dyspnea or orthopnea, and signs of obstructive uropathy (oliguria and azotemia) at each clinic visit.	1. Hydramnios may result in preterm labor. Amniocentesis provides dramatic relief of the patient's symptoms, but the fluid quickly reaccumulates.
2. Schedule sonogram every 4 weeks after 20 weeks. Plot head and chest circumference.	2. Serial assessment assists in recognition of discordant growth.
3. Additional individualized interventions: _____ _____	3. Rationales: _____ _____

Nursing diagnosis: *High risk for injury related to preterm labor and delivery (2 goals)*

GOAL 1: Minimize the risk of initiating preterm labor.

Interventions	**Rationales**
1. Reinforce the need for rest. Bed rest and hospitalization may be required during the third trimester.	1. Bed rest may increase uterine perfusion. Decreased mechanical force on the cervix may delay dilatation.

Interventions

2. Instruct patient to avoid coitus, enemas, and cathartics during the third trimester.

3. Additional individualized interventions: _____

Rationales

2. These activities may trigger uterine contractions.

3. Rationales: _____

GOAL 2: Promote safe delivery of preterm infants.

Interventions

1. Confirm number of fetuses evidenced in sonography.

2. Prepare the patient for vaginal delivery or cesarean section.

3. Notify obstetric and neonatal teams. Have on hand routine delivery room equipment as well as resuscitative equipment for each of the deliveries anticipated.

4. Additional individualized interventions: _____

Rationales

1. Duration of gestation is inversely proportionate to the number of fetuses. Preparation for delivery includes expert care for each of the infants delivered.

2. Vaginal delivery may be attempted if a cephalic presentation of the presenting twin exists. Cesarean section is indicated with fetal distress, hypotonic uterine dysfunction, placental anomalies, severe hypertension, or marked difference between size of fetuses.

3. Preterm delivery of multiple infants requires coordinated, aggressive treatment.

4. Rationales: _____

Nursing diagnosis: *Ineffective individual coping related to dramatic increase in family size*

GOAL: Increase patient's ability to cope.

Interventions

1. Accept patient's response to pregnancy outcome. Answer any questions the patient may have directly and honestly. Include the patient's mate in interactions.

2. Provide opportunity as soon as feasible for handling infants. Arrange for child care classes that include care of twins.

3. Refer to social service, as indicated.

4. Additional individualized interventions: _____

Rationales

1. Response to pregnancy outcome is highly individual. Acceptance of the patient's response and inclusion of significant others facilitates ability to cope.

2. Handling facilitates maternal-infant bonding. Classes give a frame of reference for care of multiple infants, providing practice and opportunity for reinforcement.

3. Increased or unexpected family needs may trigger a financial crisis.

4. Rationales: _____

ASSOCIATED PLANS AND APPENDICES
• Cesarean Section Birth
• Inappropriate Size or Weight for Gestational Age, Small
• Normal Antepartum
• Preterm Infant, Less Than 37 Weeks
• Aspects of Psychological Care—Maternal (Appendix 4)
• Preparing for Nonemergency Surgery (Appendix 5)

ADDITIONAL NURSING DIAGNOSES
• Activity intolerance related to anatomic and physiologic demands of multifetal pregnancy
• Ineffective breathing pattern related to uterine pressure against the lungs

Placenta Previa

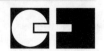

DEFINITION

Placenta previa is low placental attachment over or near the internal cervical os. The degrees of placental placement, from least to greatest severity, respectively, are:
• low implantation or low-lying placenta, in which the placenta is implanted in the lower uterine segment close to the os
• marginal placenta previa, in which the placenta encroaches upon but does not occlude the os
• partial or incomplete placenta previa, in which the placenta partially occludes the os
• total or central placenta previa, in which the placenta completely occludes the os.

Uterine segment differentiation in later pregnancy causes the lower section to lengthen and thin. Placental villi tear and bleeding occurs from open uterine sinuses. Maternal complications include hemorrhage and shock and may necessitate preterm delivery. No associated pain in this third trimester event occurs unless it occurs simultaneously with the onset of labor. Confirmed placenta previa associated with minimal vaginal bleeding early in the third trimester may be treated conservatively with bed rest to allow the fetus time to mature. Uncontrolled vaginal bleeding, fetal distress, or loss of fetal viability warrant delivery; labor may be spontaneous or induced by amniotomy and vaginal delivery accomplished if the following conditions exist: gestational age of 37 weeks or more or fetal lung maturity established by lecithin sphingomyelin ratio, cervix partially dilated, low presenting fetal part, or minimal or controlled bleeding. Cesarean section delivery is performed if the placenta is felt on cervical examination; with massive, uncontrolled bleeding; or in case of fetal distress.

ETIOLOGY AND PRECIPITATING FACTORS
• etiology unknown
• patient at risk: increased parity, advancing age, multiple pregnancy, uterine scarring associated with surgery, and erythroblastosis fetalis

PHYSICAL FINDINGS
Cardiovascular
• tachycardia
• hypotension
• vertigo
• syncope
• diaphoresis
• pallor
• cyanosis

Genitourinary
• painless, bright red, scant to profuse vaginal bleeding in third trimester
• normal uterine tone
• soft, nontender uterus
• fetal malpresentation: oblique, breech, or transverse
• fundal height greater than gestational age would warrant; placenta hindering fetal descent
• oliguria or anuria

Integumentary
• cold, moist skin
• dry mucous membranes

Neurologic
• restlessness
• lethargy
• confusion
• somnolence

Respiratory
• tachypnea

Subjective
• feelings of thirst, cold, apprehension

DIAGNOSTIC STUDIES
• Ultrasonography reveals placental implantation site, fetal viability, gestational age, position, and station.
• X-ray studies may reveal soft tissue density in front of presenting fetal part.
• Isotope scanning or localization locates the placenta.
• Vaginal or rectal examinations are contraindicated because manipulation of the cervix may initiate massive bleeding. If patient is at or near term, if labor has begun, or if bleeding threatens maternal welfare, the physician may perform a vaginal examination in an operating room where setups for both vaginal and cesarean section deliveries are immediately available.

Laboratory data
• hemoglobin (Hb) and hematocrit (HCT) values—decrease
• coagulation factors—usually within normal limits

Collaborative problem: *Fluid volume deficit related to bleeding (3 goals)*

GOAL 1: Identify signs of bleeding.

Interventions

1. Assess bleeding every 15 minutes or as patient's condition warrants:

• Note onset and amount of vaginal bleeding before admission.

• Monitor vaginal bleeding: color, number of perineal pads used, degree of saturation, and weight.

• Assess vital signs, capillary refill time, and pulse pressure; compare with baseline.

• *Do not* perform vaginal examinations.

2. Monitor Hb and HCT values.

3. Additional individualized interventions: _____

Rationales

1. Blood loss may occur at rest or during activity; it may be characterized as spotting, gushing, or continuous.

• Painless, bright red vaginal bleeding in the third trimester characterizes placenta previa.

• Accurate assessment helps estimate blood loss and estimate replacement needs. (*Note:* 1 gram of blood by weight equals 1 ml; saturated pad is approximately 100 ml.)

• A decreased refill time in the capillary blanch test indicates decreased peripheral circulation. A narrowing pulse pressure indicates early shock. Maternal hypervolemia and initial compensatory mechanisms may mask signs of shock: tachycardia, hypotension, tachypnea, and restlessness.

• Vaginal examination may trigger severe hemorrhage.

2. Decreasing Hb and HCT values are consistent with blood loss.

3. Rationales: _____

GOAL 2: Restore and maintain normovolemia.

Interventions

1. Maintain hydration.

• Administer I.V. infusion of lactated Ringer's solution, using a large-bore needle.

• Monitor hourly fluid intake and output.

• Perform central venous pressure (CVP) monitoring.

2. Administer whole blood.

3. Additional individualized interventions: _____

Rationales

1. Rapid fluid replacement is necessary to correct hypovolemia.

• Fluids and venous access are provided while awaiting typing and crossmatching of blood products. Food and water are withheld in anticipation of delivery.

• Minimum physiologically acceptable urine output is 30 ml/hour. Output reflects renal perfusion.

• Normal CVP readings during pregnancy are 8 to 10 cm H_2O. Readings of 15 to 20 cm H_2O indicate circulatory overload. Monitoring trend response and adjusting I.V. flow rates facilitates safe, accurate replacement therapy.

2. Large volumes may be required to replace loss.

3. Rationales: _____

GOAL 3: Optimize tissue perfusion.

Interventions

1. Maintain bed rest in left lateral position.

2. Administer oxygen by mask at 7 to 10 liters/minute, as patient condition warrants.

Rationales

1. Bed rest decreases physiologic and metabolic demands. The left side-lying position promotes blood flow to the uterus and fetus.

2. Supplemental oxygen enhances tissue perfusion at alveolocapillary membrane.

Interventions	Rationales
3. Additional individualized interventions: _____	3. Rationales: _____

Collaborative problem: *High risk for maternal injury related to uteroplacental insufficiency (2 goals)*

GOAL 1: Detect early signs of fetal distress.

Interventions	Rationales
1. Assess fetal status (with external fetal monitor only) with each maternal assessment, noting fetal heart rate (FHR) patterns, variability, fetal activity, and comparison with baseline.	1. Indications of fetal distress include fetal tachycardia and decreased baseline variability with late onset and recovery deceleration times. Cessation of FHR warrants immediate surgical intervention.
2. Additional individualized interventions: _____	2. Rationales: _____

GOAL 2: Promote safe delivery of preterm infant.

Interventions	Rationales
1. Prepare for cesarean section.	1. Prompt delivery of a compromised fetus is critical to survival.
2. Notify perinatal team of impending delivery and have operative, resuscitative equipment at hand.	2. Survival of preterm infant is dependent on aggressive resuscitation and sustained intensive care.
3. Additional individualized interventions: _____	3. Rationales: _____

Nursing diagnosis: *Fear related to unknown fetal outcome*

GOAL: Decrease fear.

Interventions	Rationales
1. Provide information in a clear, forthright manner; ascertain patient's understanding of information given.	1. Open communication gives patient a sense of control and helps decrease fear. Infant survival depends on gestational age, maturity, and amount of blood lost.
2. Permit presence of significant others. Keep them informed of patient's progress, allowing phone calls and visits as appropriate.	2. Interaction utilizes already established support system.
3. Additional individualized interventions: _____	3. Rationales: _____

ASSOCIATED PLANS AND APPENDICES
• Cesarean Section Birth
• Inappropriate Size or Weight for Gestational Age, Small
• Labor and Vaginal Birth
• Preterm Infant, Less Than 37 Weeks
• Aspects of Psychological Care—Maternal (Appendix 4)

ADDITIONAL NURSING DIAGNOSES
• Knowledge deficit related to impending emergency surgery
• Self-esteem disturbance related to inability to give birth vaginally and to preterm delivery

Pregnancy Complicated by Cardiac Disease

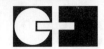

DEFINITION

Anatomic and physiologic changes of the cardiovascular system occur throughout pregnancy. Normal compensatory mechanisms include—but are not limited to—increases in cardiac output, heart rate, and total blood volume. The cardiovascular system, in its normal uncompromised state, can withstand these stressors as well as those associated with labor, delivery, and the postpartum state. However, the system stressed by cardiac disease lacks the reserve to adapt to these changes. Diagnosis of cardiac disease in a pregnant patient may be difficult because of the normal changes associated with pregnancy, such as functional systolic murmurs, dyspnea, and edema. Rheumatic heart disease and congenital defects comprise the majority of cardiovascular diseases occurring during pregnancy. Surgical repairs to correct underlying defects are ideally done before conception, but may be performed during pregnancy. Obstetric care is aimed at preventing or minimizing complications. A standardized patient classification system is based on the patient's increasing disability (Classes I to IV, respectively) and reflects the functional capacity of the heart. Regardless of the cause of the cardiac disorder, management is orchestrated by classification. The gravity of each classification and the potential progression from one to the next must be recognized. Cardiac decompensation is the prime complication; it may result in spontaneous abortion, fetal growth retardation, preterm delivery, intrauterine death, and maternal death. Prognosis is usually good, but depends on the functional capacity of the heart, complications that would further stress the already compromised heart, aggressive treatment, and ability of the patient to comply with the rigid prescribed regimen.

ETIOLOGY AND PRECIPITATING FACTORS

• rheumatic heart disease; congenital heart defects; syphilis; arteriosclerosis; coronary occlusion; renal, pulmonary, and thyroid disorders; skeletal defects of the spine; peripartal cardiomyopathy

PHYSICAL FINDINGS
Cardiovascular
• vertigo
• syncope
• tachycardia
• pulse irregularities*

• progressive generalized edema*
• diastolic, presystolic, or continuous murmur†
• loud, harsh, systolic murmur, especially if associated with a thrill†
• severe arrhythmia†
• unequivocal cardiac enlargement†

Integumentary
• cyanosis*

Respiratory
• dyspnea
• orthopnea*
• cough, with or without hemoptysis*
• basilar crackles*

Subjective
• feelings of fatigue, palpitations, smothering

DIAGNOSTIC STUDIES
• Radiologic studies may reveal abnormalities in cardiac or vessel size, contour, outline, position, or density; unequivocal cardiac enlargement confirms a diagnosis of cardiovascular disease in pregnancy.
(*Note:* The necessity of X-ray studies must be carefully evaluated; if studies are performed, a lead shield should cover the abdomen and pelvis.)
• ECG may reveal hypertrophy, arrhythmias, ischemia, conduction defects, heart block, pericarditis, and electrolyte abnormalities.
• Echocardiography may reveal valvular abnormalities, ventricular dysfunction, or other cardiac disorders.
• Phonocardiography may reveal valvular abnormalities as well as other cardiac disorders.

Laboratory data
• Hemoglobin (Hb) and hematocrit (HCT) values—may decrease in response to expansion of blood volume (normal 12 to 15 g/dl and 35% to 45%, respectively). HCT may increase from constant hypoxia.
• White blood cell count—increases (normal 5,000 to 10,000/mm^3 in first trimester; 10,000 to 12,000/mm^3 by term).
• Clotting factors—decrease; depression of fibrinolytic activity is seen during normal pregnancy and during postpartum.

---

*Presenting signs and symptoms of cardiovascular disease in pregnancy, with other findings normal
†Confirms the diagnosis of cardiovascular disease in pregnancy

Collaborative problem: *Increased cardiac output related to the physiologic demands of pregnancy on an already-compromised heart (3 goals)*

GOAL 1: Recognize the cardiovascular alterations caused by pregnancy.

Interventions

1. Note at each clinic visit and compare with baseline of nonpregnant state:
- blood pressure

- heart rate

- respiratory rate.

2. Assess for benign physiologic edema, including dependent leg edema.

3. Assess for anemia, including decreased Hb and HCT values, pallor, and decreased, disproportionate activity tolerance.

4. Coordinate consultation with a cardiologist.

5. Additional individualized interventions: _____

Rationales

1. Ongoing assessment permits timely interventions, if required.

- A decrease of 5 to 10 mm Hg in both systolic and diastolic arterial pressure is seen in the first half of pregnancy and is related to peripheral vasodilation; by the third trimester, values have reverted to earlier levels.

- A gradual increase of 15 to 20 beats/minute is seen between the 14th and 20th week of pregnancy; increase persists for remainder of pregnancy and is related to increased cardiac output.

- An increase in respiratory rate of about two breaths/minute is seen concurrently with increased volume or depth of respiration and is related to increased oxygen demands; a lowered CO_2 threshold in response to hormonal changes contributes to feeling of dyspnea.

2. Pooling of fluid in the legs occurs in later pregnancy and results from pressure of the gravid uterus on blood vessels.

3. Hemoglobin and hematocrit values of 10 g/dl and 35%, respectively, indicate anemia. Symptoms result from decreased oxygen availability. Activity intolerance may indicate heart failure.

4. Care of the high-risk pregnant patient requires medical as well as obstetric management.

5. Rationales: _____

GOAL 2: Decrease stressors that would place further demands on cardiac function.

Interventions

1. Advise adequate rest. Minimum requirements include:
- 10 hours of sleep every night
- half hour rest period after each meal
- light housework, some easy walking permitted
- no lifting, straining.

2. Advise dietary control. Include the following in teaching:
- weight gain not to exceed the recommended 22 to 28 lb (10 to 13 kg) during the course of the pregnancy
- limitations on sodium intake:
   □ no high-sodium foods
   □ no added salt in food preparation or serving
- monitoring potassium intake and for symptoms of hypokalemia, which include thirst, vertigo, confusion, hypoventilation, muscular weakness, twitching, tetany, and pulse irregularities
- monitoring iron intake; nutrition teaching should include identifying foods high in iron.

Rationales

1. Rest requirements progress from Class I to IV; Classes III and IV require bed rest and hospitalization for the duration of pregnancy. Class IV patients have decompensation at rest and require aggressive medical and obstetric care.

2. Dietary control promotes decreased stress on cardiovascular system.

- Weight gain allows for optimal fetal growth and maternal changes.

- Excess weight from retained fluids increases the cardiac work load. Sodium intake tends to increase fluid retention.

- Erratic or decreased potassium levels may be associated with cardiac dysfunction or be an adverse reaction to digitalis therapy.

- Dietary iron requirements of pregnancy are approximately 18 mg/day with supplementary preparations of 200 mg of simple iron compounds recommended.

Interventions

3. Promote infection control, including prevention of respiratory and urinary tract infections. Take drug sensitivity history; administer benzathine penicillin G (Bicillin L-A) 1.2 million units I.M. each month for patients with a history of rheumatic fever or rheumatic heart disease.

4. Monitor anticoagulant (heparin) therapy, if prescribed, including the following:

• activated partial thromboplastin time (APTT)

• signs of bleeding: petechiae, ecchymosis, hematuria, tarry stools, or bleeding from any orifice.

5. Additional individualized interventions: _____

Rationales

3. Infection is implicated in triggering decompensation because it may increase metabolism and contribute to the spread of organisms to cardiac structure. Antibiotics may be given prophylactically to minimize the risk of bacterial endocarditis.

4. Heparin is the drug of choice antepartum because it does not cross the placenta.

• APTT from 1.5 to 2.5 times the control indicate accepted therapeutic anticoagulant range.

• These signs may require decreased dose or withdrawal of heparin or administration of protamine sulfate.

5. Rationales: _____

GOAL 3: Recognize the signs and symptoms of cardiac decompensation.

Interventions

1. Assess the following at each clinic visit, every 8 hours during hospitalization, or as patient condition warrants:
• patient perceptions of increasing fatigue, vertigo, difficulty breathing, palpitations, and chest pain
• generalized edema
• persistent basilar crackles, hemoptysis
• pulse irregularities.

2. Additional individualized interventions: _____

Rationales

1. Continual assessment is imperative because the onset of signs and symptoms may be gradual or abrupt. Cardiac decompensation warrants immediate medical intervention; correction is necessary for safe delivery with satisfactory maternal and fetal outcomes.

2. Rationales: _____

Collaborative problem: *High risk for maternal injury related to increased cardiac work load during labor and delivery*

GOAL: Minimize maternal injury; promote safe delivery.

Interventions

1. Monitor labor, and take these steps:

• Administer oxygen by mask.

• Withhold heparin just before delivery.

• Administer morphine if delivery is not imminent.
• Administer aqueous penicillin G and either gentamicin (Garamycin) or tobramycin (Tobrex).
• Position in side-lying position, preferably left. Elevate head and shoulders with pillows.

2. Monitor for cardiac decompensation with each labor assessment, noting pulse greater than 100 beats/minute or respirations greater than 24 breaths/minute or dyspnea.

Rationales

1. Vaginal delivery is the procedure of choice; cesarean section is usually limited to correction of an obstetric emergency.

• Supplemental oxygen enhances perfusion at the alveolocapillary membrane.

• The increased risk of hemorrhage associated with labor and delivery precludes anticoagulant use.

• Pain and anxiety increase cardiac work load.

• Antibiotics minimize the risk of bacterial endocarditis and infective arteritis.

• Position minimizes the risk of supine hypotensive syndrome and facilitates uterine perfusion.

2. These signs, when accompanied by a completely dilated cervix and engaged presenting part, are indicators of delivery. With only partial dilatation, cardiac decompensation is diagnosed and will progress with delivery.

Interventions

3. Assist with treatments for cardiac decompensation, including the following:
• Place the patient in Fowler's position and administer oxygen via intermittent positive pressure.
• Administer furosemide (Lasix) I.V.
• Administer digitalis I.V.

4. Assist with delivery, including these steps:
• Place the patient in left lateral or semirecumbent position.
• Avoid use of stirrups.
• Assist with the administration of anesthesia.

• Monitor blood pressure.

5. Additional individualized interventions: _____

Rationales

3. This enhances oxygenation and decreases the potential for pulmonary edema. Stimulation of diuresis will ultimately reduce pulmonary congestion. A rapid-acting cardiac glycoside such as digitalis increases the force and the effectiveness of the myocardial contraction.

4. Assistance promotes safe delivery.
• These positions enhance cardiac function.

• Venous compression impedes circulation.
• Besides administering analgesia, it is necessary to minimize the bearing down reflex and resulting multi-factor cardiac stressors. Epidural anesthesia may be indicated.

• Hypotension associated with anesthesia poses grave maternal risks.

5. Rationales: _____

Nursing diagnosis: *High risk for fetal injury related to uteroplacental insufficiency (2 goals)*

GOAL 1: Detect early signs of fetal distress.

Interventions

1. Starting in last half of pregnancy, instruct patient to count daily fetal movements and to report any sudden decreases in or cessation of movement.

2. Starting at 32 weeks' gestation, perform nonstress test (NST) with each clinic visit.

3. Assess fetal status with each maternal assessment, including FHR patterns and variability and fetal activity. Compare with baseline.

4. Additional individualized interventions: _____

Rationales

1. Fetal activity is highly variable. Consistent movement later in pregnancy is one indicator of fetal health. Sudden decreases in activity portend fetal jeopardy.

2. A reactive NST (fetal activity with an increase in fetal heart rate [FHR]) is one indicator of fetal well-being and is associated with fetal development and maturity.

3. Indications of fetal distress include hyperactivity; fetal heart tones that are slow, irregular, and clinically difficult to hear; late decelerations; and increased FHR with decreased variability.

4. Rationales: _____

GOAL 2: Promote safe delivery of the preterm infant.

Interventions

1. Facilitate labor and monitor its progress.

2. Notify neonatal unit of impending delivery. Obtain necessary resuscitative equipment.

3. Additional individualized interventions: _____

Rationales

1. Prompt delivery of a compromised fetus is critical to its survival.

2. Survival of preterm infant depends on aggressive resuscitation and sustained intensive care.

3. Rationales: _____

ASSOCIATED PLANS AND APPENDICES
• Inappropriate Size or Weight for Gestational Age, Small
• Normal Antepartum
• Preterm Infant, Less Than 37 Weeks
• Aspects of Psychological Care—Maternal (Appendix 4)

ADDITIONAL NURSING DIAGNOSES
• Activity intolerance related to cardiovascular stresses of pregnancy on a compromised heart
• Altered sexuality patterns related to need for family planning of future pregnancies
• Impaired home maintenance management related to decreased ability to perform usual homemaker functions
• Powerlessness related to conflicting maternal role and rigid health restrictions

Pregnancy Complicated by Diabetes Mellitus

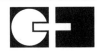

DEFINITION

Diabetes mellitus is a disorder of carbohydrate, protein, and fat metabolism. It results from abnormal insulin secretion or utilization and is characterized by fasting hyperglycemia and decreased glucose tolerance. Because pregnancy places additional stressors on carbohydrate metabolism, it is potentially diabetogenic; that is, it may trigger the syndrome. It may also aggravate pre-existing diabetes and increase the risk of certain complications associated with pregnancy. Gestational diabetes is a classification that includes glucose intolerance either induced by pregnancy or discovered during pregnancy. In general, diabetic patients are at risk for ketoacidosis associated with hyperglycemia, macrovascular and microvascular diseases, and neuropathy; hypoglycemia and resulting shock are associated with variables of insulin regulation. The diabetic patient is at greater risk for more frequent and more severe infection, pregnancy-induced hypertension, abruptio placentae, spontaneous abortion, hydramnios, dystocia and vaginal injuries associated with macrosomia (large for gestational age [LGA] infants), postpartum hemorrhage, and death. Infants of diabetic mothers are at risk for the following: being small for gestational age in mothers with advanced diabetes complicated by vascular disease; lung immaturity; respiratory distress syndrome; macrosomia (mother mild diabetic without vascular disease); multiple birth traumas associated directly with macrosomia and difficult vaginal delivery; multiple congenital anomalies; hypoglycemia, hypocalcemia, hyperbilirubinemia, a predisposition to diabetes, and death. Medical management, ranging from dietary modifications alone to control with insulin, is directed at controlling maternal glycemia throughout pregnancy to ensure maternal health, to minimize complications, and to facilitate a good fetal outcome.

ETIOLOGY AND PRECIPITATING FACTORS

• etiology: complex interplay of heredity and environment
• patient at risk: close familial history of diabetes, including twin concordance, obstetric history of hydramnios or fetal demise, previous delivery of an LGA neonate (weighing 9 lb [4,000 g] or more), or congenital anomalies
• patient profile that suggests disorder: recurrent, resistant candidal vaginitis; hydramnios; LGA fetus; persistent glycosuria

PHYSICAL FINDINGS*
Genitourinary
• fundal height greater than gestational age would warrant
• urinary frequency after the first trimester
• persistent glycosuria

Subjective
• feelings of excessive thirst or hunger

DIAGNOSTIC STUDIES
• Suspicious patient history or clinical profile warrants laboratory workup to confirm diagnosis.
• Sonography confirms fetal age and identifies hydramnios, fetal macrosomia, and intrauterine growth retardation.

Laboratory data
• fasting plasma glucose (FPG)*—increases
• glycosylated hemoglobin (HbA_{1c}) increases (values represent mean blood glucose level over previous 4 to 8 weeks; accurate only after 7th week of gestation)
• postprandial plasma glucose—increases
• oral glucose tolerance test (OGTT)*—increases
• I.V. glucose tolerance test (IVGTT)—increases
• tolbutamide tolerance test—contraindicated for both diagnosis and treatment, because the drug may have a teratogenic effect and produces hypoglycemia in the neonate

---

CRITERIA FOR DIAGNOSIS OF GESTATIONAL DIABETES USING 100-G ORAL GLUCOSE TOLERANCE TEST

Venous Plasma Glucose
The following venous plasma glucose levels confirm gestational diabetes when two or more levels are met or exceeded.

Fasting ≥ 105 mg/dl (5.8 mmol/L)
1 hour ≥ 190 mg/dl (10.6 mmol/L)
2 hours ≥ 165 mg/dl (9.2 mmol/L)
3 hours ≥ 145 mg/dl (8.1 mmol/L)

Adapted from "Classification and Diagnosis of Diabetes Mellitus and Other Categories of Glucose Intolerance," by the National Diabetes Data Group, M. Harris et al, in *Diabetes,* Vol. 28, page 1049. December 1979.

---

*Findings represent early diabetes not complicated by impending ketoacidosis or by vascular or neurologic changes.

Collaborative problem: *Alteration in carbohydrate metabolism related to normal gestation or to pregnancy-induced or overt dysfunction (3 goals)*

GOAL 1: Identify normal changes in glucose excretion during pregnancy.

Interventions

1. Monitor urine glucose level using reagent strip (Testape or Cliniustix) with each clinic visit or, if hospitalized, before meals and at bedtime. Verify fasting or preprandial status.

2. Additional individualized interventions: _____

Rationales

1. Glycosuria commonly results from a lowered renal threshold for glucose induced by pregnancy and does not necessarily indicate pathology. Testing agents are specific for glucose and bypass positive results caused by benign lactosuria.

2. Rationales: _____

GOAL 2: Identify endogenous insulin regulation and adapt exogenous insulin requirements to maternal physiologic demands.

Interventions

1. Monitor blood glucose levels, as ordered, and administer insulin accordingly.

2. Regulate insulin dosage based on physiologic needs, which vary with trimester demands. The first trimester produces lower requirements; and the second and third trimesters produce increased and highly individual requirements.

3. Monitor for sudden onset of the following signs and symptoms:
• nervousness
• shaking, trembling
• weakness
• hunger
• moist, pale skin
• normal or shallow respirations
• normal to full, bounding pulse
• headache
• diplopia, blurred vision
• disorientation
• seizures, coma.

4. Monitor for gradual onset of the following signs and symptoms:
• polyuria, polydipsia
• thirst
• nausea and vomiting
• abdominal pain
• flushed, dry skin
• weak, rapid pulse; low blood pressure
• fruity, acetone breath
• drowsiness, headache.

5. Additional individualized interventions: _____

Rationales

1. Blood glucose profile reflects glycemic state than urine more accurately. Lowered renal threshold may result in glycosuria with blood glucose levels as low as 130 mg/dl.

2. Proliferation primarily of placental hormones, human placental lactogen, estrogen, and progesterone results in insulin resistance; insulinase, a placental enzyme, increases degradation of insulin. Hormone production peaks between weeks 18 and 20.

3. These are signs and symptoms of hypoglycemia, which may result from insufficient food intake or excessive insulin administration. Blood glucose levels will be less than 60 mg/dl; no glucose will be seen in urine; and ketones will be absent (negative) to trace in blood and urine. Prompt treatment with a readily absorbable oral carbohydrate in the conscious patient or of I.V. glucagon or glucose in the unconscious patient is crucial to prevent maternal cerebral hypoglycemia, which may jeopardize fetal life.

4. These are signs and symptoms of diabetic ketoacidosis, which may result from normal or excessive food intake and insufficient insulin. Blood glucose levels will be greater than 250 mg/dl; urine glucose levels will be high; and ketone levels will be high in blood and urine.

5. Rationales: _____

GOAL 3: Control maternal glucose levels; maintain euglycemia.

Interventions	Rationales
1. Coordinate with dietitian in diet regulation, including adequate daily intake of high-quality foods, specifically: • protein: 1.3 to 1.7 grams/kg of pregnant body weight; add 1 oz (30 grams) to current diet • carbohydrate: 5 to 7 oz (150 to 200 grams) of complex starches; avoid concentrated sweets • fat: 2 to 3 oz (60 to 80 grams).	1. Balanced diet promotes fetal growth and maternal changes. Control of maternal glucose levels early in pregnancy minimizes risk of congenital fetal anomalies.
2. Regulate weight gain: • 13.5 to 18 kcal/lb (30 to 40 kcal/kg) • weight reduction or calorie restriction in obese patient not advisable • pattern of weight gain: 2 to 4 lb (1 to 2 kg) during first trimester; 0.9 lb (0.4 kg) per week afterward • meal spacing: three meals, with three equally spaced snacks.	2. Caloric intake supports fetal growth, enlargement of the breast and uterus, and production of amniotic fluid, blood, and extracellular fluid. Inadequate caloric intake may result in nutritional deficiencies and catabolism of maternal tissue. Food intake should parallel peaks of insulin activity. Spacing of meals minimizes risk of hypoglycemia and promotes euglycemia.
3. Monitor exercise regimen; avoid spurts of activity or sporadic exercising. Adjust program in view of pre-pregnancy endurance levels, trimester, glucose levels, and insulin requirements.	3. Blood glucose levels usually decrease with exercise, decreasing the need for insulin. Insulin dosage may need to be altered to parallel maternal glucose levels. Complex carbohydrate intake before exercise reduces risk of hypoglycemia. Sporadic, inconsistent exercise causes fluctuations in blood glucose levels that are difficult to control.
4. Monitor the patient for the following: • upper respiratory infection: throat soreness, nasal congestion, sneezing, rhinorrhea, watery eyes • urinary tract infection: urinary frequency and nocturia combined with urgency and dysuria • candidiasis: scant white or yellow vaginal discharge; vulval edema, erythema, and pruritus; possibly white, cheesy patches on vaginal walls; dyspareunia.	4. Infections in the pregnant diabetic are more frequent, severe, and resistant to treatment. The physiologic stressors of infection, compounded by insulin resistance associated with infection during pregnancy, may trigger hyperglycemia.
5. Additional individualized interventions: _____	5. Rationales: _____

Nursing diagnosis: *Anxiety related to maternal diagnosis*

GOAL: Minimize anxiety.

Interventions	Rationales
1. Provide information on diabetes and diabetes control in a clear, forthright manner. Ascertain patient's comprehension of information and introduce new information slowly and sequentially.	1. Open communication helps establish trust and good rapport.
• Include information on diet, blood and urine testing, insulin administration and glucose monitoring, hypoglycemic reactions and remedies, and infection control; stress prevention.	• Accurate information gives patient a sense of control over disorder.
• Demonstrate blood or urine testing and insulin administration.	• Skills are essential in maintaining consistent blood levels.
• Ask patient to give return demonstrations on blood or urine testing and insulin administration.	• Demonstrations objectively validate patient competency.
2. Refer patient to diabetes support group.	2. Identification with others with similar problems offers a forum for information sharing and provides support.

Interventions

3. Additional individualized interventions: _____

_____

Rationales

3. Rationales: _____

_____

Nursing diagnosis: *Powerlessness related to fetal outcome*

GOAL: Minimize powerlessness.

Interventions

1. Accept patient as member of health care team; keep her informed of fetal status.

2. Reinforce teaching on diabetes control.

3. Additional individualized interventions: _____

_____

Rationales

1. Providing information on test results and options for self-care gives patient a sense of control.

2. Control of blood glucose level in early pregnancy is associated with lowered risk of congenital anomalies.

3. Rationales: _____

_____

Collaborative problem: *Ineffective breathing pattern related to uterine enlargement and excessive amniotic fluid*

GOAL: Facilitate effective breathing.

Interventions

1. Monitor patient's color, activity tolerance, and vital signs.

2. Maintain patient in upright position.

3. Assist physician with amniocentesis.

4. Additional individualized interventions: _____

_____

Rationales

1. Comprehensive assessment is necessary to rule out other causes of dyspnea.

2. The upright position decreases mechanical pressure of uterus on adjacent organs.

3. Release of fluid provides immediate relief.

4. Rationales: _____

_____

Collaborative problem: *High risk for fetal injury related to dependence on maternal glycemic states (2 goals)*

GOAL 1: Minimize potential for injury.

Interventions

1. Monitor maternal insulin requirements and glucose level control; correlate with trimester.

2. Starting in second half of pregnancy, instruct patient to count daily fetal movements and to report any sudden decreases in or cessation of movements.

Rationales

1. Initial decreases in insulin requirements, followed by increases in second and third trimesters, imply placental function.

2. Fetal activity is highly variable. Consistent movement in later pregnancy is one indicator of fetal health; sudden decreases in activity portend fetal jeopardy.

Interventions

3. Starting at 32 weeks' gestation, perform nonstress test (NST) at each clinic visit.

4. Additional individualized interventions: _____

Rationales

3. A reactive NST (fetal activity with an increase in fetal heart rate) is one indicator of fetal well-being and is associated with fetal development and maturity.

4. Rationales: _____

GOAL 2: Promote safe delivery of the infant.

Interventions

1. Assess fetal lung maturity, using the lecithin/sphingomyelin (L/S) ratio

2. Assist with labor induction, augmentation, vaginal delivery, or cesarean section, as follows:

• Withhold food and beverages.

• Administer an I.V. of 10% dextrose in water.
• Monitor blood glucose level hourly.

• Administer regular insulin I.V.; do not give long or intermediate-acting insulins.

3. Notify neonatal unit of impending delivery. Have necessary resuscitative equipment on hand.

4. Additional individualized interventions: _____

Rationales

1. An L/S ratio of 2.5 or greater indicates fetal lung maturity.

2. Safe delivery requires precise nursing actions based on the expected type of delivery. A planned delivery date is determined by an estimation of fetal age and maturity and an evaluation of the potential risks of acidosis or placental insufficiency.
   A vaginal delivery is attempted when the following criteria are met: cephalopelvic disproportion has been ruled out; vertex presentation is fixed in pelvis; and the cervix is ripe, soft and moderately effaced, and dilated.
   A cesarean section delivery is indicated in macrosomia or with complications necessitating preterm delivery.

• Vomiting and resulting aspiration are a significant source of maternal morbidity and mortality.

• I.V. infusion is a source of fluid and calories.

• Euglycemia during the work of labor or stress of surgery is promoted by frequent evaluation of blood glucose level and highly individualized doses of insulin.

• Regular insulin is the drug of choice because it is rapid acting and has a short duration of effect; it is the only insulin that can be administered I.V.

3. The infant of a diabetic mother, even if near term, may be subject to various complications or to congenital malformation. Sustained, coordinated aggressive care may be warranted.

4. Rationales: _____

ASSOCIATED PLANS AND APPENDICES
• Abortion
• Abruptio Placentae
• Birth Trauma
• Cesarean Section Birth
• Hemorrhage
• Hyperbilirubinemia
• Hypocalcemia
• Hypoglycemia
• Inappropriate Size or Weight for Gestational Age, Large
• Inappropriate Size or Weight for Gestational Age, Small
• Labor and Vaginal Birth
• Normal Antepartum
• Oxytocin-Induced or Oxytocin-Augmented Labor
• Pregnancy-Induced Hypertension
• Aspects of Psychological Care—Maternal (Appendix 4)
• Preparing for Nonemergency Surgery (Appendix 5)

ADDITIONAL NURSING DIAGNOSES
• High risk for trauma associated with delivery of large fetus
• Knowledge deficit related to preconception diabetic regulation before future pregnancies

ANTEPARTUM
Pregnancy-Induced Hypertension

DEFINITION
Preeclampsia, currently known as pregnancy-induced hypertension (PIH), is a syndrome characterized by hypertension, proteinuria, and, frequently, edema. Pathophysiologic processes include—but are not limited to—vascular constriction and vasospasm, increased pressor responses to angiotensin II, decreased normal hypervolemia (hypovolemia), hemoconcentration, coagulopathy, and renal and hepatic dysfunction. PIH may be mild or severe. The preeclamptic condition usually appears at or after the 20th week of gestation and continues into the postpartum period; it may occur in later pregnancy, during labor, or during the first 48 hours postpartum. Symptoms may occur earlier with proliferating chorionic villi, as is found in hydatidiform mole, or marked molar degeneration. Preeclampsia may progress until eclampsia—that is, seizures—occur. Maternal complications partly include cerebrovascular accidents, cerebral edema, coagulopathies, abruptio placentae, renal and hepatic dysfunction, and a fetus that is small for gestational age or stillborn. Management is directed at controlling preeclampsia, minimizing the risk of eclampsia, delivering a viable fetus as close to term as possible, and restoring maternal homeostasis.

ETIOLOGY AND PRECIPITATING FACTORS
• The cause of vasospasm and hypertension in response to chorionic villi is unknown.
• Patient at risk: primigravida, maternal age less than 17 or greater than 35, familial history of PIH, presence of multiple fetuses or hydramnios, diabetes mellitus, chronic vascular or renal disease, hydatidiform mole, or hydrops fetalis.

PHYSICAL FINDINGS
Cardiovascular
• systolic blood pressure of 140 mm Hg or more or any increase of 30 mm Hg or more over predetermined baseline; diastolic blood pressure of 90 mm Hg or more or any increase of 15 mm Hg or more over predetermined baseline
• edema of hands and face, present on arising

Genitourinary
• proteinuria
• oliguria (severe PIH)

Neurologic
• headache (severe PIH)
• visual disturbances (severe PIH)
• hyperflexia (severe PIH)
• seizures (severe PIH)

Subjective
• epigastric or right upper abdominal pain (severe PIH)

DIAGNOSTIC STUDIES
• Ultrasonography may reveal intrauterine growth retardation (IUGR).

Laboratory data
• Urinalysis—protein present.
• Serum total protein and albumin levels—decrease.
• Hematocrit (HCT) value—increases.
• Uric acid level—increases (thiazide therapy may cause independent hyperuricemia).
• Blood urea nitrogen (BUN) and creatinine levels—increase in severe PIH.
• Aspartate aminotransferase (AST) and lactic dehydrogenase levels—increase in severe PIH.
• Bilirubin levels—increases in severe PIH.
• Platelet count—decreases in severe PIH.

Nursing diagnosis: *High risk for maternal injury related to organ or system dysfunction as a sequela of vasospasm and increased blood pressure (5 goals)*

GOAL 1: Recognize the early signs of pregnancy-induced vasospasm and increased blood pressure.

Interventions
1. Monitor blood pressure at each clinic visit.

Rationales
1. Blood pressure normally does not change during pregnancy; slight decreases are seen during the second and early third trimesters. Psychosocial variables that may increase blood pressure (clinic visit itself, noise, small children, lack of support system) should be evaluated. Hypertension exists if blood pressure is elevated on two separate readings taken at least 6 hours apart.

Interventions

- Ensure patient is in same position each time blood pressure is taken.

- Confirm prepregnant baseline values and monitor trends; integrate risk profile with clinical findings.

- Perform roll-over or pressor response test in at-risk primigravida from weeks 28 to 32. Take blood pressure in left lateral recumbent position; repeat blood pressure after turning to supine position.

2. Monitor the patient for proteinuria, defined as 300 mg protein or greater in 24-hour urine specimen or 1 g/liter concentration or greater in a minimum of two random urine specimens taken 6 or more hours apart. Use clean-catch, midstream urine.

3. Monitor for nondependent pathologic edema, especially of hands and face, and integrate finding into complete clinical profile.

4. Additional individualized interventions: _____

Rationales

- Position affects blood pressure readings. Brachial readings vary as follows:
  □ Highest: patient sitting
  □ Intermediate: patient supine
  □ Lowest: patient lying in left lateral position.

- A differential diagnosis of hypertensive states assists in proper management. Chronic, preexisting hypertension must be considered. Eclampsia may rapidly develop in pregnancy-aggravated hypertension; significant increases in blood pressure, without any other symptom, may trigger eclampsia.

- Diastolic increases of 20 mm Hg or more may be predictive of PIH.

2. Proteinuria is seen in approximately 20% of all pregnant patients. It develops later in the course of PIH and may be the last of the triad of symptoms to appear. Proteinuria associated with hypertension is associated with a significant rate of fetal demise. Use clean-catch specimen to avoid a false-positive reading from vaginal secretions or presence of red blood cells.

3. Dependent edema is a common finding in uncomplicated pregnancies. Generalized edema is one of the first of the triad of symptoms to appear. Severity bears little relationship to fetal outcome.

4. Rationales: _____

GOAL 2: Minimize or control progression of dysfunction.

Interventions

1. Institute weight controls, including these steps:

- Instruct patient to weigh daily at home; confirm weight at bimonthly or weekly clinic visits; note dramatic as well as progressive changes.

- Increase protein intake from suggested pregnancy diet of 1 gram/kg/day to 1.5 gram/kg/day.

- Maintain normal sodium intake (2 to 6 grams daily); avoid excessive intake. Avoid use of diuretics.

2. Assess edema at each clinic visit, keeping these guidelines in mind:
- 1+ (2 mm) — minimal edema of pedal and pretibial areas
- 2+ (4 mm) — marked edema of lower extremities
- 3+ (6 mm) — edema of hands, face, lower abdominal wall, and sacrum
- 4+ (8 mm) — severe generalized edema with ascites.

3. Institute bed rest measures at home or in the hospital, recommending the left lateral recumbent position when appropriate.

Rationales

1. A gradual total weight gain of 22 to 28 lb (10 to 13 kg) is optimal for fetal growth and maternal changes.

- Sudden increases of more than 2 lb (0.9 kg)/week or 6 lb (2.3 kg)/month suggest sodium and water retention related to PIH. Sudden and pronounced weight gain usually precedes overt nondependent edema.

- Protein deficiency has been hypothesized as a cause of PIH; dietary increase may be used to replace urinary loss of protein.

- Body fluid loss may exacerbate PIH hemoconcentration and decreased placental perfusion. Diuretics have been implicated in decreased renal and uteroplacental perfusion. Potassium and sodium depletion may occur as a result of thiazide therapy.

2. Decreased renal perfusion and glomerular filtration and fluid volume shifts from vascular to interstitial spaces cause sudden, excessive weight gain and edema.

3. Bed rest decreases metabolic and physiologic demands. Left lateral positioning facilitates uterine and renal perfusion.

Interventions

4. Teach homebound patient and family to report any signs of increased PIH severity, including:
• headache, often frontal or occipital and unrelieved by common analgesics
• visual disturbances, from blurring to overt blindness
• hyperreflexia
• markedly decreased urine output
• epigastric or right upper abdominal pain
• altered sensorium
• vaginal bleeding, abdominal or uterine tenderness or pain; significant changes in fetal activity.

5. Additional individualized interventions: _____

Rationales

4. These signs indicate worsening of the condition, which requires immediate hospitalization and intensive management to prevent eclampsia.

5. Rationales: _____

GOAL 3: Recognize the signs and symptoms of PIH progression and minimize their sequelae.

Interventions

1. Monitor blood pressure every 4 hours, or as patient condition warrants, using same size cuff, with the patient in the same position, and using the same arm.

2. Start an I.V. line, using a large-gauge needle; infuse a balanced saline solution.

3. Weigh patient daily, and monitor for edema.

4. Insert indwelling urinary (Foley) catheter.

5. Monitor renal function hourly, by noting the following:
• urine output

• specific gravity

• protein level, measured by dipstick:
    1+: 30 mg/dl
    2+: 100 mg/dl
    3+: 300 mg/dl
    4+: 2,000 mg/dl or more.

6. Monitor laboratory values, including creatinine, BUN, and AST; platelet count; and HCT.

7. Monitor for ominous signs of deteriorating condition, including:
• headache

• visual disturbances

• hyperreflexia (3+ or 4+) of brachial, wrist, patellar, or Achilles tendons
• markedly decreased urine output

Rationales

1. Diastolic pressure of 110 mm Hg or greater indicates severe PIH. A systolic pressure of 140 mm Hg or greater or a diastolic pressure of 90 mm Hg or greater warrants hospitalization. Rapid fluctuation may occur.

2. An I.V. line provides immediate venous access. Fluids may be given to correct hypovolemia associated with PIH.

3. Sudden weight gain indicates water and sodium retention.

4. Catheterization facilitates frequent renal assessment, which is critical in advanced dysfunction.

5. Renal funtion is evaluated by the following measures:
• Output of 400 ml/day indicates severe PIH. Minimum acceptable physiologic urine output is 30 ml/hour.
• Increased urine specific gravity is consistent with oliguria.
• Persistent readings of 2+ or greater indicate severe PIH.

6. Increased HCT value is an indicator of increased hemoconcentration; thrombocytopenia, of coagulopathy. Increases in creatinine and BUN values show reduced renal perfusion and glomerular filtration; increased AST level shows altered hepatic function.

7. A deteriorating condition is evaluated by the following factors:
• The first episode of eclampsia is commonly preceded by headache.
• Retinal arteriolar spasm (visible on funduscopic examination), ischemia, and edema are thought to be responsible for visual disturbances.
• Brisk, hyperactive neurologic responses may be related to cerebral edema or hemorrhagic lesions.
• Decreased output indicates compromised renal function.

Interventions

- epigastric or right upper abdominal pain
- crackles, rhonchi, dyspnea
- vaginal bleeding, abdominal or uterine tenderness or pain, significant change in fetal activity, and coagulopathy.

8. Administer the vasodilator hydralazine (Apresoline) I.V. and monitor the following:

- fetal heart tones

- maternal blood pressure

- maternal pulse rate.

9. Additional individualized interventions: _____

Rationales

- Edema or bleeding may engorge the hepatic capsule.
- These symptoms indicate pulmonary edema.
- Abruptio placentae, disseminated intravascular coagulation, and HELLP syndrome (**H**emolysis, **E**levated **L**iver enzymes, and **L**ow **P**latelet count) are potential complications of PIH.

8. Vasodilation results in lowered blood pressure.

- Small, incremental doses of hydralazine have few untoward effects on the fetus.
- Uteroplacental blood flow is adequate with diastolic levels of 90 to 100 mm Hg.
- Tachycardia may result from drug therapy.

9. Rationales: _____

GOAL 4: Prevent or control seizures.

Interventions

1. Administer I.V. magnesium sulfate by continuous or intermittent piggyback infusion; follow with I.M. injection per protocol or physician's order.

2. Monitor these factors during magnesium sulfate therapy:

- blood pressure—continuously during I.V. administration; every 15 minutes after I.M. administration
- magnesium sulfate blood levels

- patellar reflexes; if absent, do not give drug

- respiratory rate; if depressed (less than 16 breaths/minute), do not give drug
- urine output.

3. Have these items ready for immediate use:
- 1.5 ml of 10% solution I.V. calcium gluconate
- oxygen and suctioning equipment
- resuscitative equipment.

4. Maintain seizure precautions:
- Place patient in quiet, dimly lit room; limit visitors.
- Secure and pad side rails.

- Have bite block, padded tongue depressors, and airway available.

5. Additional individualized interventions: _____

Rationales

1. Magnesium sulfate blocks neuromuscular transmission and prevents or stops seizures.

2. Assessment assists in evaluating therapeutic response and adverse reactions.
- Vasodilation may cause marked hypotension.

- Magnesium blood levels between 4 and 7.5 mEq/liter indicate therapeutic values and almost always prevent seizures.
- Magnesium blood levels of 8 to 10 mEq/liter indicate toxicity manifested by loss of deep tendon reflexes.
- Respiratory depression and possibly cardiac arrest develop with magnesium blood levels of 12 to 15 mEq/liter.
- Renal function must be determined because the drug is excreted almost exclusively by the kidneys; 30 ml/hour is the minimum acceptable level.

3. Calcium acts as an antagonist to magnesium sulfate and is the treatment of choice for respiratory depression. Administer it slowly for about 3 minutes concurrently with oxygen. Endotracheal intubation and artificial ventilation are necessary in cases of respiratory or cardiac arrest.

4. Seizure precautions ensure patient safety.
- A quiet room reduces stimuli that may trigger a seizure.
- This precaution reduces the potential for trauma or injury during tonic-clonic seizure or during the combative stage.
- These are inserted only before the patient's jaw is clenched. The block may prevent injury to the mouth and tongue and help maintain airway.

5. Rationales: _____

GOAL 5: Maintain patient safety during and after a seizure.

Interventions

1. Position patient on side, if possible. Do not restrict activity; administer oxygen, and suction, as necessary.

2. Remain with patient after seizure.

3. Monitor patient for rales, rhonchi, dyspnea, and hemoptysis; note amount of I.V. fluid infused.

4. Additional individualized interventions: _____

_____

Rationales

1. The side-lying position reduces the risk of airway occlusion and aspiration. Restriction of forceful, almost violent muscular movement may result in injury. Supplemental oxygen is necessary to reverse hypoxia, and suctioning removes secretions.

2. Cessation of tonic-clonic movement may be followed by varying degrees of consciousness, combativeness, impaired vision, further seizures, or coma.

3. These symptoms are consistent with pulmonary edema, which may be compounded by fluid overload from I.V. fluids used to correct hemoconcentration.

4. Rationales: _____

_____

Nursing diagnosis: *High risk for fetal injury related to impaired maternal-placental perfusion (2 goals)*

GOAL 1: Recognize alterations in fetal well-being.

Interventions

1. Assess the following at each clinic visit:
• fundal height — correlate with last menstrual period and estimated date of confinement
• fetal activity — compare with maternal diary of fetal movement and with fetal heart rate (FHR).

2. Assist with maternal ultrasonography.

3. Assess serial maternal tests for plasma or urine estriol and human placental lactogen.

4. Assist with nonstress test.

5. Additional individualized interventions: _____

_____

Rationales

1. Lack of appropriate growth or smaller uterine growth than gestational age would indicate may suggest intra-uterine growth retardation (IUGR). Significant decrease in fetal activity may indicate uteroplacental insufficiency.

2. Ultrasonography identifies fetal and placenta size and may reveal IUGR or grade III placenta (acceleration of the maturational process of the placenta) associated with PIH.

3. Decreasing values may be consistent with an impaired fetoplacental unit.

4. Acceleration of FHR in response to fetal movement is somewhat predictive of fetal well-being and of how the fetus will react to labor and delivery.

5. Rationales: _____

_____

GOAL 2: Promote safe delivery of a viable infant.

Interventions

1. Continue maternal assessments. If preeclampsia is severe, prepare for and assist with amniotomy and oxytocin-induced labor and delivery if cervix is ripe.

2. Prepare for cesarean section birth if induction is not successful.

Rationales

1. Fetal survival may be more jeopardized by continuation of the pregnancy than by preterm delivery.

2. An unfavorable cervix or failure to progress in labor requires surgical intervention.

Interventions

3. Notify obstetric and neonatal teams of anticipated delivery. Have resuscitative equipment immediately available for use.

4. Additional individualized interventions: _____

_____

Rationales

3. The preterm, immature infant will need aggressive and protracted treatment for survival.

4. Rationales: _____

_____

ASSOCIATED PLANS AND APPENDICES
• Abruptio Placentae
• Cesarean Section Birth
• Hydatidiform Mole (Molar Pregnancy)
• Labor and Vaginal Birth
• Multiple Gestation
• Normal Antepartum
• Preterm Infant, Less Than 37 Weeks
• Aspects of Psychological Care—Maternal (Appendix 4)

ADDITIONAL NURSING DIAGNOSES
• Altered nutrition: less than body requirements related to low protein intake
• Fluid volume deficit related to fluid shift from intravascular to extravascular spaces
• Sensory-perceptual alteration (visual) related to retinal edema

Premature Rupture of Membranes

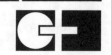

DEFINITION

Premature rupture of membranes (PROM) is the usually spontaneous rupture of the amniochorionic sac remote from term. Labor frequently begins within 24 to 48 hours and delivery is effected within days, whether or not attempts at labor suppression occur. Complications may include maternal or fetal infection, prolapsed cord resulting from fetal malpresentation or small presenting part, or delivery of a preterm infant.

ETIOLOGY AND PRECIPITATING FACTORS

• Etiology is unknown, but PROM is occasionally the result of labor induction when the patient is incorrectly assessed as gestationally ready.
• Patient at risk: multiple gestation, hydramnios, less than optimal maternal weight gain, maternal history of incompetent cervix or cervical manipulation before pregnancy, fetal malpresentation.

PHYSICAL FINDINGS
Genitourinary

• amniotic fluid in the vagina

Subjective

• feeling of fluid gushing or leaking from vagina

DIAGNOSTIC STUDIES
Laboratory data

• Fern test—positive, showing: crystalline frondlike or fern pattern that indicates amniotic fluid; neither urine, blood, nor vaginal secretions elicit this configuration.
• pH of vaginal secretions (nitrazine paper test)—7.0 to 7.5; blood, cervical mucus, and some vaginal infections are also alkaline and may invalidate this test.

pH TEST FOR INTACT MEMBRANES

	pH	Color
Membranes probably intact	5.0	Yellow
	5.5	Olive-yellow
	6.0	Olive-green
Membranes probably ruptured	6.5	Blue-green
	7.0	Blue-gray
	7.5	Deep blue

Collaborative problem: *High risk for intrauterine infection related to disruption of amniochorionic barrier (2 goals)*

GOAL 1: Identify PROM.

Interventions

1. Review and document time of rupture, color of fluid, estimation of amount, odor, and patient's subjective sensations.

2. Review menstrual history, including regularity, duration, characteristics of each menses, and date of last menstrual period.

3. Measure fundal height.

4. Assist physician with sterile vaginal examination, taking the following steps:

• Use sterile water as lubricating fluid.
• Confirm presence of amniotic fluid and its characteristics, especially pH.

Rationales

1. Accurate database assists in formulation of diagnosis and subsequent treatment modalities.

2. Accurate history assists in establishing gestational age and fetal maturity.

3. Fundal height is used to estimate gestational age; however, fetal size does not necessarily correspond with fetal age.

4. Vaginal inspection should be kept to a minimum. Sterile speculum examination minimizes the introduction or spread of organisms.

• Water will not alter pH of secretions.

• Urine and vaginal secretions are acidic. Amniotic fluid is neutral or mildly alkaline (as evidenced by turning nitrazine strip blue). Microscopic crystalline fern configuration confirms amniotic fluid. Bloody show may render a false-positive reading because blood is alkaline.

Interventions

5. Additional individualized interventions: _____

Rationales

5. Rationales: _____

GOAL 2: Prevent or minimize potential for infection after PROM.

Interventions

1. Determine if patient is a candidate for home management. Patient should be afebrile with normal white blood cell count, absence of labor, gestational age 33 weeks or less, and absence of maternal or fetal dysfunction or disease that would warrant immediate delivery.

2. Enact conservative treatment modalities at home. Tell the patient the following:
• The patient should forego coitus and douching.

• The patient should immediately report signs of infection to appropriate personnel:
   □ temperature greater 100.4° F (38° C)
   □ thick or foul-smelling vaginal discharge.
• The physician may institute prophylactic antibiotic therapy.

3. If gestational age is greater than 33 weeks, prepare for delivery. Induced labor or cesarean section bith may be necessary.

4. Additional individualized interventions: _____

Rationales

1. If no infection is present, conservative management may be enacted to allow time for in utero fetal development and maturity.

2. The patient whose condition is managed at home needs specific guidelines.
• Vaginal penetration of any kind may be a source of infection.
• Pyrexia or thick, foul-smelling discharge indicates active infection.

• The effectiveness of prophylactic antibiotic therapy is suspect.

3. Gestational age and consequent fetal maturity is associated with lower neonatal mortality. Oxytocin may be necessary if spontaneous labor has not begun 24 hours after PROM. Cesarean section birth is indicated if induction is not successful or with a transverse lie or breech presentation.

4. Rationales: _____

Nursing diagnosis: *Fear related to PROM and possible fetal jeopardy*

GOAL: Minimize fear.

Interventions

1. Speak calmly and deliberately. Explain procedures and examinations before they are done and keep patient and mate informed of their outcomes.

2. Additional individualized interventions: _____

Rationales

1. Fear of fetal jeopardy is real, and fetal outcome may be compromised. A realistic appraisal of maternal condition and the implications for the fetus may give the patient some sense of control, may decrease fear, and allow for possible anticipatory grieving for preterm infant.

2. Rationales: _____

ASSOCIATED PLANS AND APPENDICES

• Cesarean Section Birth
• Inappropriate Size or Weight for Gestational Age, Small
• Labor and Vaginal Birth
• Normal Antepartum
• Oxytocin-Induced or Oxytocin-Augmented Labor
• Preterm Infant, Less Than 37 Weeks
• Preterm or Premature Labor
• Sepsis Neonatorum and Infectious Disorders
• Aspects of Psychological Care—Maternal (Appendix 4)

ADDITIONAL NURSING DIAGNOSES

• Altered sexuality patterns related to medically prescribed sexual abstinence
• High risk for fetal trauma related to cord compression
• Self-esteem disturbance related to inability to carry fetus to term

Preterm or Premature Labor

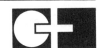

DEFINITION

Premature labor is the onset of the first phase of labor before the 38th week of gestation and after the 20th. Delivery before the 20th week is considered a spontaneous abortion. Good fetal outcome is enhanced when delivery occurs after the 37th week and infant weight is 5.5 lb (2,500 g) or greater. Preterm infants are at increased risk for mental and physical impairment and death. Every effort should be made to continue the pregnancy as long as it does not jeopardize maternal well-being and as long as the uterine environment is more favorable to the fetus than delivery.

ETIOLOGY AND PRECIPITATING FACTORS

• Etiology unknown in most instances.
• Predisposing conditions include:
   □ Maternal factors: premature rupture of membranes, incompetent cervix, preeclampsia or eclampsia, cardiovascular or renal disease, diabetes, infection, injury, abdominal surgery, uterine anomalies, history of previous preterm labor and delivery, or retained intrauterine device (IUD).
   □ Placental factors: abruptio placentae, placenta previa, placental malformation, or malnutrition.
   □ Fetal factors: multiple gestation, hydramnios, fetal anomaly or infection, or fetal death.

PHYSICAL FINDINGS
Genitourinary
• uterine contractions before 37th week of gestation that occur at least every 10 minutes and last for 30 or more seconds for 1 hour or more
• cervical dilatation and effacement
• possibly ruptured membranes

Subjective
• pain or pressure in lower back and abdomen

DIAGNOSTIC STUDIES
• Accurate and complete history and physical examination may furnish enough data for a definitive diagnosis.
• Ultrasonography may be employed to reveal gestational age of fetus(es), fetal maturity, presentation, position, viability, placental abnormalities, hydramnios, or retained IUD.

Collaborative problem: *High risk for premature labor and delivery (2 goals)*

GOAL 1: Recognize signs of preterm labor.

Interventions

1. Review menstrual history, including regularity, duration, characteristics of each menses, and date of last menstrual period.

2. Measure fundal height.

3. Monitor for signs of false labor, including contractions that occur at irregular, long intervals and do not increase in regularity, intensity, or duration; localized lower abdominal discomfort; nondilated cervix; and contractions that are unaffected or ameliorated by walking and are relieved, usually, by sedatives.

4. Recognize signs of true labor, including regular contractions that increase in frequency and intensity; back and abdominal discomfort; cervical dilation; and contractions usually intensified by walking and not halted by sedatives.

5. Additional individualized interventions: _____

Rationales

1. Accurate history assists in establishing precise gestational age.

2. Fundal height is used to estimate gestational age; however, fetal size does not necessarily correspond with fetal age.

3. False labor is a common phenomenon and requires no intervention.

4. Proper and early identification of labor status facilitates successful tocolysis (suppression of labor).

5. Rationales: _____

GOAL 2: Arrest spontaneous, preterm labor.

Interventions

1. Enact conservative treatment methods, including bed rest, with head of bed slightly elevated and patient preferably in left side-lying position. Coitus and enema administration are prohibited.

2. Determine if patient and fetus are candidates for tocolytic therapy. Tocolytic therapy may be effective in the following:
• viable fetus of 20 to 35 weeks' gestation with good fetal heart tones, no distress or disease
• true labor
• intact membranes with no bulging
• cervix dilated no more than 4 cm
• cervical effacement less than 50%
• absence of maternal bleeding or outstanding medical disorders.

3. Start an I.V. line. Maintain hydration and strict fluid intake and output monitoring.

4. Have magnesium sulfate I.V. available.

• Monitor for intact deep tendon reflexes, respiratory rate greater than 16 breaths/minute, urine output greater than 30 ml/hour; note blood magnesium levels.
• Have I.V. calcium gluconate on hand.

5. Have available ritodrine (Yutopar) I.V., I.M., and P.O., and assess patient for severe preeclampsia and eclampsia, cardiac dysfunction, hypertension, thyroid dysfunction, and chorioamnionitis; also, diabetes mellitus or concurrent glucocorticoid therapy. Note restlessness, dyspnea, cyanosis, sense of suffocation, and rales; also note chest pain or tightness, tachycardia, hypotension, widened pulse pressure, hypokalemia, hyperglycemia, hyperinsulinism, acidosis, decreased hematocrit value, and subsequent headache, nausea, and vomiting.

6. Have beta-blocking agent, such as propranolol (Inderal), on hand.

7. Additional individualized interventions: _____

_____

Rationales

1. Without bleeding or ruptured membranes, bed rest is effective in arresting labor in 50% of cases; it minimizes the gravitational pull of the fetus on the cervix. Left side-lying position facilitates uterine perfusion. Coitus or enema administration may initiate or stimulate labor.

2. Tocolytic agents inhibit labor and permit continuation of fetal growth and development. If spontaneous, preterm labor advances further, labor would be difficult to stop. Tocolytes are contraindicated in those conditions, such as hemorrhage, where continuation of the pregnancy would jeopardize maternal or fetal health.

3. An I.V. line provides venous access. Premature labor is associated with dehydration; fluid intake and output monitoring facilitates ongoing evaluation of renal function.

4. As a tocolytic agent, magnesium sulfate decreases myometrial contractility.
• Depressed respirations and hyporeflexia indicate magnesium toxicity. Intact renal function is needed to excrete magnesium.
• Calcium is the antagonist of magnesium.

5. As a tocolytic agent, ritodrine is beta-adrenergic agonist that relaxes the smooth muscle of the uterus. It is contraindicated in patients with hypertensive conditions, cardiac and thyroid dysfunction, and chorioamnionitis; it should be used with caution in those with diabetes mellitus or ongoing glucocorticoid therapy. After administering watch for signs of pulmonary edema, which may indicate toxicity. The other symptoms may warrant discontinuation of ritodrine.

6. A beta blocker may be necessary to antagonize drug action.

7. Rationales: _____

_____

Collaborative problem: *High risk for fetal injury related to maternal premature labor status and imminent delivery*

GOAL: Decrease or minimize potential for injury.

Interventions

1. Review maternal history and confirm gestational age.

Rationales

1. Preterm birth is implicated in over two-thirds of all neonatal deaths.

Interventions

2. Review amniotic fluid analysis for fetal lung maturity, noting rapid surfactant test (shake, bubble, or foam test) and the following:

• lecithin/sphingomyelin (L/S) ratio

• phosphatidylglycerol
• creatinine

• bilirubin
• lipids

• color.

3. Monitor fetal heart rate and report rate greater than 160 beats/minute.

4. Prepare for glucocorticoid drug therapy:

• Assess for diabetes, maternal hypertension, infection, peptic ulcer, and imminent delivery.
• Review hospital and drug manufacturers' protocols for administration, including fetal age less than 34 weeks; administer upon initiation of tocolytic therapy and again in 24 hours. Retreatment may be indicated if delivery does not occur within 7 days.

5. Prepare for vaginal or cesarean section birth; alert obstetric and neonatal teams. Have resuscitative equipment ready for use.

6. Additional individualized interventions: _____

Rationales

2. In this practical, bedside version of L/S analysis, bubbles present 15 minutes after vigorous shaking indicate fetal lung maturity.
• The L/S ratio can be used to determine fetal lung maturity: less than 1—immaturity (less than 30 weeks); 1—borderline; and greater than 2—maturity (35 weeks or more).
• Absence indicates immaturity.
• Creatinine levels of 1.8 to 2 mg/dl indicate maturity (more than 36 weeks). Note maternal hypertensive and renal status because these diseases will cause deceptive increases.
• Bilirubin is not present after 36 weeks.
• A level greater than 20% indicates maturity (more than 36 weeks).
• Meconium staining possibly indicates fetal hypoxia.

3. Fetal tachycardia is associated with use of tocolytics; drug dose may be reduced or discontinued depending on patient response.

4. Betamethasone (Betatrex), dexamethasone (Decadron), or hydrocortisone (Hydrocortone), when administered to the mother, may stimulate fetal lung maturity and decrease the frequency of respiratory distress syndrome; Food and Drug Administration approval has not yet been given because long-term effects are not known.
• Adrenocorticosteroids are contraindicated under these conditions.
• Increased surfactant levels associated with steroid use are transitory; return to uncorrected levels occurs in 8 to 10 days.

5. If rupture of membranes occurs, labor will probably continue. The preterm infant will require intensive and long-term care.

6. Rationales: _____

Nursing diagnosis: *Pain related to uterine contractions*

GOAL: Decrease or minimize pain.

Interventions

1. Establish rapport with patient and significant others.

2. Assess for pain and its characteristics.

3. Perform comfort measures, including position changes, relaxation techniques, rubdowns, effleurage, and pharmacologic analgesia.

Rationales

1. A positive relationship facilitates trust and decreases anxiety.

2. Typically, pain in lower back radiates to abdomen and increases in intensity, frequency, and duration.

3. Increased tissue perfusion, plus stimulation of large afferent, sensory fibers decrease perception of pain; analgesics are given cautiously. Their depressive characteristics may compromise fetal status.

Interventions

4. Keep patient informed of fetal status. Allow her to listen to fetal heart tone during assessment.

5. Additional individualized interventions: _____

_____

Rationales

4. Anxiety related to fetal outcome may intensify perception of pain.

5. Rationales: _____

_____

ASSOCIATED PLANS AND APPENDICES
• Abruptio Placentae
• Cesarean Section Birth
• Inappropriate Size or Weight for Gestational Age, Small
• Labor and Vaginal Birth
• Multiple Gestation
• Placenta Previa
• Pregnancy Complicated by Diabetes Mellitus
• Pregnancy-Induced Hypertension
• Premature Rupture of Membranes
• Preterm Infant, Less Than 37 Weeks
• Aspects of Psychological Care—Maternal (Appendix 4)
• Parent Teaching Guides (Appendix 12)

ADDITIONAL NURSING DIAGNOSES
• Anxiety related to unknown fetal outcome
• Knowledge deficit related to preterm labor and use of tocolytic drugs
• Spiritual distress related to perception that some activity may have triggered preterm labor

Prolapsed Umbilical Cord

DEFINITION
Prolapsed umbilical cord is an emergency condition in which the umbilical cord is displaced between the presenting fetal part and the maternal bony pelvis. Cord compression ensues and results in fetal hypoxia and, if not immediately corrected, fetal death.

ETIOLOGY AND PRECIPITATING FACTORS
• Etiology: Any condition that prevents proper engagement of the presenting fetal part snugly into the maternal pelvis may result in prolapsed umbilical cord.
• Patients at risk: patient with fetal malpresentation, unengaged fetal head, contracted maternal inlet, premature rupture of the membranes, placenta previa, small fetus, multiple (and therefore smaller) fetuses, longer umbilical cords.

PHYSICAL FINDINGS
Genitourinary
• bradycardia or absent fetal heart tones (FHT)
• ruptured membranes
• cord palpable on vaginal examination
• cord protrusion from vagina

Subjective
• sensation of cord passage

DIAGNOSTIC STUDIES
• Ultrasonography may reveal those conditions that may predispose to prolapsed umbilical cord.

Nursing diagnosis: High risk for fetal injury (hypoxia) related to cord compression (3 goals)

GOAL 1: Recognize early signs of cord compression.

Interventions

1. Monitor fetal presentation and position.

2. Monitor FHT and electronic tracings throughout labor, especially when membranes rupture and immediately after amniotomy. Monitor for baseline bradycardia or prolonged variable decelerations.

3. Additional individualized interventions: _____

Rationales

1. Breech and shoulder presentations and transverse lies may predispose to cord prolapse.

2. Rupture of the membranes is commonly followed by prolapse when the presenting part is not complementary to maternal structure. Variable deceleration may indicate cord compression.

3. Rationales: _____

GOAL 2: Minimize or prevent further cord compression.

Interventions

1. Perform sterile vaginal examination. If umbilical cord is felt, position fingers to move presenting part off the cord. Maintain position until emergency delivery can be performed.

2. Place patient in knee-chest or the Trendelenburg position. Support with pillows.

3. Administer oxygen.

4. Do not reinsert externally prolapsed umbilical cord.

Rationales

1. Manipulation reduces the compression and facilitates circulation through the cord.

2. Gravitational release of the presenting fetal part reduces cord compression.

3. Administration facilitates oxygenation, which may be compromised when position further pushes uterus against ventilatory structures.

4. Reinsertion may twist or kink the cord and exacerbate the compression.

Interventions	**Rationales**
5. Apply warm sterile saline solution compresses to umbilical cord if it is externally prolapsed.	5. Compresses may help keep cord pulsating.
6. Additional individualized interventions: _____	6. Rationales: _____

GOAL 3: Promote safe delivery of a jeopardized fetus.

Interventions	**Rationales**
1. Monitor the patient for ruptured membranes, ripe cervix (dilated fully, spontaneously, and progressively), cephalopelvic proportion, occiput presentation, and uteroplacental adequacy.	1. Patients meeting these criteria may be delivered vaginally.
2. Do not administer oxytocin.	2. Forceful uterine contractions may bottleneck fetal head against maternal bony pelvis with dire consequences for patient and fetus.
3. Prepare for cesarean section birth.	3. If the above criteria cannot be met, cesarean section is the method of delivery; in either case, delivery must be rapid to prevent fetal hypoxia, central nervous system impairment, or death.
4. Additional individualized interventions: _____	4. Rationales: _____

Nursing diagnosis: *High risk for intrauterine infection related to exposure of externally prolapsed cord to perineal area*

GOAL: Minimize potential for infection.

Interventions	**Rationales**
1. Do not reinsert umbilical cord.	1. The cord may be grossly contaminated with organisms or pathogens from the vulva, anus, skin, or the bedclothes.
2. Completely cover protruding cord with sterile saline solution dressing or perineal pad.	2. The dressing acts as a barrier, minimizing risk of further contamination; the sterile saline solution minimizes risk of cord vessel atrophy.
3. Additional individualized interventions: _____	3. Rationales: _____

Nursing diagnosis: *Fear related to fetal outcome*

GOAL: Minimize fear.

Interventions	**Rationales**
1. Calmly explain procedures and their rationale. Repeat as necessary. Keep patient advised of fetal status.	1. Fear is realistic, and explanation may give patient a sense of control, decrease fear, and enhance compliance.

Interventions

2. Additional individualized interventions: _____

_____

Rationales

2. Rationales: _____

_____

ASSOCIATED PLANS AND APPENDICES
• Multiple Gestation
• Placenta Previa
• Premature Rupture of Membranes
• Aspects of Psychological Care—Maternal (Appendix 4)

ADDITIONAL NURSING DIAGNOSES
• Ineffective breathing pattern related to therapeutically imposed knee-chest position
• Knowledge deficit related to diagnosis and emergency procedures
• Powerlessness related to fetal outcome

Rh Isoimmunization

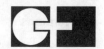

DEFINITION

Rh isoimmunization is an antigen-antibody sensitization response that causes the development of maternal antibodies to fetal red blood cells (RBCs). Placental transfer of antibodies to the fetus lyses fetal RBCs and produces hemolytic anemia and hyperbilirubinemia.

Several antigens may evoke this incompatibility response (ABO group; Rh D, C, c, e; other blood groups); but the Rh genotype D carries the most severe antigenic potential. If untreated, fetal effects include death, erythroblastosis fetalis, choreoathetosis, or neurologic and sensory deficits. Prognosis for the fetus or neonate used to be grim, but identification of nonsensitized patients and pharmacologic prophylaxis have dramatically improved this outcome.

ETIOLOGY AND PRECIPITATING FACTORS

• Etiology: Rh antibody production in the Rh-negative pregnant patient is stimulated by exposure to the Rh antigen during the pregnancy of a Rh-positive conceptus, incompatible blood transfusion, or fetomaternal bleeding associated with abruptio placentae or placenta previa. The first pregnancy, whether full term, stillborn, aborted, ectopic, or molar, is usually unaffected. The risk of sensitization increases with each subsequent pregnancy.
• Patient at risk: Rh-negative patient with Rh-positive sexual partner; Basque ethnicity.

PHYSICAL FINDINGS
• none (maternal)

DIAGNOSTIC STUDIES
Laboratory data
• Rh and ABO screening—identifies blood type and Rh.
• Maternal antibody titers—positive indirect Coombs' test indicates the presence of maternal Rh-positive antibodies.

Collaborative problem: *High risk for fetal injury related to fetomaternal blood incompatibility (4 goals)*

GOAL 1: Identify patient who is at risk for fetomaternal incompatibility.

Interventions

1. At first clinic visit, review:
• ABO blood group and Rh of patient and sexual partner
• maternal history, including history of blood or blood product transfusion, plasmapheresis, or amniocentesis; previous Rh immune globulin injections after delivery or abortion.

2. Refer Rh-negative patient and Rh-positive sexual partner for analysis of blood group, Rh, and zygosity.

3. Additional individualized interventions: _____

Rationales

1. Immediate identification of at-risk population assists in early management. Introduction of fetal erythrocytes into the maternal circulation may occur at delivery, usually during separation of the placenta; ill-matched blood transfusions may introduce the antigen, as may any procedure or condition that may leak blood from fetal to maternal circulation.

2. Laboratory data confirms history.

3. Rationales: _____

GOAL 2: Prevent isoimmunization in the Rh_o(D)-negative, nonsensitized patient.

Interventions

1. Determine whether the patient is a candidate for immune globulin prophylaxis. Such candidates include Rh_o(D)-negative, nonsensitized patient with an Rh-positive mate or who delivered an Rh_o(D)-positive neonate with a negative direct Coombs' test (both determined from cord blood).

Rationales

1. Rh_o(D) immune globulin (RhoGAM) provides temporary passive immunity by preventing the formation of maternal antibodies in the Rh-negative patient with an Rh-positive infant.

Interventions

2. Administer Rh$_o$(D) immune globulin I.M., using the following guidelines:

• Administer to the mother only (never to the father or infant).

• Administer 300 mcg within 72 hours of each delivery or abortion.

• Administer 300 mcg per protocol or order at these times:
  □ 28 and 34 weeks' gestation
  □ when amniocentesis is performed
  □ with vaginal bleeding associated with placental abruption.

• Individualize dosage after a large fetomaternal bleed or transfusion accident.

3. Additional individualized interventions: _____

Rationales

2. I.M. administration of Rh$_o$(D) immune globulin accomplishes the following:

• Administration to Rh-positive persons results in lysis of RBCs.

• One 300-mcg dose will suppress the maternal immune response to 15 ml of Rh-positive RBCs.

• Prenatal administration has been suggested to reduce the incidence of isoimmunization associated with silent fetomaternal bleeding.

• Dosage calculation for bleeds can be determined by laboratory techniques, such as Kleihauer-Betke acid elution technique.

3. Rationales: _____

GOAL 3: Identify the Rh$_o$(D)-negative, sensitized patient with a jeopardized fetus.

Interventions

1. Continually monitor antibody titers for degree of maternal sensitization monthly through 24th week of gestation, biweekly 25th through 40th week of gestation, and 1 week before estimated date of confinement.

2. Assist with amniocentesis if titers are greater than 1:16.

3. Monitor spectrophotometric measures of the delta optical density of amniotic fluid.

4. Additional individualized interventions: _____

Rationales

1. Detection of sensitization is critical because, if untreated, it is associated with a 30% perinatal mortality rate.

2. Increased titers indicate that marked hemolytic disease of the fetus may already exist.

3. Spectrophotometric readings indicate bilirubin levels; the severity of fetal hemolytic disease is indicated by the following zones:
A — mild or no disease
B — moderate
C — severe.

4. Rationales: _____

GOAL 4: Prevent or minimize fetal injury.

Interventions

1. Confirm zone A or B spectrophotometric readings of amniotic fluid.

2. Prepare for intrauterine fetal transfusions which require the following:

• Perform ultrasound study of fetus.

• Infuse crossmatched, fresh Rh-negative type O packed RBCs into fetal peritoneal cavity that has been identified by X-ray visualization or a radio-opaque contrast agent.

• Repeat transfusion procedure every 2 weeks.

Rationales

1. Delivery of fetus can be delayed until fetal maturity can be established, usually after 36th week of gestation.

2. The immature fetus between 23 and 32 weeks' gestation with severe hemolysis (zone C) will require transfusion to correct anemia resulting from RBC hemolysis.

• This procedure identifies placental site and fetal position and location.

• RBCs are absorbed into fetal circulation.

• Treatment is continued until fetal maturity is attained.

Interventions

3. Monitor fetal heart tones, sinusoidal fetal heart rate, and repetitive decelerations.

4. Prepare for induced delivery or cesarean section birth.

5. Additional individualized interventions: _____

_____

Rationales

3. These patterns have been associated, in part, with erythroblastosis fetalis; delivery is usually warranted.

4. Cesarean section birth is indicated when delivery is required remote from term. Manual removal of the placenta is contraindicated.

5. Rationales: _____

_____

ASSOCIATED PLANS AND APPENDICES
• Cesarean Section Birth
• Hyperbilirubinemia
• Inappropriate Size or Weight for Gestational Age, Small
• Labor and Vaginal Birth
• Oxytocin-Induced or Oxytocin-Augmented Labor
• Preterm Infant, Less Than 37 Weeks
• Aspects of Psychological Care—Maternal (Appendix 4)

ADDITIONAL NURSING DIAGNOSES
• Fear related to intrauterine blood transfusion and effects on fetus
• Ineffective individual coping related to bimonthly invasive procedure to gravid uterus
• Knowledge deficit related to blood type, Rh type, and zygosity of self and partner and implications for fetus

Sexually Transmitted Diseases/ TORCH

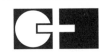

DEFINITION
Pathogenic invasion of a microorganism or virus into the pregnant patient may cause injury to the mother, fetus, or both. Invasion may occur before conception, during the insemination that causes pregnancy, or during pregnancy. Transmission to the fetus occurs via transplacental inoculation, fetal contact with the infected maternal genitalia, or both. The following sexually transmitted diseases (STDs) will be considered: syphilis, gonorrhea, chlamydia, and the TORCH conditions: toxoplasmosis (TO), rubella (R), cytomegalovirus (C), and herpes simplex (H). TORCH categorization may vary; the O may include other diseases, such as syphilis, varicella, group B beta-hemolytic streptococcus, and chlamydia.

ETIOLOGY AND PRECIPITATING FACTORS
- syphilis: the spirochete *Treponema pallidum*
- gonorrhea: the bacterium *Neisseria gonorrhoeae*
- chlamydia: the bacterium *Chlamydia trachomatis*
- toxoplasmosis: the protozoa *Toxoplasma gondii*
- rubella: the virus rubella
- cytomegalovirus: the virus cytomegalovirus (CMV)
- herpes simplex type II (HSV-II): the virus *Herpesvirus hominis*

PHYSICAL FINDINGS
Syphilis
- Primary
  - □ painless chancres at entry point
  - □ painless, single enlarged lymph node
  - □ low-grade fever
  - □ weight loss
  - □ malaise
  - □ transient alopecia
- Secondary
  - □ symmetric, well-defined rash over body
  - □ condylomata on moist surfaces
  - □ malaise, headache, anorexia, nausea, myalgia, and fatigue
- Tertiary
  - □ local or diffuse gummas
  - □ periostitis or osteitis
  - □ cardiovascular syphilis
  - □ neurosyphilis

Gonorrhea
- Early
  - □ frequently asymptomatic
  - □ mucopurulent or purulent, foul-smelling cervical or rectal discharge
  - □ gray vulval exudate or condylomata; vulvovaginitis

  - □ cervical edema, erosion, and tenderness
  - □ urinary frequency and dysuria
- Late
  - □ lower abdominal pain, distention, and chronic pelvic pain
  - □ pyrexia, cervical tenderness, nausea, and emesis

Chlamydia
- frequently asymptomatic
- occasional cervicitis and urethritis with urinary frequency and dysuria
- pelvic pain, dyspareunia

Toxoplasmosis
- possibly asymptomatic
- myalgia
- malaise
- diffuse maculopapular rash
- splenomegaly
- posterior, cervical lymphadenopathy

Active rubella
- prodromal headache
- malaise
- anorexia
- low-grade fever
- coryza
- lymphadenopathy
- conjunctivitis
- maculopapular rash on face, trunk, and extremities
- Forcheimer petechial macules on soft palate
- photophobia

CMV
- asymptomatic
- possible mononucleosis-like cluster of symptoms
- cervical discharge

HSV-II
- Painless vesicles rupture followed by:
  - □ recurrent itchy, purulent, painful vesicles of external genitalia, vagina, and cervix
  - □ pyrexia, malaise, and anorexia
- genital irritation and pruritus
- foul-smelling, profuse vaginal and urethral discharges
- painful inguinal lymphadenopathy
- dysuria

DIAGNOSTIC STUDIES
Laboratory data
- Syphilis: positive darkfield microscopy for *T. pallidum* from chancre exudate or secondary lesion; weakly reac-

tive or reactive Veneral Disease Research Laboratory (VDRL) test; positive fluorescent treponemal antibody absorption (FTA-ABS) test
• Gonorrhea: identification of gonococcus by Gram stain of exudate and confirmation by bacterial culture
• Chlamydia: positive culture of *C. trachomatis;* Gram stain may reveal numerous leukocytes
• Toxoplasmosis: identification of protozoa with Wright or Giemsa stain; Sabin-Feldman dye titers greater than 1:1,000; presence of IgM-fluorescent antibodies to evaluate recent acquisitions
• Rubella: acute sample antibody titer greater than

1:10; previous infections and, therefore, immunity evidenced by hemagglutination inhibition (HAI) titer greater than 1:10 to 1:20 or positive complement fixation
• CMV: intranuclear inclusions in epithelial cells in urine sediment; complement fixation in sera during acute and convalescent phases
• HSV-II: positive cytopathic effect on culture from exudate; smear may contain large, multinucleate cells with eosinophilic viral inclusion bodies; concurrent rise in antibody titer may be seen

---

Collaborative problem: *High risk for maternal infection related to exposure to pathogens (2 goals)*

GOAL 1: Identify exposure to infection or early infection.

Interventions

1. Screen for syphilis. Administer VDRL test on first clinic visit, to be confirmed by FTA-ABS if positive. Repeat in third trimester and on all umbilical cord bloods in high-risk patients (those with infected, multiple, or casual sexual partners).

2. Screen for gonorrhea, including cervical, urethral, or rectal discharge; cervical edema, tenderness, or erosion; urinary frequency, urgency, and dysuria; and pelvic or abdominal discomfort. Culture all exudates; repeat in third trimester in high-risk patients.

3. Screen for asymptomatic chlamydia, including history of PID or genital infection; high-risk populations including teens and pregnant women whose partners have a history of nongonococcal urethritis (NGU). Culture any exudates.

4. Screen for toxoplasmosis, including rash, lymphadenopathy, constitutional symptoms, history of foreign travel, eating raw or uncooked meats, and exposure to cats and cat excreta.

5. Screen for exposure to rubella, including confirmed history of disease, recent exposure to disease, rash, and constitutional symptoms.

6. Screen for CMV, including mononucleosis-like or constitutional symptoms; complement fixation, IgM antibody titer, or neutralization test may be recommended.

7. Screen for HSV-II, including painful vesicles, genital irritation and pruritus, lymphadenopathy, dysuria, and pyrexia; culture active lesions.

8. Additional individualized interventions: _____

Rationales

1. Syphilis transmission to the fetus may cause mid-trimester abortion, stillbirth, or preterm or term delivery of an infant with congenital syphilis. Maternal implications include progression to tertiary syphilis with cardiovascular and neurologic involvement.

2. Gonorrhea transmission to the fetus may cause ophthalmia neonatorum, gonococcal pneumonia, or neonatal sepsis. Maternal implications include salpingitis, chronic pelvic inflammatory disease (PID), gonococcal arthritis, or disseminated infection with bacteremia.

3. Chlamydia transmission to the fetus may cause ophthalmia neonatorum, chlamydial pneumonia, preterm birth, stillbirth, or neonatal demise. Maternal implications include PID and NGU.

4. Toxoplasmosis transmission to the fetus may cause preterm birth, stillbirth, or congenital toxoplasmosis. Maternal implications include localized or massive generalized infection.

5. Rubella transmission to fetus during first trimester may cause marked congenital anomalies of heart, brain, eyes, and ears and death; second-trimester exposure is associated with hearing impairment.

6. CMV transmission to the fetus may result in abortion, stillbirth, or delivery of an infant who is small for gestational age and who has active disease.

7. First-trimester HSV-II transmission to the fetus may result in abortion; later infection is associated with preterm birth, neonatal vesicular lesions, and overwhelming infection.

8. Rationales: _____

GOAL 2: Prevent or minimize infection.

Interventions

1. To treat syphilis infection, have I.M. penicillin G benzathine (Bicillin L-A) or I.M. aqueous penicillin G procaine (Wycillin) on hand for patients not allergic to penicillin; or erythromycin (Erythrocin), doxycycline (Vibramycin), or ceftriaxone (Rocephin) for allergic patients.

2. To treat gonorrhea infection, have amoxicillin, probenecid (Benemid), spectinomycin (Trobicin), and ceftriaxone on hand.

3. To treat chlamydial infection, have erythromycin base (Robimycin), erythromycin ethylsuccinate (Wyamycin E), or amoxicillin on hand. Culture exudate, if possible.

4. To prevent or treat toxoplasmosis infection, have pyrimethamine (Daraprim) and sulfonamides on hand; discontinue sulfonamides before delivery. Instruct patients to avoid cats, to never handle litter boxes or cat excreta, and to eat only thoroughly cooked meats.

5. To prevent rubella infection, have live rubella vaccine on hand for:
• postpartum mothers with HAI titers less than 1:8
• prepubertal children older than 15 months
• sexually active, susceptible women who are not pregnant and are using contraceptives.

6. Tell high-risk patient that CMV can neither be prevented nor treated at present. The virus, present in urine, saliva, cervical mucus, semen, and breast milk, can be spread by close as well as intimate contact.

7. To treat HSV-II infection, encourage partner's use of condom, whether he is symptomatic or not. Also:
• Administer acyclovir (Zovirax) in severe disseminated infection.
• Prepare for cesarean section birth if genital lesions are present or suspected in the genital tract, or if culture reveals presence of virus.

8. Additional individualized interventions: _____

Rationales

1. Protocols have been recommended by the Centers for Disease Control and Prevention. Treatment of partner minimizes the risk of reinfection. Continual monitoring is necessary to assess recurrences.

2. Treating partner minimizes reinfection risk. Culture results indicate efficacy of drug therapy.

3. Culture may not be widely available or cost may be prohibitive. Drugs listed are appropriate for a partner who is culture positive or exhibits symptoms of NGU.

4. Patient activities are prophylactic in nature. Pyrimethamine is the drug of choice, although its use is limited because of its teratogenic effects, most notably in early pregnancy. Increased bilirubin level is associated with sulfonamide use.

5. No treatment exists for rubella, and prophylaxis has been most effective in controlling disease. The vaccine is contraindicated in pregnancy because the fetus can be affected by it in early pregnancy. Pregnancy is not advised for 3 months after inoculation because of possible effects on the fetus.

6. CMV transmission to the fetus across the placenta or through contact with the genital tract mainly affects the fetal blood, brain, and liver.

7. Viral shedding persists even without overt symptoms.

• Acyclovir reduces maternal viral shedding time; it is not routinely recommended.
• Fetal contact with the infected genital tract is the major source of transmission. Delivery by cesarean section may prevent transmission.

8. Rationales: _____

ASSOCIATED PLANS AND APPENDICES
• Cesarean Section Birth
• Inappropriate Size or Weight for Gestational Age, Small
• Normal Antepartum
• Preterm Infant, Less Than 37 Weeks
• Sepsis Neonatorum and Infectious Disorders
• Aspects of Psychological Care—Maternal (Appendix 4)
• The Family and Home Assessment (Appendix 7)

ADDITIONAL NURSING DIAGNOSES
• Activity intolerance related to prodromal symptoms or subclinical disease
• Altered sexuality patterns related to required condom use or safer sex practices to reduce genital reinfection of partner
• Spiritual distress related to guilt for having acquired disease and its possible repercussion on fetus or infant

Vaginal and Urinary Infections

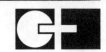

DEFINITION
The pregnant patient may contract various vaginal infections. Conditions discussed here include candidal (monilial) vaginitis, trichomonal vaginitis, and condyloma acuminatum. See *Description and management of common vaginal infections.*

Lower urinary tract infections (cystitis and urethritis) are common in pregnancy and are associated with recent instrumentation or bacteriuria. Physical alterations related to normal pregnancy, lower gastrointestinal (GI) tract and subsequent ascending genitourinary (GU) infection place the patient at risk for acute pyelonephritis.

ETIOLOGY AND PRECIPITATING FACTORS:
• Etiology: most commonly, the gram-negative bacteria *E. coli*; also, *Klebsiella, Proteus, Enterobacter, Pseudomonas,* and *Serratia.*

• Patient at risk: lower socioeconomic status, high parity, previous urinary tract infection (UTI), sickle cell trait, undiagnosed obstructive lesions, congenital abnormalities of GU tract.

PHYSICAL FINDINGS
Genitourinary
• urinary frequency and urgency; dysuria, especially at end of micturition

DIAGNOSTIC STUDIES
Laboratory data
• clean-catch urinalysis—positive, for organisms greater than 100,000/ml or too numerous to count
• red blood cells in urine or gross hematuria

Collaborative problem: *High risk for urinary infection related to physiologic maternal adaptations to pregnancy and to pathogenic invasion (2 goals)*

GOAL 1: Identify signs of early infection.

Interventions

1. Perform clean catch, midstream urinalysis for bacteria at first clinic visit. Use dipstick to test for nitrites.

2. Additional individualized interventions: _____

Rationales

1. Clean-catch urine renders a characteristic sample without risk of infection.

2. Rationales: _____

GOAL 2: Prevent infection or minimize its progression.

Interventions

1. Instruct patient on hygienic and prophylactic practices:
• Wipe from front to back after voiding.
• Void after coitus.
• Void as the urge presents.

2. Assure adequate hydration; baseline fluid requirements in absence of cardiovascular or renal disease, illness, or trauma are:
• 100 ml/kg of actual weight/day—first 10 kg
• 50 ml/kg of actual weight/day—second 10 kg
• 20 ml/kg of actual weight/day—remaining weight.
Double this amount with actual urinary infection, screening first for cardiovascular or renal impairment.

Rationales

1. Proper hygiene and prophylaxis minimize the risk of transmitting organisms from the GI to the GU tract. Voiding washes secretions from external urethra. Stasis facilitates growth and multiplication of organisms.

2. A dilute urine results in a lowered colony count per milliliter and promotes more frequent urination.

DESCRIPTION AND MANAGEMENT OF COMMON VAGINAL INFECTIONS

	Candidal vaginitis	Trichomonal vaginitis	Condyloma accuminatum (genital warts)
Causative Organism	Fungus: *Candida albicans*	Protozoa: *Trichomonas vaginalis*	Virus: papilloma virus
Predisposing and Causative Factors	• Sexual transmission • Diabetes: Glycosuria provides a medium for growth of pathogen. • Antibiotics suppress normal flora and foster superinfection. • Steroids and immunosuppressive drugs suppress immune function.	• Asymptomatic males with trichomonal infection of the genitourinary tract may infect sexual partner. • Concurrent gonorrheal infection is common.	• Protracted incubation period of 1 to 6 months. • Perirectal and rectal involvement common in homosexual and bisexual men.
Signs and Symptoms	• Scant, thick white or yellow-white vaginal discharge with cheeselike material adhering to vaginal walls • Vaginal irritation and pruritus • Vulval edema; erythema • Excoriation	• Profuse, foamy, green-yellow vaginal discharge • Vulval pruritus, irritation, edema, and excoriation with irritation from perineum to thighs • Strawberry appearance of cervix and vagina • Dysuria • Dyspareunia	• Small, soft, painless pink or red raised areas that quickly grow to gray pedunculated warts; multiple growths render a cauliflower-looking appearance
Diagnosis	• Positive Gram stain smear, culture of organism	• Dark-field, phase contrast, or ordinary microscopy for organism • Positive culture revealed on Papanicolaou smear • Possible positive gonorrhea and other sexually transmitted disease smears	• Identification by inspection • Workup for syphilis necessary to rule out condylomata lata of second-stage syphilis
Management	• Nystatin (Mycostatin) vaginal suppositories: Use one suppository (100,000 units) for 7 to 14 days. • Postinsertion: Apply nystatin, miconazole (Monistat), or clotrimazole (Mycelex) creams to perineum and perianal area.	• Metronidazole (Flagyl) 250 mg P.O. after meals t.i.d. for 7 days after first trimester; teratogenic effect inconclusive to date.	• During pregnancy, trichloracetic acid applied to condyloma weekly. • Topical podophyllin, the drug of choice, usually deferred until after delivery because it has been associated with marked toxicity and fetal demise. • Electrocauterization, excision.
Implications	• Relapse or reinfection is common: Sexual partner must also be treated to prevent back-and-forth transmission. • Full course of drug therapy must be completed even though symptoms may subside within a few days.	• Avoid coitus until infection is controlled. • Sexual partner must be treated. • Avoid alcoholic beverages (adverse reactions associated with drug therapy). • Discontinue if central nervous system side effects appear.	• Sexual partners must be examined. • Relapses are not uncommon and require treatment.

Interventions

3. Monitor for urinary frequency, urgency, and dysuria and correlate with gestational status. Note history of UTI or diabetes mellitus. Perform smear for *Chlamydia trachomatis* in high-risk patients.

4. Be prepared to administer one of the following medications after a drug history and urine culture have been performed:

• nitrofurantoin (Nitrofan) 100 mg four times daily with food for 10 days (in all but term pregnancies)

• sulfisoxazole (Gantrisin) 1 gram four times daily for 10 days (in all but term pregnancies)

• ampicillin (Omnipen) 500 mg four times daily for 10 days.

5. Monitor the patient for signs of acute pyelonephritis, including:
• frequency, urgency, and dysuria
• abrupt onset of pyrexia, chills, unilateral or bilateral flank pain, or lumbar aching or pain; possible nausea, emesis, or anorexia
• tenderness at costovertebral angles
• leukocytes in urine and bacteriuria.

6. Perform clean-catch urinalysis for culture at completion of drug therapy and every 1 to 2 months thereafter.

7. Additional individualized interventions: _____

Rationales

3. Urinary frequency alone in the first and third trimesters is a result of uterine pressure on the urinary bladder. Past UTI and urinary stasis of normal pregnancy predispose patient to infection. Glycosuria associated with diabetes provides a good medium for growth and multiplication of bacteria. Chlamydial infection may be asymptomatic.

4. Drug therapy is usually successful in infection control. History exposes sensitivity profile to each drug. Culture and sensitivity identifies organism susceptibility to various antibiotics. Safety of these medications in pregnancy has not been fully established and the risks must be weighed against the benefits.
• Nitrofurantoin poses risk of hemolytic anemia to the immature enzyme system of the neonate.
• Sulfisoxazole crosses the placental barrier and may result in kernicterus.
• Ampicillin is contraindicated if allergy to penicillin has been established.

5. Labor, appendicitis, abruptio placentae, or myomal infarction may be mistakenly diagnosed. Careful assessment facilitates proper diagnosis and management.

6. Analysis confirms success of treatment and screens for asymptomatic or symptomatic recurrence.

7. Rationales: _____

Collaborative problem: *Pain related to bladder spasms during micturition*

GOAL: Prevent or minimize pain.

Interventions

1. Advise patient to take warm sitz baths after voiding, when possible.

2. Increase fluid intake (see Goal 2 of Collaborative problem "High risk for urinary infection"). Encourage use of cranberry juice.

3. Have on hand phenazopyridine HCl (Pyridium) 200 mg for use three times daily after meals or atropine sulfate-methylene blue (Urised), two tablets P.O. four times daily as symptoms persist.

Rationales

1. Heat decreases spasms and promotes relaxation. Also, cleaning of perineum will reduce pathogenic population.

2. Cranberry juice acidifies the urine; although the effectiveness may be suspect, the additional fluid is desirable.

3. Topical analgesia on urinary tract mucosa by phenazopyridine and the antiseptic and parasympatholytic actions of atropine sulfate-methylene blue may relieve the symptoms of infection. Inform patient that phenazopyridine will turn urine red-orange. Atropine sulfate-methylene blue will color urine blue to blue-green. As with all drugs administered during pregnancy, the risk-to-benefit ratio must be evaluated carefully.

Interventions	Rationales
4. Additional individualized interventions: _____	4. Rationales: _____

Nursing diagnosis: *Pain (perineal) related to vulval inflammation, pruritus, and excoriation*

GOAL: Minimize discomfort and facilitate healing.

Interventions	Rationales
1. Take medical, gynecologic, and obstetric histories and monitor patient for perineal edema, erythema, pruritis, excoriation, discharge, and pain or discomfort (See *Description and management of common vaginal infections,* page 81.)	1. Assessment facilitates diagnosis and appropriate therapy and management.
2. Instruct patient on the following comfort measures:	2. Teaching the patient hygiene measures promotes patient comfort and healing.
• Wearing cotton underwear; avoiding tight undergarments, slacks, or hose; applying small amount of cornstarch to external genitalia and thighs, if desired	• Synthetic or tight clothing help retain perineal moisture. Cornstarch is nonirritating and absorbs moisture.
• washing perineum two or more times a day with a mild, nonperfumed, nondeodorant soap	• Washing minimizes irritating secretions or discharge.
• taking warm sitz or tub baths twice daily	• Vasodilation produced by warm bath increases blood and lymph flow to area and promotes healing.
• after elimination, wiping perineum from front to back; avoiding scratching perineum; and washing hands thoroughly after touching genitals	• Wiping action minimizes transfer of anal contaminants to urethra and vagina. Soiled hands are a major factor in infection spread or recurrence.
• avoiding use of feminine hygiene sprays, perfumed soaps, bubble bath, or perfumed, colored toilet tissue	• Use of these products may produce perineal irritation.
• performing perineal hygiene before using prescribed perineal or vaginal suppositories	• Secretions may interfere with absorption.
• avoiding douching.	• Douching has been associated with air embolism.
3. Additional individualized interventions: _____	3. Rationales: _____

ASSOCIATED PLANS AND APPENDICES
• Normal Antepartum
• Sepsis Neonatorum and Infectious Disorders
• Sexually Transmitted Diseases/TORCH
• Aspects of Psychological Care — Maternal (Appendix 4)

ADDITIONAL NURSING DIAGNOSES
• Altered sexuality patterns related to medically imposed sexual abstinence
• Altered urinary elimination related to physiologic maternal adaptation to pregnancy and infection
• Knowledge deficit related to feminine hygiene practices

SECTION II
INTRAPARTUM

Cesarean Section Birth   85
Labor and Vaginal Birth   92
Oxytocin-Induced or Oxytocin-Augmented Labor   103

INTRAPARTUM
Cesarean Section Birth

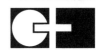

DEFINITION
Cesarean section birth is an alternative birthing method in which the fetus is delivered through incisions made into the abdominal and uterine walls (see *Cesarean section procedures*). It is indicated for any condition in which maternal or fetal health is jeopardized and for which postponement of delivery or vaginal birth itself would compromise the patient's safety. Indications for cesarean section birth may include—but are not limited to—these conditions: a compromised fetus; previous cesarean section birth; dystocia; fetopelvic disproportion; breech, shoulder, or compound presentations; abruptio placentae; placenta previa; prolapsed umbilical cord; prolonged rupture of membranes; preeclampsia or eclampsia; insulin-dependent diabetes mellitus; spinal or pelvic fractures; pelvic tumors; gonorrhea; or genital herpes. For more detailed information on each condition, see the appropriate plans of care.

The surgical procedure may be an emergency procedure or it may be anticipated. If cesarean section is anticipated, the parents are given greater latitude about birthing and anesthesia options, as well as the opportunity for comprehensive preoperative teaching. Presented here are physical findings associated with fetal distress, types and implications of cesarean section procedures, and postpartum considerations that are specific to patients who have undergone cesarean section birth. Review of the normal postpartum experience is essential.

PHYSICAL FINDINGS
Common indications of fetal distress:
- ☐ sudden decrease or cessation of fetal movement
- ☐ meconium-stained amniotic fluid (without breech presentation)
- ☐ fetal heart rate (FHR) persistently less than 120 or greater than 160 beats/minute
- ☐ baseline variability less than 5 beats/minute
- ☐ repetitive early, late, or variable patterns of deceleration with poor recovery to baseline
- ☐ variable decelerations greater than 1 minute duration or less than 60 beats/minute
- ☐ absence of beat-to-beat variability
- ☐ sinusoidal FHR pattern
- ☐ pH of fetal scalp (capillary) blood 7.25 or lower
- ☐ nonreactive nonstress test
- ☐ positive oxytocin challenge test

Nursing diagnosis: *Ineffective individual coping related to surgical intervention, perceived loss of the birthing experience, and fatigue*

GOAL: Bolster patient's coping mechanisms.

Interventions

1. Accept patient's reaction to cesarean section birth. Note isolation, lack of concentration, silence, regressive behaviors, or repeatedly asked questions. Integrate with prepregnancy and prenatal behavior described by partner.

2. Allow patient to verbalize feelings. Reinforce preparatory teaching of prenatal classes, if applicable. Focus on birth experience and commonalities between vaginal and cesarean section births.

3. Cluster nursing assessments and activities. Allow intervals of inactivity.

4. Perform or review family and home assessments and include patient and significant others in discharge planning.

Rationales

1. Inability to cope may take various forms; subtle manifestations may be equally representative of the perceived trauma as are the more overt behaviors of verbalizing, moaning, or crying.

2. Although prenatal classes include information on cesarean section birth, many patients cannot relate to it. Patients completing their first pregnancy or who have had repeat cesarean sections may be especially disappointed in not having delivered vaginally. Focusing on the birth rather than the surgical experience is a positive activity and may lessen disappointment and guilt.

3. Fatigue lessens the patient's ability to cope.

4. Care of the infant and home maintenance may be especially difficult if the patient has limited assistance and multiple responsibilities. Discharge planning that begins on admission may prevent, improve, or resolve home problems.

CESAREAN SECTION PROCEDURES

	Classic	Low Classic	Low Transverse
Description	• Vertical incision made into the body of the uterus above the lower uterine segment and up into the uterine fundus; rarely used	• Vertical incision made into lower uterine segment (Kroenig technique)	• Transverse incision through lower uterine segment (Kerr technique); most commonly used

uterus ——

bladder ——

	Classic	Low Classic	Low Transverse
Advantages	• Used with anterior implantation of placenta, transverse lie, shoulder presentation, or with adhesions	• Vertical extension possible if delivery warrants	• Procedure of choice for cephalic presentation • Decreased blood loss • Requires less bladder dissection from myometrium • Ease of repair • Rarely ruptures in subsequent pregnancies • Adhesions less likely • Peritonitis risk decreased • Cosmetic appeal
Disadvantages	• Greater blood loss • Increased risk of scar rupture in subsequent pregnancy • No attempt for vaginal delivery with subsequent pregnancy would be made • Adhesions likely	• Increased bladder dissection needed to keep within lower uterine segment • Downward extension may result in cervical, vaginal, or bladder tears • Upward extension into uterine body causes more difficult closure and less satisfactory reperitonealization • Risk of rupture in subsequent pregnancy, especially labor, more likely than in low transverse	• Size limitation for extension; possible lacerations occurring during lateral extension may involve large branches of uterine artery and vein • Decreased uterine visibility; compounded in obese patient

Interventions	**Rationales**
5. Reassure patient that subsequent deliveries may include vaginal birth.	5. Patient may feel that future deliveries must be by cesarean section; the resulting anxiety may interfere with her ability to cope with the present situation.
6. Additional individualized interventions: _____	6. Rationales: _____

Collaborative problem: *Pain related to surgical incision*

GOAL: Minimize pain.

Interventions	**Rationales**
1. Assess pain for location, severity, duration, and defining characteristics. Ascertain that incision site is not infected and bladder not distended.	1. Assessment confirms pain is related to surgical incision.
2. Administer meperidine (Demerol) I.M. or morphine S.C. every 3 to 4 hours, noting degree of relief obtained. Administer before pain becomes too intense and when indicated by patient's verbal request and nonverbal cues.	2. Pharmacologic analgesia will be necessary for 48 hours or more because of surgical manipulation; weaning to oral analgesics occurs afterward. Increased ability to cope and compliance with activity usually ensue. The resulting ability to hold infant easily fosters bonding.
3. Perform comfort measures and encourage relaxation techniques.	3. These techniques enhance pharmacologic analgesia and give patient a sense of control.
4. Additional individualized interventions: _____	4. Rationales: _____

Collaborative problem: *High risk for fluid volume deficit related to blood loss associated with surgery, underlying condition that necessitated surgery, and uterine hypotonicity*

GOAL: Prevent or minimize fluid volume deficit.

Interventions	**Rationales**
1. Assess vital signs every half hour for 4 hours, every hour for 4 hours, then every 4 hours and as patient condition warrants. Correlate findings with prenatal levels. Note estimated blood loss during surgery and types of anesthesia administered.	1. Blood pressure is essentially unchanged in the postpartum period and bradycardia is common. Early indications of hemorrhage include prolonged capillary refill times on the blanch test. Significant losses may occur through unappreciated bleeding and before classic signs of hypovolemia occur.
2. Concurrently assess fundal contractility. Support incision with nondominant hand and palpate fundus from sides using dominant hand. Schedule assessment, when possible (based on patient condition), after administration of analgesics.	2. Hemorrhage is a significant source of maternal morbidity. Assessment of fundal height and contractility is commonly neglected or postponed because of discomfort to patient.
3. Concurrently assess number of perineal pads used, time interval before changing, and degree of saturation. Assess lochia for color, amount, odor, characteristics, and the presence and amount of clots. Differentiate lochia rubra from frank bleeding.	3. Significant losses may occur intrapartally. Postpartum course should be the same as for vaginal birth.

Interventions

4. Assess abdominal dressing for drainage, noting color. Circumscribe and date drainage area with pen.

5. Assess incision for active bleeding, seepage, approximation of edges, and hematoma formation.

6. Note hematocrit levels, comparing prenatal, intrapartum, and postpartum levels.

7. Determine whether patient is receiving sufficient fluids. Continue fluid administration initiated intrapartally.

8. Additional individualized interventions: _____

_____

Rationales

4. A thick abdominal dressing with multiple layers of wide adhesive may be applied immediately after surgery and, unless saturated or soiled, is not removed for 24 to 48 hours. Assessment technique must be modified but not eliminated.

5. Visualization is possible when the original dressing has been changed or removed.

6. A hematocrit of 33% or greater usually indicates maternal tolerance of blood loss.

7. Prolonged labor before surgical delivery may have caused hypovolemia. Circulating blood volume is enhanced and sequelae of loss minimized by administering I.V. fluids.

8. Rationales: _____

_____

Nursing diagnosis: *High risk for maternal infection related to delivery and secondary to surgical incision, repeated vaginal examination, sequelae of anesthesia administration, bladder intubation, or I.V. lines*

GOAL: Minimize or prevent infection.

Interventions

1. Monitor vital signs, including temperature, every 4 hours and as patient condition warrants.

2. Assess abdomen, incision, and abdominal dressing.

3. Assess perineum, noting presence of foul-smelling lochia. Continue with perineal care.

4. Assess bladder drainage; note color, amount, and odor of urine; presence of blood, clots, or sediment; and fluid input and output. Catheter care should be incorporated into perineal care. Assess for dysuria and retention after catheter is removed.

5. Assess breath sounds; note decreased or absent sounds, rales, rhonchi, and cough. Schedule coughing and deep-breathing exercises after administration of analgesics.

Rationales

1. An initial low-grade fever less than 100.4° F (38° C) is associated with parturition and inflammatory changes associated with surgery. Protracted low-grade fever or actual pyrexia is associated with infection and warrants antibiotic therapy.

2. Indications of healing include a clean, dry incision that has well-approximated edges and no erythema, edema, or drainage. Outer dressing should be clean, dry, and intact. Abdomen should be soft with well-contracted uterus at or below umbilicus as involution progresses.

3. Ascending genital tract infection may result from repeated intrapartum vaginal examinations or questionable hygienic practices. Scrupulous perineal care is indicated regardless of type of delivery.

4. An indwelling urinary (Foley) catheter is usually inserted before surgery and remains in place for 24 hours postpartum; its presence contributes to infection. The urine should be clear, amber, odorless, and free of blood, sediment, or clots. Increased output is associated with diuresis secondary to intrapartum administration of oxytocin and to normal postpartum changes. Bloody urine may indicate trauma associated with delivery and warrants immediate attention.

5. General anesthesia and voluntary immobility secondary to pain may result in accumulation of secretions and decreased ventilatory function.

Interventions	Rationales
6. Assess I.V. site for erythema, edema, induration, and infiltration. Change I.V. tubing and dressing once daily.	6. Infection at the I.V. site can cause significant maternal morbidity.
7. Additional individualized interventions: _____	7. Rationales: _____

Nursing diagnosis: *Activity intolerance related to delivery and secondary to anesthesia administration, surgical incision, and pain*

GOAL: Minimize sequelae of inactivity and assist with progressive activity.

Interventions	Rationales
1. Note type of anesthesia administered intrapartally and recovery times; reposition patient after prescribed period of bed rest.	1. General anesthesia recovery times vary. Position changes and turning are usually indicated every 2 hours during the first 24 hours of prescribed bed rest. Spinal anesthesia recovery requires lying flat in bed in the supine or side-lying position for 8 to 12 hours.
2. Demonstrate or review pulmonary hygiene measures. Assist patient with deep breathing and coughing every 2 to 4 hours, after administering analgesics if possible. Place bed in semi- to high Fowler's position. Splint incision with pillow or intertwined fingers.	2. Premedication fosters compliance by decreasing pain and anxiety.
3. While the patient is on bed rest, instruct her in leg exercises (paddling or modified knee bends, for example); schedule time for exercises and offer encouragement.	3. Blood stasis in peripheral vessels predisposes patient to thrombophlebitis.
4. Assist patient with progressive ambulation. Begin with the patient dangling her legs over the side of the bed, then progress to her sitting at bedside and taking accompanied walks over designated lengths.	4. Hypotension and resulting vertigo commonly accompany early ambulation. Actual or anticipated pain and interference from I.V. lines and urinary catheter may frighten or confuse the patient and result in reluctance to move.
5. Additional individualized interventions: _____	5. Rationales: _____

Collaborative problem: *Altered nutrition: less than body requirements related to fasting status imposed by anesthesia and surgery and by physiologic response to abdominal surgery*

GOAL: Maintain fluid requirements and facilitate diet progression.

Interventions	Rationales
1. Administer balanced electrolyte and glucose I.V. solution at rate of approximately 100 ml/hour; continue until foods are tolerated.	1. I.V. feedings supply fluid but not the caloric or nutritional requirements of postpartum course.
2. Assess abdomen, noting size, tension, and bowel sounds. Ask if flatus has been expelled.	2. Peristalsis usually returns within 24 hours and is characterized by a soft, nondistended abdomen with active bowel sounds.

INTRAPARTUM

Interventions

3. Offer water and surgical (clear) liquids, and progress diet, as tolerated. Note ability to retain food and verbalization of hunger. Keep I.V. line in place until liquids are successfully retained.

4. Assist with menu selection, encouraging foods high in protein, vitamin C, and iron.

5. Additional individualized interventions: _____

Rationales

3. Diet progression usually proceeds from surgical to full liquids, followed by soft or pureed foods to full, regular diet. Ascertaining ability to retain liquids before removing I.V. line obviates need for restarting I.V. line should dyspepsia, nausea, or emesis occur.

4. Protein and vitamin C promote in wound healing, and iron is needed to correct anemia.

5. Rationales: _____

Nursing diagnosis: *Knowledge deficit related to postpartum course and implications for subsequent pregnancies*

GOAL: Correct knowledge deficit.

Interventions

1. Decide when patient is most ready to learn, based on her freedom from discomfort and distraction and her willingness to ask questions or express her concerns or doubts. Provide privacy. Actively listen, allowing time for questions.

2. Provide information on postpartum course, including:
• hygiene: Sutures or clips are removed usually on the 4th or 5th day and before discharge. Showering is frequently allowed by the 3rd day if patient is ambulating without difficulty.
• exercise: Heavy work, including lifting of heavy objects, is not permitted until postpartum visit with practitioner, usually for 2 weeks. Driving is prohibited for 4 to 6 weeks.
• coitus: Sexual relations may safely be resumed after the postpartum examination, usually in 3 to 6 weeks. Contraception alternatives are given as part of discharge planning and during the return examination to physician at 3 to 6 weeks.
• Patient should concern herself predominantly with care of herself and the infant.

3. Provide information, as appropriate, on repeat elective cesarean section births. Using general guidelines, suggest that vaginal birth after cesarean section may be accomplished if the underlying condition has been corrected or does not recur. "Once a section, always a section" is no longer true.

4. Additional individualized interventions: _____

Rationales

1. Information is more readily received and retained if learning readiness is established.

2. Information gives patient an active role in her own care and allows time to make adaptations in home environment. Patient should be aware that heavy bleeding may occur after marked exertion. Maternal injury or pregnancy may result if sexual relations are resumed before postpartum examination. The stressors of a new infant and major surgery may easily lead to fatigue and depression; help by family members may be beneficial.

3. Certain conditions preclude vaginal birth. A trial labor may be conducted in the absence of diagnosed maternal or fetal dysfunction. Criteria for trial labor include: pelvic adequacy, preferably one prior low cervical transverse unextended uterine incision, informed consent, and immediate professional and logistical support for a cesarean section delivery should the trial fail.

4. Rationales: _____

ASSOCIATED PLANS AND APPENDICES
• Abruptio Placentae
• Hemorrhage
• Normal Antepartum
• Placenta Previa
• Pregnancy Complicated by Diabetes Mellitus
• Pregnancy-Induced Hypertension
• Prolapsed Umbilical Cord
• Puerperal Infection
• Puerperium
• Sexually Transmitted Diseases/TORCH
• Thromboembolic Disease
• Aspects of Psychological Care—Maternal (Appendix 4)
• Preparing for Nonemergency Surgery (Appendix 5)
• Selected Methods of Family Planning (Appendix 6)
• The Family and Home Assessment (Appendix 7)

ASSOCIATED NURSING DIAGNOSES
• Constipation related to anticipatory abdominal pain
• High risk for altered parenting related to postponed bonding secondary to inability to touch, hold, or care for infant because of effects of anesthesia, pain, or infant condition
• Self-esteem disturbance related to perceived inability to give birth "naturally"

INTRAPARTUM

INTRAPARTUM
Labor and Vaginal Birth

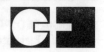

DEFINITION

Labor is a physiologic process in which the fetus, after an approximate 282-day habitus in utero, is expelled. Three distinct stages of labor are recognized, although expanded systems of categorization include prelabor and latent phases, before the first stage, and a fourth stage after delivery.

• Prelabor is a somewhat amorphous stage occurring several weeks before true labor and results in increased uterine activity, which serves to ready the cervix for its eventual effacement and dilation.

• The latent phase is characterized by irregular, infrequent contractions that may assist in eventual effacement and dilation.

• First-stage labor is characterized by cervical effacement and dilation, readying passage of the fetal head.

• Second-stage labor results in expulsion of the fetus.

• Third-stage labor results in placental separation and expulsion.

• Fourth-stage labor is the 1 to 4 hours after placental delivery in which the contracting uterus controls bleeding. During this period, the mother is at risk for hemorrhage and complications associated with uterine atony, anesthesia induction, and metabolic disorders.

Delivery in the occiput or vertex presentation accounts for 95% to 97% of all labors, and this fetal presentation is assumed in this plan. The positional changes necessary to accommodate fetal head to maternal pelvis include engagement, descent, flexion, internal rotation, extension, external rotation, and expulsion. Within 5 to 10 minutes of expulsion, placental separation usually occurs, and delivery is enacted either spontaneously or manually.

Management of the labor process is directed at maintaining optimal maternal and fetal well-being, identifying and ameliorating distress, and preventing or minimizing complications.

ETIOLOGY AND PRECIPITATING FACTORS

• Etiology: Triggering of the labor process is hypothesized to be the role of these factors: oxytocin release by the neurohypophysis; estrogen stimulation; progesterone withdrawal; increased maternal prostaglandin and fetal cortisol levels; increased uterine size; calcium release from the sarcoplasmic reticulum; pressure of presenting part on the cervix and lower uterine segment; or placental aging.

• Signs of impending labor include:
    □ "lightening" — decrease in fundal height, reshaping and enlarging of the lower abdomen, flattening of the costal region, and subjective maternal feeling of fetal "dropping" occur with descent of the fetus to or through the pelvic inlet and lower uterine development. This phenomenon occurs several weeks be-

fore true labor and is more pronounced in primigravid patients.
    □ "false labor" — irregular, brief uterine contractions of the lower abdomen and groin that do not progress and do not result in cervical dilation. These contractions, more common in patients of high parity and during late pregnancy, should be considered harbingers of true labor and monitored closely.
    □ "bloody show" — the vaginal discharge of blood-tinged mucus is a precursor of labor, which may occur hours to days before actual labor. It represents the mucous plug of the cervical canal and should be differentiated from frank bleeding.

PHYSICAL FINDINGS
Stage 1: Latent phase

• cervical dilation: 0 to 3 cm

• cervical effacement in primiparous patient is usually complete before dilation; in multiparous patient, it occurs with dilation

• duration of latent phase: 8 to 10 hours

• uterine contractions are mild, 5 to 30 minutes apart, and last 10 to 30 seconds

• membranes ruptured or intact

• scant brown or pink vaginal discharge or mucus plug

• station: primiparous patient — usually 0; multiparous patient — 0 to −2

• fetal heart tones (FHT): clearest at level of or below umbilicus, dependent on fetal position

Stage 1: Active phase

• cervical dilation: 4 to 7 cm

• duration of active phase: approximately 6 hours

• uterine contractions are moderate, 3 to 5 minutes apart, and last 30 to 45 seconds

• scant to moderate bloody mucus

• station: 0 to +1

• FHT: heard slightly below umbilicus or lower abdomen

Stage 1: Transition phase

• cervical dilation: 8 to 10 cm

• duration of transition phase: 1 to 2 hours

• uterine contractions of transition phase: strong, 2 to 3 minutes apart, and last 45 to 60 seconds

• copious bloody mucus

• station: +2 to +3

• FHT: clearest directly above symphysis pubis

Stage 2: Expulsion of fetus

• cervical dilation complete at 10 cm

• cervical effacement 100%

• duration of Stage 2: 20 to 50 minutes

• uterine contractions are strong, 2 to 3 minutes apart, and last 60 to 90 seconds; fetal bradycardia during

contraction may occur
• membranes may rupture
• copious bloody mucus
• station: fetal descent continues at a rate of 1 cm/hour in primiparous patient and 2 cm or more in multiparous patient until perineal floor is reached
• urge to push begins
• perineum bulges, flattens
• crowning occurs
• infant is born

Stage 3: Expulsion of placenta
• usually within 5 to 10 minutes of delivery
• uterine shape globular, usually firmer; fundus rises
• dark vaginal bleeding—gush or trickle
• umbilical cord protrudes further from introitus
• placenta intact: shiny presentation of fetal side of placental separation occurs from inner to outer margins (Schultze mechanism); rough presentation of maternal side of placental separation occurs from outer margins inward (Duncan mechanism)

• placenta, membranes, and umbilical cord intact and free of anomaly

Stage 4
• fundus firm or becomes firm when massaged, midline at level of umbilicus
• moderate lochia rubra
• episiotomy and laceration repair clean without ecchymosis or discharge, minimal edema; tenderness commensurate with analgesia, usually mild; edges well approximated
• possible extrusion of hemorrhoids

DIAGNOSTIC STUDIES
• Diagnosis is based on physical findings. Little testing is done unless maternal or fetal disorder or disease is suspected.
• Fern test identifies integrity of membranes; crystalline frondlike or fern pattern (arborization) indicates amniotic fluid; neither urine, blood, nor vaginal secretions elicit this configuration.

Collaborative problem: *Onset of true labor related to hormonal and physical changes*

GOAL: Identify contractions of true labor and establish obstetric baseline.

Interventions

1. Assess contractions for location, regularity, intensity, duration, time of relaxation between contractions, and relief from analgesics. Also assess degree of cervical dilation.

2. Upon admission to obstetric unit, review patient profile for:
• last menstrual period (LMP) and estimated date of confinement (EDC)
• pelvic adequacy—pelvic size is identified by the physician and includes diagonal conjugate (distance of sacral promontory to lower margin of symphysis pubis), ischial spines, pelvic walls, and sacrum
• obstetric, gynecologic, and outstanding medical histories
• age
• height, weight
• blood type and Rh of patient and sexual partner
• medications being taken
• allergies
• prenatal care and progress
• prenatal preparation for childbirth
• patient concerns and perceptions about pregnancy and labor.

3. If there is no gross or frank bleeding, use strict aseptic technique to perform a vaginal examination, assessing the following:
• status of membranes and presence of amniotic fluid

Rationales

1. True labor is characterized by regular contractions of increasing intensity and with gradually shortened intervals between. Pain is perceived in back and abdomen and is not stopped by analgesics. Cervical dilation is progressive.

2. Profile establishes data base and assists in prevention or early identification of patient problems.

3. Bleeding may indicate previa or premature separation, and manipulation may further compromise patient status.

• Nitrazine paper test or the more reliable fern test confirms rupture of membranes. Pale, straw-colored fluid with a pH of 6.5 to 7.5 is the norm.

Interventions	Rationales
• cervical dilation and effacement	• Softness and degrees of dilation and effacement assist in staging labor. Cervical location with reference to vagina and presenting part may identify preterm labor by its posterior position. *Note:* Dilation reflects the average diameter of the cervical opening; a diameter of 10 cm is considered complete or fully dilated and should allow passage of a full-term fetus. Effacement reflects cervical thinning and shortening that occurs in late pregnancy or during actual labor; complete effacement obliterates the cervical canal and transforms the 2 cm cervical length to a paper-thin, circular orifice.
• identification of presenting part	• Part identification is essential to safe labor management. Position, which is changeable, may also be identified by Leopold's maneuvers.
• station.	• Station relates the level of the presenting fetal part to an imaginary line between the maternal ischial spines.
4. Take vital signs, including temperature, pulse rate, respirations and blood pressure; compare with pre-pregnancy and prenatal levels. Assess for peripheral edema and reflexes; note any abnormalities. Integrate findings with history and physical examination.	4. Information establishes database, identifies high-risk patients, and aids in early recognition of complications and their management.
5. Apply external fetal monitor; note FHT.	5. Fetal status and database are established (see *Fetal heart activity*). External (indirect) electronic fetal monitoring typically is used for patients with low-risk pregnancies. Transducers applied to the abdomen measure fetal heart activity as well as the frequency and duration of uterine contractions. External monitoring is non-invasive, easily applied, and independent of cervical dilation, membrane rupture, or fetal head engagement. Related nursing responsibilities include assessing, monitoring, and documenting fetal heart and uterine activity, performing appropriate and timely independent nursing actions, and reporting nonreassuring and ominous fetal heart patterns to the physician.
6. Draw blood for:	6. Profile of blood analysis establishes database.
• hematocrit and hemoglobin values	• Hematocrit and hemoglobin values assess oxygen-carrying capacity and identify anemia and possible blood loss.
• serology	• Serology determines exposure to sexually transmitted disease.
• type and crossmatch if at greater risk for bleeding.	• A sample is needed to confirm blood type and Rh and possible holding of blood for emergency use.
7. Obtain clean-catch urine sample for protein, glucose, and bacteria.	7. Small amounts of urine glucose (1+) are normal and attributed to an increased glomerular filtration rate and impaired tubular reabsorption; some proteinuria (1+) may be seen in vigorous labor as a result of protein catabolism. Bacteriuria may indicate infection. Aberrations warrant further analysis and remediation.
8. Additional individualized interventions: _____	8. Rationales: _____

FETAL HEART ACTIVITY

Evaluation of fetal heart activity provides valuable information for fetal assessment. This chart describes baseline fetal heart rate and variations of fetal heart activity. Fetal heart patterns that restore confidence about fetal status are called *reassuring;* those that fail to remove doubt about fetal status are called *nonreassuring.*

Term	Description	Implication
Baseline fetal heart rate (FHR)	Mean FHR, measured between contractions or during intervals between periodic changes. Ranges from 120 to 160 beats per minute (bpm) in normal term fetus. May fluctuate 5 to 15 bpm normally.	• Decreased FHR suggests fetal sleep. • Increased FHR suggests fetal movement.
Tachycardia	Persistent (≥10 minutes) FHR above 160 bpm. Generally associated with loss of variability. Mild tachycardia: FHR 161 to 180 bpm; severe tachycardia: FHR >180 bpm.	• May indicate maternal fever, amnionitis, maternal use of parasympatholytic agents (such as atropine) or beta sympathomimetic agents (such as ritodrine [Yutopar]), maternal hyperthyroidism, early fetal hypoxia, fetal anemia, fetal infection, fetal tachyarrhythmias, or fetal heart failure. • Indicates fetal compromise when associated with decelerations or absence of variability; less serious when periodic changes are absent.
Bradycardia	Persistent (≥10 minutes) FHR below 120 bpm. Mild bradycardia: FHR 80 to 100 bpm; severe bradycardia: FHR <80 bpm.	• May indicate fetal head compression from occiput posterior or occiput transverse fetal position, especially during second stage of labor. • May indicate fetal hypoxia, maternal use of beta blockers (such as propranolol [Inderal]), maternal connective tissue disease, maternal hypothermia, congenital or acquired fetal heart block, or post-term pregnancy. • May signal fetal compromise if associated with loss of variability and decelerations. • Reassuring if associated with good variability.
Variability	Normal cyclic irregularity in cardiac rhythm. Short-term variability: beat-to-beat (R-wave-to-R-wave) change of consecutive cardiac cycles, generally 3 to 8 bpm. Long-term variability: cyclic fluctuations or ''waviness,'' generally 3 to 5 cycles per minute. Normal variability is single most reliable predictor (among FHR characteristics) of fetal status.	• Baseline variability is associated with fetal wakefulness. • Increased variability is associated with mild and early fetal hypoxia, fetal activity or stimulation, and uterine manipulation. • Decreased variability is associated with fetal sleep, hypoxia or acidosis, extreme prematurity, maternal use of CNS depressants (such as analgesics, narcotics, barbiturates, and tranquilizers) or parasympatholytics (such as atropine), general anesthesia, congenital anomalies of cardiac and central nervous systems, and fetal tachycardias. When preceded by late decelerations, decreased variability indicates fetal compromise.
Acceleration	Transient increase in FHR baseline (generally above 15 bpm) lasting 15 to 20 seconds.	• May indicate partial umbilical cord occlusion, uterine contractions, fetal movement, or fetal stimulation during pelvic examination • Reassuring, signalling fetal well-being, when associated with fetal movement and normal variability
Early deceleration	Transient decrease in FHR below baseline. (FHR rarely falls below 100 or 110 bpm, or 20 to 30 bpm below baseline.) Concurrent with uterine contractions; uniformly shaped; associated with average baseline variability.	• May indicate fetal head compression, associated with active phase of labor and cervical dilation of 4 to 7 cm. • Reassuring; not associated with tachycardia, hypoxia, or loss of variability.

FETAL HEART ACTIVITY *(continued)*

Term	Description	Implication
Late deceleration	Transient repetitive FHR decrease below baseline. Occurs late in contraction phase; nadir of deceleration occurs after acme of uterine contraction. Return and descent typically are smooth and gradual. Commonly associated with loss of variability and increasing baseline FHR. Rarely precedes or follows acceleration.	• May indicate uteroplacental insufficiency resulting from maternal hypotension, uterine hypertonicity, hyperactivity (such as from oxytocin augmentation or labor induction), epidural or spinal anesthesia, hypertensive disorders, abruptio placentae, placenta previa, amnionitis, diabetes mellitus, collagen vascular disease, intrauterine growth retardation, postmaturity, or fetal hypoxia. • Nonreassuring; indicates fetal compromise when persistent or associated with elevated baseline FHR and loss of variability.
Variable deceleration	Abrupt, transient decrease in FHR. Variable in duration, intensity, and timing relative to uterine contraction. Often preceded or followed by small, transient acceleration. Return to baseline is rapid. Significant when lasting more than 60 seconds with FHR below 70 bpm.	• May indicate oligohydramnios and umbilical cord compression from short, knotted, or prolapsed cord; cord wrapped around fetal body part; or cord between fetus and maternal pelvis. • Reassuring if baseline FHR and short-term variability of baseline FHR are normal and if pattern lasts no more than 30 to 45 seconds and exhibits rapid return from nadir to baseline. • Indicates fetal hypoxia and acidosis if pattern becomes progressively more severe and prolonged or sustained. Seen late in labor with fetal descent and maternal pushing.

Nursing diagnosis: *High risk for ascending genital tract infection related to vaginal insult secondary to multiple vaginal examinations, proximity to rectum, normal nonsterile environment of pudenda, and access provided by rupture of membranes before labor*

GOAL: Prevent or minimize infection.

Interventions

1. Perform all vaginal assessments using strict aseptic technique.

2. Administer a cleansing disposable enema of sodium phosphate (rarely done).

3. Clean external genitalia and perineum. Wash with antiseptic solution while protecting introitus every 4 hours, after defecation. Change underpad regularly and whenever it becomes wet or soiled.

4. Monitor vital signs. Note early rupture of membranes; presence of meconium; and odor, color, and consistency of amniotic discharge. Correlate findings with white blood cell count. Note FHT.

Rationales

1. Pathogenic bacterial invasion through the dilating cervix is minimized.

2. Protocol varies among hospitals. If the patient has not had recent diarrhea, enemas may be given to minimize the fecal contamination that occurs when maternal pushing ensues. Stimulation of the bowel may stimulate the uterus.

3. These interventions remove contaminants and minimize vaginal exposure to pathogens.

4. Indications of infection include temperature elevation greater than 100.4° F (38° C); thick, yellow, and foul-smelling amniotic fluid; and a history of early membrane rupture. Meconium-stained fluid may indicate a compromised fetus. Leukocytosis is a normal occurrence during labor, and its presence does not necessarily indicate infection.

Interventions

5. Additional individualized interventions: _____

Rationales

5. Rationales: _____

Collaborative problem: *Increased myometrial activity and cervical changes associated with Stage 1 labor*

GOAL: Identify progression from latent to transition stages.

Interventions

1. Using palpation or external monitoring, assess uterine contractions for location, intensity, duration, and resting intervals. Perform hourly; as labor progresses, perform every hour, every 30 minutes, every 15 minutes, then after every contraction. Refer to "Physical Findings," page 92, for normal progression. Allow for individual variation. If a fetal monitor is unavailable, assess FHT after every contraction when patient is completely dilated.

2. Assess cervical dilation and effacement and fetal station. Use Friedman graph to correlate cervical dilation, fetal descent, and duration of labor. Include significant activities and occurrences (for example, amount, type, and dosage of medications; artificial or spontaneous rupture of membranes; color and amount of amniotic fluid; and marked change in fetal status). Note fetal heart rate (FHR) and variability.

3. Assess bloody show and passage of mucous plug. Concurrently evaluate for cord prolapse.

4. Assess amniotic fluid for color, amount, and odor. Assist physician with amniotomy.

5. Monitor vital signs hourly and temperature every 4 hours if membranes have not ruptured; otherwise, every 1 to 2 hours. If blood pressure is elevated or analgesia has been administered, monitoring every 10 to 15 minutes may be warranted. Perform between contractions. Integrate findings with medical history and significant physical findings. Check FHT every 15 minutes.

6. Transfer to delivery suite when patient exhibits perineal bulging or when contractions result in display of occiput: +1 to +2; or when multiparous patient has advanced to 0 to +1 station.

7. Additional individualized interventions: _____

Rationales

1. Relationship between factors assists in monitoring progression of labor.

2. Cervical dilation and fetal descent are more reliable measures of labor progression. The Friedman graph serves as an objective tool for monitoring labor, as well as a medicolegal chronology.

3. Early in labor, the cervical mucous plug may be passed. As labor progresses, bloody show becomes more copious. Bright red bleeding in any amount or umbilical cord protrusion warrants immediate evaluation and intervention.

4. Rupture of the membranes usually occurs spontaneously during labor. The decision to rupture the membrane is a medical one. The ensuing benefits of a more rapidly progressing labor and availability of amniotic fluid to monitor fetal well-being must be weighed against the potential for ascending genital tract infection and prolapsed umbilical cord.

5. Findings assist in evaluating maternal and fetal responses to labor and to increased risks posed by actual or incipient hypertensive and cardiac disorders.

6. These signs indicate that delivery is imminent.

7. Rationales: _____

Nursing diagnosis: *Anxiety related to unknown surroundings and hospital procedures, absent or minimal childbirth preparation, fatigue or excitement*

GOAL: Minimize anxiety.

Interventions	Rationales
1. Introduce self as primary caregiver to patient and significant others. Give factual information. Explain hospital's admission policies and procedures that can be anticipated; listen to concerns and allow time for questions.	1. Identification of the caregiver and establishment of rapport decrease anxiety. Factual information minimizes fear of the unknown.
2. Ascertain the patient's level of childbirth preparation, then review, reinforce, or teach, as appropriate. Have patient give brief demonstration of breathing and relaxation techniques.	2. Activities give patient and partner a sense of control.
3. Ascertain patient's age, marital status, previous childbearing experiences, ethnicity and degree of acculturation, use of personal space, and response to teaching. Be nonjudgmental.	3. Information provides a data base for psychosocial needs.
4. Ensure privacy during examination; drape and minimize exposure.	4. Respect for the patient is demonstrated by these interventions.
5. Allow for cultural or religious rituals or practices for patient and partner when medically possible.	5. Incorporation of symbolic practices may be a source of comfort and strength, and may enchance coping with labor and delivery.
6. Additional individualized interventions: _____	6. Rationales: _____

Nursing diagnosis: *Decreased cardiac output related to uterine contractions with diversion of blood from uterine artery, to position, and to use of Valsalva's maneuver*

GOAL: Minimize sequelae secondary to labor-induced alterations in cardiac output.

Interventions	Rationales
1. Monitor maternal vital signs every hour and FHT every 15 minutes as patient's condition warrants.	1. Evaluation of levels assists in determining maternal and fetal status.
2. Assist, teach, or reinforce measures that allow patient to relax between contractions.	2. Uteroplacental blood flow is reestablished between contractions.
3. Monitor the patient for supine hypotensive syndrome (vena cava syndrome), including hypotension and tachycardia. Encourage left lateral or semi-Fowler's position; avoid supine position.	3. Compression of the ascending vena cava results in decreased cardiac output and, ultimately, in decreased placental perfusion. Left recumbent position facilitates uterine perfusion.
4. Additional individualized interventions: _____	4. Rationales: _____

Collaborative problem: *High risk for fluid volume deficit related to decreased gastric motility and to subsequent medical limitation of oral intake and to diaphoresis associated with the work of labor*

GOAL: Identify signs of dehydration and intervene accordingly.

Interventions

1. Monitor hydration status, including condition of skin, mucous membranes, and eyes, and subjective feelings of thirst.

2. Continue to restrict oral intake; ice chips may be allowed.

3. Monitor fluid intake and output. Note amount of diaphoresis.

4. Administer an I.V. infusion of balanced salt solution with glucose to a fasting patient in advanced labor.

5. Additional individualized interventions: _____

_____

Rationales

1. A well-hydrated state is characterized by smooth, supple skin; moist mucous membranes; and absence of thirst.

2. Prolonged gastric emptying occurs during labor. Vomiting may result in aspiration, a significant source of obstetric morbidity.

3. Renal function is evaluated; minimal satisfactory output is 30 to 50 ml/hour.

4. I.V. fluid administration prevents dehydration and acidosis; provides a vehicle for glucose and insulin administration in a diabetic patient; and allows prophylactic oxytocin administration.

5. Rationales: _____

_____

Nursing diagnosis: *Altered urinary elimination related to pressure of the presenting fetal part and to regional anesthesia*

GOAL: Maintain or restore bladder function.

Interventions

1. Assess for filling bladder by palpating above symphysis pubis.

2. Assist patient to bathroom or toilet every 2 to 4 hours. Perform nursing measures to promote voiding (for example, running water and putting patient's hands in water).

3. Catheterize, if necessary, between contractions with a small, well-lubricated catheter.

4. Additional individualized interventions: _____

_____

Rationales

1. Urge to void may be absent. Using the symphysis pubis as an anatomic landmark assists in locating organ.

2. Bladder distention may interfere with fetal descent and contribute to postpartum uterine atony. Decreased bladder tone, urine retention, and infection may result.

3. Using such a catheter minimizes trauma from catheter insertion.

4. Rationales: _____

_____

Collaborative problem: *Pain related to uterine hypoxia, pressure of presenting part, and cervical dilation*

GOAL: Minimize, manage, or control pain.

Interventions

1. Monitor contractions for frequency, intensity, and duration; correlate with cervical dilation, effacement, and station.

Rationales

1. Assessment monitors progression of labor.

Interventions

2. Keep patient informed of her progress. Allow her to listen to fetal heart beat.

3. Encourage ambulation if the following criteria can be met:
• latent or active Stage 1 labor
• no analgesia administration
• intact membranes
• no vaginal bleeding
• no fetal distress.

4. When patient is confined to bed, minimize discomfort in the following ways:
• Allow her to find comfortable position.
• Tell her to avoid the supine position.
• If she lies in supine position, place wedge under her left hip.
• Encourage left lateral or semi-Fowler's position.

5. Encourage use of distraction techniques, including talking, watching TV, reading, and playing board games, and encourage patient to focus on past experiences or on an object in a room away from her.

6. Promote comfort measures, encouraging the patient to use pelvic rocking, administering back rubs and effleurage, and applying cold or warm compresses to the back.

7. Cluster nursing activities so patient can rest. Keep room quiet and free of distracting stimuli.

8. Coach the patient through controlled breathing techniques, progressing through the following levels as Stage 1 progresses:
• Level 1—slow, deliberate inhalations through the nose; exhalation through nose or mouth
• Level 2—shallow, rapid inhalations through the nose, slowing as contraction wanes; exhalation through the mouth
• Level 3—increasingly rapid and shallow respirations; inhalations and exhalation through the mouth; mold mouth during exhalation to hee-hoo configuration.

9. Administer analgesics (if patient desires), most commonly, meperidine with promethazine (Mepergan) when active labor has been established and cervix is dilated 4 to 5 cm or more.

10. Assist practitioner with single injection or indwelling catheter insertion for paracervical or peridural block. Continue with frequent monitoring of maternal vital signs and electronic monitoring of FHR.

11. Additional individualized interventions: _____

Rationales

2. These interventions include the patient in the health care team and involve her in her own care.

3. Ambulation provides diversion and offers psychological comfort.

4. The left recumbent position facilitates uterine perfusion and ultimately, labor progression.

5. These distraction techniques ensure that contractions do not become the focus of the patient's attention.

6. These activities reduce abdominal and back discomfort.

7. Fatigue diminishes the patient's ability to cope.

8. Controlled breathing facilitates relaxation, distraction, and coping abilities.

9. Once contractions become intense, analgesics may be given to control pain and allow patient to rest between contractions. Analgesics cannot be given too early, because they may slow labor process; nor can they be given within 1 hour of delivery because of their depressant effect on the fetus.

10. No drug has a single action; although maternal analgesia may be affected, adverse reactions may affect patient or fetus.

11. Rationales: _____

Nursing diagnosis: *High risk for fetal injury related to uteroplacental insufficiency*

GOAL: Minimize or prevent injury.

Interventions

1. Review prenatal record for date of LMP and EDC. Note pelvimetry measurements and any sonographic or radiologic readings.

2. Assess fetal position and presentation by abdominal and vaginal palpation. Auscultate FHT to confirm findings.

3. Establish baseline FHR. Assess FHR on admission, after rupture of membranes every 15 minutes for 45 minutes, and as patient's condition warrants (every 15 minutes through first stage, every 5 minutes or after each contraction during second). Auscultate FHR for 30 seconds or more after a contraction; electronically monitor for 15 minutes.

4. While monitoring FHR, note these factors: bradycardia (less than 120 beats/minute), tachycardia (more than 160 beats/minute), late decelerations, variable decelerations, and variability less than 5 beats/minute.

5. Assist physician with fetal scalp sampling when acid-base balance must be ascertained.

6. Additional individualized interventions: _____

_____

Rationales

1. These interventions establish gestational maturity and determine the adequacy of maternal pelvis to accommodate fetal head.

2. Indications for cesarean section delivery include transverse lie and most breech presentations.

3. Assessment evaluates fetal well-being in response to labor. Norms include a FHR of 120 to 160 beats/minute, transient decelerations or accelerations associated with contractions or fetal movement, early decelerations, and average variability.

4. Levels indicate fetal distress and warrant intervention to increase uteroplacental functioning, including:
• continual monitoring for FHR change
• administration of oxygen to patient and placement in left recumbent position
• rehydration
• discontinuance of oxytocin infusion
• emergency treatment of prolapsed umbilical cord
• control of pyrexia.

5. Fetal blood pH levels of 7.25 or higher are considered normal during labor; levels between 7.20 and 7.24 are considered preacidotic. Serial fetal blood pH determinations in tandem with complete clinical profile are better determinants of fetal acidosis.

6. Rationales: _____

_____

Nursing diagnosis: *High risk for maternal injury and infection related to expulsive stage of labor*

GOAL: Minimize or prevent injury or infection and facilitate fetal expulsion.

Interventions

1. Increase frequency of maternal and fetal assessments. Transfer to delivery suite using physiologic guidelines listed in Intervention 6 on page 97.

2. Assist patient to delivery table, elevating head 30 to 60 degrees. Assist to lithotomy position, taking care to avoid pressure in popliteal area.

3. Assist scrubbed and gowned physician or nurse midwife with patient preparation, including perineal scrub and sterile draping. Practitioner may choose to wear double gloves.

Rationales

1. Greater physiologic stress on mother and fetus warrants evaluation of their well-being. Infection control procedures require wearing scrub suit, mask, and cap.

2. Elevation facilitates use of abdominal muscles for pushing. Pressure on popliteal area may compromise peripheral circulation.

3. A sterile environment must be maintained. Wearing double gloves may be employed for patients at high risk for acquired immunodeficiency syndrome (see Appendix 14: CDC Guidelines for Preventing HIV Transmission in Health Care Settings, page 337).

INTRAPARTUM

Interventions

4. Coach patient through expulsive, bearing-down efforts and with controlled breathing during contractions. Repeat instructions frequently. Allow patient to rest between contractions. Keep her appraised of her progress as infant's head, shoulder, and body are delivered.

5. Assist with clamping of the umbilical cord. Note fundal height and consistency. Keep hand on abdomen. Do not massage.

6. Monitor patient for globular configuration of uterus, rise of uterus in abdomen, and gush of blood from vagina and protrusion of umbilical cord.

7. Additional individualized interventions: _____

Rationales

4. Pushing is involuntary and assists in expulsion. Recovery time is needed between contractions to reestablish uteroplacental circulation.

5. A firm, contracted uterus will not bleed. Examiner's hand will facilitate immediate assessment of atony.

6. These signs are indications of placental separation. Spontaneous delivery of placenta usually occurs in 5 to 10 minutes. Evaluation of integrity of placenta minimizes potential for retained fragments.

7. Rationales: _____

Nursing diagnosis: *High risk for altered parenting related to delayed bonding*

GOAL: Promote early bonding.

Interventions

1. Allow mother to see infant immediately after delivery. After clamping of cord, place infant on mother's abdomen or put to breast, if she is breast-feeding.

2. Additional individualized interventions: _____

Rationales

1. While episiotomy is being repaired, ample time is available to acquaint the mother with infant. Greeting, touching, caressing, and examining the newborn infant are common behaviors that facilitate bonding.

2. Rationales: _____

ASSOCIATED PLANS AND APPENDICES
• Normal Antepartum
• Puerperium
• Aspects of Psychological Care—Maternal (Appendix 4)

ADDITIONAL NURSING DIAGNOSES
• Ineffective individual coping related to fatigue
• Knowledge deficit related to lack of childbirth preparation
• Sleep pattern disturbance related to regular, intense uterine contraction

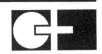

Oxytocin-Induced or Oxytocin-Augmented Labor

DEFINITION

Oxytocin injection functions exactly as the naturally occurring endogenous hormone oxytocin produced by the posterior pituitary gland. It stimulates uterine contractions. This oxytocic effect is greatest at term. Its ability to induce or stimulate labor and to augment a labor characterized by inadequate uterine contractions is addressed here. Management is directed at stimulating a labor as close to normal as possible, ensuring maternal and fetal well-being and preventing complications associated with oxytocin induction.

ETIOLOGY AND PRECIPITATING FACTORS

• Etiology: Not applicable.
• Precipitating factors: Conditions that warrant labor augmentation include hypotonic uterine dysfunction during active phase of first stage of labor or during the second stage. Conditions that warrant labor stimulation include medical conditions that necessitate early delivery, such as maternal history of precipitate labor in multigravid patient, Rh isoimmunization, severe preeclampsia near or at term, prolonged premature rupture of membranes, diabetes, abruptio placentae, gestational age greater than 42 weeks, incomplete or inevitable abortion, or fetal death.

PHYSICAL FINDINGS
Genitourinary
• uterine dysfunction: prolonged phase or stage of labor beyond expected norms, lack of progress in dilatation or effacement, or lack of descent of presenting fetal part
• uterine contractions infrequent and of short duration and mild intensity
• maternal exhaustion

DIAGNOSTIC STUDIES
• Fetal sonography evaluates fetal size and position.
• Radiologic pelvimetry, although rarely performed, may be used to evaluate fetal size and position and to rule out cephalopelvic disproportion.

Laboratory data
• Fern test—confirms rupture of membranes.
• Blood glucose level—provides database for glucose and insulin management of diabetic patient.

Collaborative problem: *High risk for maternal injury related to inadequate uterine contractions or to necessity for medically indicated oxytocin induction (3 goals)*

GOAL 1: Identify sources of injury.

Interventions

1. Review patient history, including estimated date of confinement, gynecologic and obstetric histories, and electronic fetal and uterine contraction record.

2. Assess whether the patient is a candidate for oxytocin use. Note the following:
• parity fewer than 5
• no uterine overdistention or previous scarring
• no mechanical obstruction or cephalopelvic disproportion
• active labor that has progressed to 50% effacement and 2 to 3 cm dilatation
• near term fetus, vertex presentation, good fetal heart tones (FHT).

3. Additional individualized interventions: _____

Rationales

1. Augmentation is considered only after a trial of labor has failed to progress. Information provides a database for care planning and early identification of problems.

2. The potency of oxytocin precludes its use in various conditions. The profile enhances the scenario for a normal vaginal birth and good maternal and fetal outcomes.

3. Rationales: _____

GOAL 2: Minimize injury while stimulating or augmenting uterine contractions.

Interventions	**Rationales**
1. Before induction, reassess uterine contractions. Assess patient's blood pressure and pulse rate. Monitor fetal heart rate (FHR) with a minimum tracing of 15 minutes.	1. Baseline data is established.
2. Start a primary I.V. line of physiologic electrolyte solution. Use an infusion pump and piggyback oxytocin with secondary I.V. set.	2. Electrolyte solution minimizes oxytocin's antidiuretic effect. Hemodynamic changes associated with the drug demand controlled flow rate to minimize potential for overdose. Piggybacking allows for emergency discontinuance of drug in cases of drug-induced tetany or hypersensitivity without compromising venous access.
3. Upon initiation of oxytocin induction, patient must be constantly attended. FHT and uterine contractions must be continuously electronically monitored and charted every 15 minutes and at each increase in dosage.	3. Oxytocin is rapid-acting and has a half-life of approximately 3 minutes when administered I.V. Fetal distress or uterine hyperactivity warrant immediate discontinuance of drug infusion.
4. Administer oxytocin per order and protocol, using the following guidelines:	4. One syringe (Tubex) contains 10 units/ml, the pharmacologic equivalent of 10 USP posterior pituitary units.
• 1 ml (10 units) of oxytocin/1,000 ml dilutant	• The infusion will contain 10 mU of oxytocin/ml.
• infuse 1 to 2 mU/minute; slowly increase dosage by 1 to 2 mU/minute until contractions of moderate intensity (50 to 75 mm Hg) occur every 2 to 3 minutes and are of 45 to 60 seconds' duration.	• These findings indicate that the pattern of normal labor has been established. Response time is variable. If progressive cervical changes have not occurred and delivery is imminent with the prescribed parameters, labor induction has failed and surgical delivery may be appropriate.
5. Additional individualized interventions:_____	5. Rationales: _____

GOAL 3: Identify early signs of oxytocin-induced uterine hyperactivity and intervene accordingly.

Interventions	**Rationales**
1. Continue assessments of maternal vital signs and frequency, intensity, and duration of contractions, and the interval between contractions. Note all significant patient activities and procedures on tracing strip.	1. Assessment assists in monitoring drug response and labor progression.
2. Monitor for signs of hyperstimulation, including: • contraction frequency greater than every 2 minutes • sustained or prolonged contractions greater than 75 to 90 seconds • resting uterine tone of 15 to 20 mm H_2O or more between contractions • intrauterine pressure greater than 75 mm Hg.	2. Hyperstimulation may result from overdose or uterine hypersensitivity to oxytocin given in therapeutic amounts. Regardless of cause, hyperstimulation, with its strong or protracted contractions, may cause abruptio placentae, uterine rupture, cervical and vaginal lacerations, impaired uteroplacental blood flow with resulting fetal hypoxia, postpartum hemorrhage, or death.
3. Immediately stop oxytocin drip and infuse primary I.V.	3. Plasma concentrations of short-lived oxytocin quickly drop with drug discontinuance.
4. Have magnesium sulfate 1 to 2 grams I.V. available.	4. Although management of hyperstimulation is usually palliative, magnesium sulfate may be given to relieve uterine tetany.
5. Additional individualized interventions:_____	5. Rationales: _____

Nursing diagnosis: *High risk for fetal injury related to uteroplacental insufficiency* (2 goals)

GOAL 1: Identify signs of uteroplacental insufficiency.

Interventions

1. Electronically monitor FHT 15 minutes before induction and before increasing oxytocin dosage. Monitor for insufficiency, following these guidelines:
• FHR less than 120 or more than 160 beats/minute (bradycardia or tachycardia, respectively)
• repetitive late or variable decelerations
• baseline variability less than 5 beats/minute
• meconium staining of amniotic fluid.

2. Monitor maternal vital signs, especially blood pressure.

3. Additional individualized interventions:_____

Rationales

1. Hypertonic or tetanic contractions impair uteroplacental blood flow. Fetal hypoxia and distress follow.

2. Epidural anesthesia may cause hypotension, resulting in decreased blood flow to the placenta and subsequent fetal hypoxia.

3. Rationales: _____

GOAL 2: Minimize injury.

Interventions

1. Stop oxytocin drip and infuse primary I.V. if uteropleurtal insufficiency should occur. Notify physician.

2. Position patient in left recumbent position and administer oxygen by mask at 4 to 7 liters/minute.

3. Additional individualized interventions: _____

Rationales

1. If effects of oxytocin are not quickly reversed, emergency surgical delivery of a compromised infant may be necessary.

2. This position facilitates uterine perfusion. Supplemental oxygen enhances capillary-alveolar perfusion.

3. Rationales: _____

Nursing diagnosis: *Pain related to oxytocic effect*

GOAL: Minimize pain.

Interventions

1. Establish rapport with patient and significant other.

2. Before induction, explain procedure, rapidity of onset, and anticipated progression of labor. Encourage questions. Review breathing and relaxation techniques.

3. Assess pain and its characteristics, including quality, frequency, location, and intensity. Keep patient informed of her progress.

4. Perform comfort measures, position changes, relaxation techniques, rubdowns and effleurage, and pharmacologic analgesia.

Rationales

1. A positive relationship facilitates trust and decreases anxiety.

2. Fear of the unknown increases patient's perception of pain. Oxytocin's rapid and pronounced onset and course of action may leave patient little time to garner her resources.

3. A pain profile monitors, in part, how labor is progressing.

4. Increased tissue perfusion plus the stimulation of the large, afferent sensory fibers decreases sensation of pain. Analgesics may be given after active labor has been clearly established; if given earlier, their depressive characteristics may compromise fetal status.

INTRAPARTUM

Interventions	**Rationales**
5. Additional individualized interventions: _____	5. Rationales: _____
_____	_____

ASSOCIATED PLANS AND APPENDICES
- Abortion
- Abruptio Placentae
- Cesarean Section Birth
- Labor and Vaginal Birth
- Pregnancy Complicated by Diabetes Mellitus
- Pregnancy-Induced Hypertension
- Premature Rupture of Membranes
- Rh Isoimmunization
- Aspects of Psychological Care — Maternal (Appendix 4)

ADDITIONAL NURSING DIAGNOSES
- High risk for ascending genital tract infection related to premature rupture of membranes
- High risk for fluid volume deficit related to hemorrhage secondary to uterine abruption
- High risk for fluid volume excess related to potent antidiuretic effect of oxytocin

SECTION III
POSTPARTUM

Puerperium   108
Hemorrhage   116
Puerperal Infection   119
Thromboembolic Disease   123

POSTPARTUM

POSTPARTUM
Puerperium

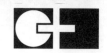

DEFINITION
The puerperium usually includes the period after the third stage of labor to 6 weeks after delivery. Physiologically, it represents a reversal of the anatomic and functional changes of pregnancy. Management is directed at monitoring these changes, minimizing the discomfort associated with them, and preventing conditions responsible for maternal morbidity and mortality, such as hemorrhage, thromboembolic disease, and infection.

ETIOLOGY AND PRECIPITATING FACTORS
• Not applicable.

PHYSICAL FINDINGS
See *Normal postpartum findings,* page 110.

DIAGNOSTIC STUDIES
Laboratory data
• In the absence of pathology, trauma, or complications, few tests are conducted.

Collaborative problem: *Altered genitourinary function related to completion of pregnancy process and to delivery*

GOAL: Identify normal alterations associated with puerperium.

Interventions

1. Assess delivery data, including:
• vital signs
• medical and obstetric histories; blood type and Rh factor
• maternal age, parity, and delivery outcome
• course of labor and delivery
• anesthesia, drugs, and parenteral fluids administered
• time of delivery
• genitourinary (GU) and abdominal assessments
• urine output.

2. Assess vital signs every 15 minutes for 1 hour, every 30 minutes for 1 hour, every hour for 4 hours, then every 4 hours for remainder of hospital stay or as patient condition warrants. Perform physical examination concurrently.

3. Assess uterus every 15 minutes for the 1st hour, every 30 to 60 minutes for the next 4 hours, then every 4 hours for remainder of hospital stay or as patient condition requires. Have the patient empty bladder before examination. Monitor fundal height, position, and tone.

4. Assess vaginal discharge, noting the following: frank bleeding and passage of clots, and color, amount, consistency, and odor of lochia.

Rationales

1. The course of the puerperium may be altered or affected by various physiologic and psychological factors.

2. Besides the physiologic adaptations noted in *Normal postpartum findings,* page 110, only mild fluctuations should be seen. Increased temperature may indicate infection (in most cases, GU infection or thrombophlebitis). Increased pulse may be associated with blood loss. Rise in blood pressure may indicate pregnancy-induced hypertension or a chronic hypertensive state.

3. A firm, contracted uterus that regresses along its predesigned course is exhibiting normal involutional changes. A distended bladder may distort findings by displacing uterus upward.

4. Frank bleeding requires immediate intervention. Small occasional clots result from pooled vaginal blood associated with the recumbent position; large or multiple clots, especially with frank or large amounts of bleeding, require immediate intervention. Lochial discharge contains red blood cells, decidual shreds, epithelial cells, multiple microorganisms, and, later, white blood cells. Alteration in predesignated flow from rubra to alba may indicate placental subinvolution, retained placental fragments, or infection.

Interventions

5. Assess episiotomy and perineum for erythema, edema, ecchymosis, pain, discharge, and approximation of suture edges.

6. Assess fluid intake and output, including time, amount, and color of each voiding for 24 hours.

7. Assess breasts for size, temperature, tenderness, discharge, and fissures.

8. Assess calves bilaterally for color, size, temperature, pulses, pain, Homans' sign, paresthesias, and paralysis.

9. Assess prepregnancy, actual, and desired weights. Note type and amount of foods consumed and cultural preferences.

10. Additional individualized interventions: _____

_____

Rationales

5. Minimal edema, tenderness, and occasional ecchymosis are expected. Pronounced pain accompanied by ecchymosis and edema may indicate perineal hematoma or trauma. Drainage or tension along the episiotomy line may portend infection.

6. Large volumes of urine can be anticipated for approximately 24 hours while extracellular fluid associated with normal pregnancy is diuresed. Monitoring of each voiding validates degree of bladder emptying.

7. Assessment provides the framework for management of the lactating patient as well as the patient who chooses to bottle-feed.

8. Assessment establishes baseline and facilitates early diagnosis of thromboembolic dysfunction related to position, immobility, and increased coagulation factors associated with pregnancy.

9. Appetite is usually excellent and intake greater than usual for several days. Observations provide a framework for diet teaching.

10. Rationales: _____

_____

Nursing diagnosis: *High risk for fluid volume deficit related to blood loss secondary to uterine atony or retained placental fragments*

GOAL: Prevent or minimize uterine atony and stimulate uterine tone.

Interventions

1. Gently massage the boggy uterus at fundus while supporting lower uterine segment.

2. Assist patient with bladder training every 3 hours if micturition is not spontaneous and complete.

3. Put suckling infant to breast.

4. Have on hand oxytocic, ergot alkaloids.

5. Administer analgesics for "afterpains."

6. Additional individualized interventions: _____

_____

Rationales

1. Gentle massage stimulates uterine contraction, assists in expulsion of retained placental fragments, and restores positive uterine tone. Aggressive manipulation may tire the myometrium and result in further atony. Support minimizes the risk of uterine inversion.

2. The uterus that is displaced by a distended bladder may become atonic.

3. Suckling stimulates the release of oxytocin, which increases myometrial contractions.

4. Pharmacologic agents may be used to stimulate uterine contraction; unless there is excessive bleeding or subinvolution, their use is questionable because bleeding is neither decreased nor involution facilitated.

5. Contractions cause discomfort. Greater pain is associated with increased parity, marked intrapartum abdominal distention, retained placental fragments, and oxytocin stimulation.

6. Rationales: _____

_____

POSTPARTUM

NORMAL POSTPARTUM FINDINGS

■ **Temperature:** May increase to 100.4° F (38° C) during the first 24 hours

■ **Pulse:** Bradycardia of 50 to 70 beats/minute lasting up to 1 week

■ **Blood pressure:** Essentially unaffected and congruent with previous readings

■ **Weight:** Immediate loss of 10 to 12 lb (4.5 to 5.4 kg); additional 5 lb (2.3-kg) loss during 1st week

■ **Uterus:** Firm and nontender; fundus midline located midway between the symphysis pubis and umbilicus after third-stage labor; at or 1 cm (1 finger) above umbilicus within 12 hours, persisting 48 hours; then regresses at a rate of 1 cm/day; prepregnant size attained within approximately 4 weeks

■ **Lochia:** Musky, fleshy, or earthy aroma; rubra for several days; progresses to serosa after 3 or 4 days, to alba after 10 days; combined volume equals approximately 100 ml

■ **Perineum:** Episiotomy and sutured lacerations clean, dry, and odorless; edges well approximated, with minimal edema and some tenderness

■ **Rectum:** Hemorrhoids may extrude

■ **Abdomen:** Soft, somewhat flabby, red or purple striae prominent, possible distasis recti abdominis (separation of abdominal recti muscles)

■ **Breasts:** Initially soft, nontender, and without erythema or discharge; colostrum secretion begins by second day postpartum, with subsequent tenderness and engorgement that persist for approximately 3 days

■ **Blood:** Increased white blood cell count, primarily granulocytes (as high as 30,000/mm³), up to 1st or 2nd postpartum day; increased hematocrit value and sedimentation rate varying with degree of diuresis and hemoconcentration

■ **Urine:** Proteinuria for up to 3 days; lactosuria persisting for several weeks

---

Collaborative problem: *High risk for injury or trauma related to hematoma formation secondary to blood vessel injury during delivery*

GOAL: Recognize hematoma formation and intervene appropriately.

Interventions

1. Assess perineum for signs of hematoma, including tense vaginal growth, ecchymosis, and severe pain. Also note possible inability to void, increased pulse, increased respiration, decreased blood pressure, and decreased hematocrit and hemoglobin values.

2. Prepare for incision and drainage of hematoma, possible blood replacement, and antibiotic therapy.

3. Additional individualized interventions: _____

Rationales

1. These signs and symptoms represent pressure of entrapped blood in confined vaginal or vulvar spaces. Vital signs and lowered blood values assist in quantifying actual amount of blood loss.

2. Large and enlarging hematomas require surgical intervention, replacement of blood loss, and antimicrobial prophylaxis or treatment. Peritoneal and retroperitoneal hematomas may require laparotomy for evacuation.

3. Rationales: _____

Nursing diagnosis: *High risk for ascending genital tract infection related to vaginal tears or lacerations, surgical episiotomy, and endometrial exfoliation*

GOAL: Prevent or minimize infection.

Interventions

1. Note trends in temperature; correlate with antepartum status and presenting symptoms.

2. Instruct patient to wash perineum with mild soap and water daily and to use peri bottle after each elimination.

Rationales

1. Persistent low-grade fever for more than 24 hours postpartum or actual pyrexia suggests infection.

2. Washing removes secretions and contaminants.

Interventions

3. Instruct patient to wipe perineum from front to back and to apply perineal pads front to back.

4. Replace sterile perineal pads after each elimination and at least once every 4 hours regardless of lochia flow.

5. Instruct patient to wash hands before and after touching genitals.

6. Additional individualized interventions: _____

_____

Rationales

3. These interventions reduce the risk of fecal contamination.

4. A warm, moist pad contaminated with organisms from the external genitalia and skin provides a good medium for bacterial growth.

5. Soiled hands act as vectors.

6. Rationales: _____

_____

Collaborative problem: *Altered immune system response related to Rh factor isoimmunization and to lack of rubella antibodies*

GOAL: Prevent sensitization in the nonsensitized patient and stimulate rubella antibody production.

Interventions

1. Administer Rh$_o$(D) immune globulin (RhoGAM) 300 mcg within 72 hours of delivery to Rh$_o$(D)-negative nonsensitized patient who has an Rh-positive spouse and an Rh$_o$(D)-positive neonate, having negative direct Coombs' test of umbilical cord blood.

2. Administer live rubella vaccine to patient who meets the following criteria:
• is not allergic to eggs or neomycin
• has hemagglutination inhibition titers less than 1:18
• plans to delay next pregnancy for at least 3 months.

3. Additional individualized interventions: _____

_____

Rationales

1. Formation of maternal antibodies is suppressed and a subsequent pregnancy is protected from circulatory fetomaternal incompatibility.

2. Allergy to eggs or neomycin strongly predisposes the patient to vaccine allergy. Low titers indicate lack of immunity. The vaccine renders lifelong immunity against rubella. The virus is teratogenic and can be transmitted to fetus during first trimester.

3. Rationales: _____

_____

Collaborative problem: *Pain related to episiotomy repair and to afterbirth pains of the contracting uterus*

GOAL: Prevent or minimize perineal or pelvic pain.

Interventions

1. Assess perineum (see *Normal postpartum findings*).

2. Apply ice pack to perineum immediately after delivery.

3. Assist with heat treatments beginning 12 hours postpartum to include:
• moist heat or sitz baths for 20 minutes three times daily with water temperature of 100° to 110° F (37.8° to 43.3° C)
• dry heat or heat lamp to exposed perineum for 20 minutes twice daily with heat source 18" to 24" (46 to 61 cm) from perineum.

Rationales

1. This assessment validates expected response and eliminates other causative factors such as hematoma or infection.

2. Cold minimizes edema and provides local anesthesia.

3. Heat soothes and assists in tissue healing by increasing blood and lymph flow to area; concurrently, moist heat cleans area, decreasing risk of infection.

POSTPARTUM

Interventions	**Rationales**
4. Teach patient to sit with less discomfort by contracting buttocks before sitting.	4. This maneuver supports underlying structures.
5. Apply local anesthetic to affected area after every perineal cleaning and pad change.	5. Local anesthetic sprays and ointments have an immediate, numbing effect.
6. Offer analgesia to patient complaining of afterbirth pains or who gives nonverbal cues of need. If patient is receiving I.V. oxytocin, check the flow rate.	6. Uterine contractions are a normal postpartum occurrence and a cause of discomfort that may require analgesia. I.V. oxytocin may be infusing too rapidly, causing increased contractions.
7. Additional individualized interventions: _____	7. Rationales: _____

Collaborative problem: *Rectal pain related to anorectal varicosities*

GOAL: Prevent or minimize rectal pain.

Interventions	**Rationales**
1. Assess anorectal area and integrate physical findings with prepregnant history.	1. Assessment identifies problems and possible established treatment modalities.
2. Apply covered ice pack or cold witch hazel compresses directly to hemorrhoids for 20 minutes every 4 hours for 24 hours immediately postpartum.	2. Cold minimizes edema and provides local anesthesia.
3. Tell patient to take warm 20-minute sitz baths of 100° to 110° F (37.8° to 43.3° C) 20 minutes after defecating.	3. Heat reduces discomfort and increases blood flow that will facilitate healing.
4. Advise use of side-lying position and avoidance of protracted sitting or standing.	4. These actions will minimize rectal pressure.
5. Demonstrate how to digitally replace externally protruding hemorrhoids.	5. This maneuver will reduce the pressure caused by the hemorrhoids.
6. Instruct the patient on diet and bowel hygiene to establish regular bowel habits. Include information on drinking adequate fluids and eating high-fiber foods.	6. Anticipation of or actual passage of a hardened stool may result in holding back, which further aggravates condition.
7. Administer pharmacologic agents, as indicated, including creams, ointments, stool softeners, laxatives, and analgesics.	7. Local anesthetics produce an immediate numbing effect. Stool softeners and laxatives facilitate painless passage of a soft stool. Analgesia may be required for perineal discomfort.
8. Additional individualized interventions: _____	8. Rationales: _____

Collaborative problem: *Altered urinary elimination related to pregnancy-induced hypervolemia, birth-induced trauma, overdistention, and the effects of anesthesia*

GOAL: Maintain or restore urinary tract function.

Interventions	**Rationales**
1. Monitor fluid intake and output for 24 to 48 hours.	1. Fluid output reflects renal function.

Interventions

2. Weigh daily and correlate with anticipated diuresis.

3. Note time, amount, and color of each elimination.

4. Assist patient to void spontaneously:
• Encourage toileting with urge to void.
• Medicate every 3 to 4 hours as necessary for pain, before ambulation.
• Suggest running tap water while in bathroom, pouring clean water over perineum while toileted.
• Encourage voiding during sitz bath or shower if elimination is difficult.

5. Assess for urinary urgency, frequency, dysuria, hematuria (differentiate from urine contaminated with vaginal discharge), and possible pyrexia.

6. Catheterize only if absolutely necessary, when there is an inability to void every 6 to 8 hours, or persistent urine retention with overflow. Use an indwelling urinary (Foley) catheter to measure residual urine; if more than 50 ml, keep in place. Continue with perineal care while catheter is in place.

7. Teach Kegel exercises as soon as anesthetic agent has worn off and patient receptivity has been ascertained. Instruct patient to mimic holding back urine for 10 seconds, then release; perform 10 exercises consecutively four times daily.

8. Additional individualized interventions: _____

_____

Rationales

2. An approximate 5-lb (2.3-kg) loss during first postpartum week represents loss (1-liter of retained fluid equals 2.2 lb [1 kg] by weight) caused by decrease in plasma volume, by involutional changes, and by normal postpartum diuresis.

3. Optimally, patient should void every 3 to 4 hours. Symptoms of incomplete emptying and retention with overflow (voiding small amounts frequently) imply poor bladder tone and predispose to GU infection as well as uterine atony.

4. Measures act as physical and occasional psychological impetus to voiding.

5. Urinary tract infection warrants antimicrobial therapy.

6. Catheterization further predisposes to GU system infection. The GU system is compromised by a traumatized, edematous, and hyperemic bladder, neural impairment associated especially with size of gravid uterus, and conduction anesthesia. Traumatic reintubation is avoided.

7. Exercise strengthens the pubococcygeal muscles and prevents or ameliorates pelvic floor relaxation and urinary stress incontinence.

8. Rationales: _____

_____

Collaborative problem: *Breast engorgement in nonnursing patient related to milk production secondary to prolactin secretion*

GOAL: Prevent or minimize breast engorgement and milk production.

Interventions

1. Assess the patient's breasts immediately postpartum and every 8 hours, noting colostrum secretion for 2 to 3 days, initial diffuse breast nodularity followed by tense, warm, engorged, and painful breasts, and low-grade fever.

2. Support breasts with a firm, well-fitted bra or breast binder.

3. Teach patient to avoid self-breast stimulation or stimulation from the infant or sexual partner, from breast pump or manual milk expression, or from hot showers or baths.

Rationales

1. Colostrum is the first lacteal secretion to present itself. Engorgement and resulting symptoms are the product of venous and lymphatic stasis.

2. Successful mechanical suppression of lactation is usually accomplished in 2 to 3 days.

3. These actions stimulate milk production.

Interventions	Rationales
4. Institute pain-relief measures: apply an ice bag to breasts, and provide oral analgesics (most commonly codeine and aspirin).	4. These measures produce local and central pain control.
5. Upon stabilization of vital signs, and at least 4 hours or more postpartum, administer one of the following: • bromocriptine (Parlodel), a dopamine agonist • testosterone enanthate with estradiol valerate (Deladumone), an estrogen • chlorotrianisene (Tace), an estrogen.	5. Pharmacologic suppression of lactation is effected by inhibition of prolactin secretion. *Note:* Bromocriptine may cause hypotension.
6. Additional individualized interventions: _____	6. Rationales: _____

Collaborative problem: *Breast engorgement in lactating patient related to milk production secondary to prolactin secretion*

GOAL: Minimize engorgement and facilitate milk production.

Interventions	Rationales
1. Assess the patient's breasts as for nonnursing patient.	1. The physiologic course, uninterrupted by mechanical or drug suppression, is the same. Engorgement is the harbinger of lactation and does not represent an aberration.
2. Provide pain-relief measures, including breast support, hot soaks, and analgesics.	2. Palliative measures that do not inhibit milk secretion may be necessary until symptoms subside.
3. Massage breasts, followed by manual milk expression or use of breast pump.	3. Mechanical expression may be necessary until symptoms abate.
4. Put infant to breast as soon as comfortable and empty breasts regularly.	4. Further engorgement is minimized and prolactin secretion is enhanced.
5. Additional individualized interventions: _____	5. Rationales: _____

Nursing diagnosis: *Knowledge deficit related to postpartum sexual activity*

GOAL: Facilitate learning through planned instruction on sexual matters.

Interventions	Rationales
1. Assess the patient's knowledge base. Allow patient to ask questions. Anticipate and prepare scenario for teaching. Perform teaching in a quiet area when patient is rested, relaxed, and free of pain.	1. Milieu facilitates rapport and learning.
2. Provide factual information on resumption of sexual activities, including the following: • Episiotomy is usually healed by 3rd postpartum week. Intercourse should not be resumed until the patient has been examined by the physician, usually 4 to 6 weeks postpartum. • Menses usually resume in nonnursing puerpera in 6 to 8 weeks.	2. Involution of the placental site is probably not complete until the 6th postpartum week. Intercourse before healing may lead to infection or pregnancy.

Interventions

3. Additional individualized interventions: _____

Rationales

3. Rationales: _____

ASSOCIATED PLANS AND APPENDICES
• Selected Daily Dietary Allowances—Maternal (Appendix 2)
• Aspects of Psychological Care—Maternal (Appendix 4)
• Selected Methods of Family Planning (Appendix 6)
• The Family and Home Assessment (Appendix 7)
• Parent Teaching Guides (Appendix 13)

ADDITIONAL NURSING DIAGNOSES
• Fear related to perceived inability to care for infant
• Ineffective individual coping related to hormonal processes and fatigue
• Ineffective thermoregulation related to postpartum chill secondary to postdelivery vasomotor response

POSTPARTUM

POSTPARTUM
Hemorrhage

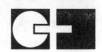

DEFINITION
Hemorrhage is blood loss of 500 ml or more after delivery. Excessive loss most commonly occurs in the early puerperium, usually within the first 24 hours, although hemorrhage may occur 4 to 6 weeks postpartum.

Management is ideally prophylactic and is directed at recognition and control of predisposing conditions, and scrupulous management of labor and delivery. Recognition and correction of hypovolemia is essential.

ETIOLOGY AND PRECIPITATING FACTORS
• Etiology: Early hemorrhage is associated with uterine overdistention and atony; lacerations, with or without hematoma formation; retained placental fragments; or hypofibrinogenemia. Late hemorrhage is associated with subinvolution, the retained products of conception, myomatas, or infection.
• Patient at risk: patient with history of postpartum uterine atony or hemorrhage, with overdistended uterus associated with hydramnios, with infant who is large for gestational age, or with multiple gestation; protracted labor or precipitate labor and delivery, high parity, prolonged relaxant anesthesia, placenta previa, abruptio placentae, medically complicated pregnancy, oxytocin augmentation or induction, or prolonged retention of a dead fetus after intrauterine death.

PHYSICAL FINDINGS
Cardiovascular
• hypotension
• tachycardia
• tachypnea
• pallor, cyanosis, and cold and clammy skin

Genitourinary
• Uterine atony
  □ soft, boggy uterus that does not or will not stay contracted
  □ bright red vaginal bleeding; amount varying from continual trickle to profuse
  □ passage or expression of multiple or large clots
  □ distended bladder
• Laceration
  □ continued bright red vaginal bleeding despite a well-contracted uterus; no clots passed
  □ possible visible tear of cervix, external genitalia, or anus
• Hematoma
  □ perineal, vaginal, urethral, bladder, or rectal pressure
  □ tense, severely painful vaginal protrusion
  □ ecchymotic perineum; purple cast to vaginal mucosa
  □ possible inability to void

• Hypofibrinogenemia
  □ multisite bleeding from any orifice or invasive site
  □ frank vaginal bleeding without clotting
• Retained placenta
  □ uterine tone dependent on amount of retention; may range from firm and contracted to somewhat boggy
  □ fragmented or missing cotyledons or membranes immediately after delivery
• Subinvolution (late hemorrhage, most commonly 4 to 6 weeks postpartum)
  □ fundal height greater than postpartum stage would warrant; poor uterine tone
  □ persistent or recurrent lochia; persistent lochial flow
  □ possible leukorrhea

Subjective
• pain with lacerations and hematoma
• apprehension, restlessness, and anxiety with hypovolemia

DIAGNOSTIC STUDIES
• Accurate and complete history and physical examination may furnish enough data for a definitive diagnosis of hypovolemia and may make diagnostic studies unnecessary.
• Ultrasonography may identify larger retained placental fragments.

Laboratory data
• Hemoglobin and hematocrit values—decrease.
• Coagulation factors—decreased fibrinogen and increased activated partial thromboplastin time.

Collaborative problem: *Fluid volume deficit related to blood loss secondary to uterine atony or to retained placental fragments or lacerations (2 goals)*

GOAL 1: Recognize signs of early uterine atony and of hemorrhage.

Interventions

1. Ascertain from delivery room personnel the following:
• outstanding medical and obstetric histories
• length and characteristics of labor
• type of delivery
• course and outcome of placental delivery
• postdelivery assessment, including estimated blood loss.

2. Perform postpartum assessment every 30 minutes for 1 hour, then every 4 hours and as patient condition warrants, noting the following:
• fundal height and tone
• amount and characteristics of vaginal discharge and bleeding
• signs of hematoma on perineum
• presence and number of clots
• presence of bladder distention.
Note pad count and weight. Save all clots and tissue passed.

3. Concurrently, monitor capillary refill time and vital signs and integrate with physical examination findings.

4. Note trends in hemoglobin and hematocrit values, compare with prenatal and intrapartum values, and integrate with estimated blood loss.

5. Monitor fluid intake and output every 8 hours; perform hourly in overt bleeding and constitutional signs of deterioration.

6. Additional individualized interventions: _____

Rationales

1. Information assists in identification of high-risk patient. Anticipated loss with vaginal birth is approximately 200 to 500 ml; with cesarean section birth, 700 to 1,000 ml.

2. Assessment provides database and facilitates early recognition of aberration. Pad count assists in estimation of blood loss and replacement needs. (*Note:* 1 ml of blood weighs 1 gram.) Identification of tissue samples may assist in medical diagnosis and thereby facilitate early treatment. A distended bladder prevents effective uterine contraction.

3. Increased capillary refill time and restlessness are indicators of early shock. Extensive blood loss may occur before the classic signs of hemorrhage (hypotension, tachycardia, tachypnea, and pallor) occur.

4. A 500-ml blood loss is usually mirrored by a 4-point decrease in hematocrit value.

5. Fluid output reflects renal function; levels of 30 to 50 ml/hour are minimally adequate.

6. Rationales: _____

GOAL 2: Minimize further dysfunctional bleeding and restore normovolemia.

Interventions

1. Evaluate bladder for distention and catheterize if distended.

2. Gently massage the boggy uterus at fundus while supporting lower uterine segment.

3. Start an I.V. infusion of a balanced solution using a large-bore needle. Type and crossmatch for blood products.

4. If atony and hemorrhage are present, administer methylergonovine (Methergine) I.M. 0.2 mg to normotensive patient or 10 to 40 units of oxytocin I.V. in 1,000 ml of a physiologic electrolyte solution. Note uterine tone. Monitor blood pressure carefully.

Rationales

1. Distended bladder displaces uterus and prevents uterine contraction.

2. Gentle massage stimulates uterine contraction, and assists in expulsion of retained placental fragments and in restoration of uterine tone. Aggressive or forceful manipulation may tire the myometrium and result in further atony. Support minimizes the risk of uterine inversion.

3. The I.V. line provides venous access before peripheral vasoconstriction associated with shock occurs and an immediate infusion site for replacement of products.

4. Oxytocics stimulate uterine contractions and therefore control postpartum bleeding. Uterine hyperactivity may result with overdose.

POSTPARTUM

Interventions

5. After delivery, administer one of the following oral oxytocic agents to the normotensive patient:
• ergonovine (Ergotrate), 0.2 to 0.4 mg two to four times daily for 2 days
• methylergonovine, 0.2 mg three or four times daily for up to 7 days.

6. Administer whole blood, plasma, or platelets.

7. Prepare patient for surgery for diagnosed lacerations, hematoma, or retained placenta.

8. Additional individualized interventions: _____

_____

Rationales

5. Oxytocics control atony and hemorrhage; if patient was hypertensive during pregnancy, ergonovine may be contraindicated.

6. Whole blood replaces actual losses and assists in restoring normovolemia. Plasma contains fibrinogen necessary to correct defects associated with disseminated intravascular coagulation. Platelets assist in coagulation to treat coagulopathies.

7. Lacerations require surgical ligations; larger hematomas require evacuation. Nonadherent, retained placenta, may require dilatation and curettage. Adherent, retained placenta (accreta) associated with profound blood loss may warrant hysterectomy.

8. Rationales: _____

_____

Collaborative problem: *High risk for genital infection related to bacterial contamination secondary to trauma and hemorrhage*

GOAL: Identify early signs of infection and intervene accordingly.

Interventions

1. Monitor for signs of infection, including the following:
• tender uterus
• chills and pyrexia
• change in lochial flow, purulent drainage, or odorous discharge
• pelvic or perineal discomfort disproportionate to type and course of delivery.
Correlate findings with intrapartum and immediate postpartum surveys.

2. Obtain sensitivity and culture on lochia or any discharge. Initiate antibiotic therapy.

3. Additional individualized interventions: _____

_____

Rationales

1. Assessment facilitates identification of high-risk patient and genesis of infection.

2. Culture and sensitivity identifies causative organism and sensitivity to various antibiotics. Cultures should be performed before administration of first dose because antibiotics may mask infection.

3. Rationales: _____

_____

ASSOCIATED PLANS AND APPENDICES
• Abruptio Placentae
• Inappropriate Size or Weight for Gestational Age, Large
• Multiple Gestation
• Placenta Previa
• Pregnancy Complicated by Diabetes Mellitus
• Puerperal Infection
• Puerperium
• Aspects of Psychological Care—Maternal (Appendix 4)

ADDITIONAL NURSING DIAGNOSES
• Altered peripheral tissue perfusion related to hypoxia secondary to blood loss
• Impaired tissue integrity related to perineal or genital lacerations

Puerperal Infection

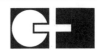

DEFINITION
Puerperal infection is postpartum infection of the genital tract. Although it may occur at any time in the puerperium, it usually occurs within 10 days after delivery. The infection may be local and involve the breasts as well as structures of delivery, including the external genitalia, vagina, uterus, and parametria; or it may progress via circulatory or lymphatic systems to pelvic cellulitis, septic thrombophlebitis, peritonitis, or bacterial shock. Aseptic technique and advances in technology have resulted in a decrease in incidence, but infection is still a leading cause of maternal morbidity. Management is ideally prophylactic, directed at early recognition of infection and prompt, aggressive antibiotic therapy. The differential diagnosis of pyrexia and careful assessment and physical examination are critical in ruling out other causes of infection, such as decreased respiratory function, pyelonephritis, thrombophlebitis, and wound infection.

ETIOLOGY AND PRECIPITATING FACTORS
• Etiology: Polymicrobial invasion by one or more of these organisms: anaerobic bacteria, including *Bacteroides, Peptostreptococcus* and *Peptococcus,* and *Clostridium;* and aerobic bacteria, including *Escherichia coli,* beta-hemolytic streptococci, *Klebsiella, Proteus mirabilis, Pseudomonas, Staphylococcus aureus,* and *Neisseria gonorrhoeae.*
• Patient at risk: anemic or poorly nourished; antenatal coitus when or after membranes have ruptured; intrapartum invasive techniques, breaks in aseptic technique, improper perineal care; prolonged labor, especially with ruptured membranes; prolonged rupture of membranes; hemorrhage, especially if greater than 1,000 ml; operative delivery; manipulation; trauma.

PHYSICAL FINDINGS
• Localized infection of external genitalia (sutured laceration or episiotomy; infected trauma of perineum, vulva, vagina, cervix, or abdominal surgical wound)
 □ low-grade fever less than 101° F (38.3° C); possible chill, possible rapid onset of pyrexia
 □ localized pain; wound pain disproportionate to extent of repair
 □ edema, erythema, necrosis of wound edges; edges no longer approximated; sanguinopurulent or purulent discharge
 □ dysuria, with or without urine retention
• Mastitis
 □ severe breast engorgement
 □ chills, rapid temperature elevation to 101° F (38.3° C) and higher; constitutional symptoms
 □ hard, red, painful breast; possible purulent discharge from nipple

• Endometritis or metritis
 □ irregular fevers, varying from 101° to 103° F (38.3° to 39.4° C), and proportionate tachycardia
 □ soft, tender uterus larger than involutional stage would warrant; protracted afterpains
 □ profuse, foul-smelling, bloody, occasionally frothy lochia; and scant, odorless lochia in beta-hemolytic streptococcal infection
• Salpingitis or oophoritis
 □ pyrexia to 103° to 104° F (39.4° to 40° C)
 □ unilateral or bilateral and lower abdominal pain
• Parametritis or pelvic cellulitis
 □ persistent pyrexia (102° to 104° F [38.8° to 40° C]), chills, and constitutional symptoms
 □ frequent unilateral or bilateral abdominal tenderness; pain on pelvic examination associated with uterine movement, possibly preceded by signs and symptoms of endometritis
 □ possible uterine fixation and pelvic mass on vaginal examination
 □ possible abscess formation that, dependent on location, may be palpated vaginally, rectally, or abdominally; inguinal focal point under skin may cause edema, erythema, tenderness
• Thrombophlebitis
 □ pyrexia 4 to 10 days postpartum
 □ pain, erythema, and edema of affected leg
 □ pelvic, lower abdominal, or flank pain; chills and spiking fevers in pelvic thrombophlebitis; fever may spike to 105° F (40.5° C), then fall precipitously
 □ decreased ventilatory function if small pulmonary emboli ensue
• Peritonitis
 □ commonly preceded by signs and symptoms of endometritis
 □ marked pyrexia, tachycardia, rapid and shallow respirations; constitutional symptoms
 □ severe abdominal pain with rigidity
 □ abdominal distention with decreased bowel sounds; nausea and vomiting (often projectile and eventually containing feces), and diarrhea
 □ excessive thirst or brown tongue and foul breath
 □ anxious expression and restlessness

Collaborative problem: *High risk for postpartum infection related to the trauma of labor, delivery, and self-inoculation, and iatrogenic introduction of pathogens (2 goals)*

GOAL 1: Prevent or minimize infection.

Interventions

1. Ascertain data from delivery room personnel, including:
• outstanding medical and obstetric histories
• course of labor and delivery and recovery time
• estimated blood loss
• anesthesia, drugs, and parenteral fluids administered.

2. Inspect perineum using good lighting. Note color, integrity of perineum, episiotomy characteristics and color, approximation of edges, and possible discharge or pain.

3. Assess fundal height and tone. Massage boggy uterus.

4. Assess lochia for type, amount, odor, and characteristics. Correlate with postpartum data.

5. Assess breast for erythema, pain, engorgement, and nipple discharge. Correlate with normal postpartum changes and note whether patient is breast-feeding.

6. Monitor vital signs, especially temperature, every 4 hours and as patient condition warrants. Note pyrexia trends (temperatures in excess of 100.4° F [38° C] on any 2 of the first 10 days postpartum, exclusive of the first 24 hours, to be taken by mouth by a standard technique at least four times daily [Joint Committee on Maternal Welfare]).

7. Note white blood cell count and integrate data into complete clinical profile.

8. Perform perineal care and hygienic measures. Enforce hand washing by patient and caregiver. Perform perineal cleaning and frequent pad changes, provide a heat lamp, and apply antibiotic creams.

9. Monitor fluid intake and output and encourage fluid intake.

10. Assist patient in selection of a balanced diet; encourage intake of protein, vitamin C, and iron.

11. Assess lung sounds, respiratory rate, and effort. Assist patient with pulmonary hygiene, including coughing and deep breathing every 4 hours.

12. Assess calves bilaterally for color, size, temperature, Homans' sign, pain, pulses, and paresthesias. Assist with progressive ambulation. Encourage frequent position change in bed.

Rationales

1. Assessment identifies high-risk patient. All puerperal patients are at risk for infection because of their denuded placental attachment sites and thin, highly vascular decidua.

2. Careful inspection provides data base and assists in early identification of hematoma or inflammation and infection.

3. Assessment confirms normal involutional processes. Massage stimulates contractility and expulsion of placental fragments. Infection is commonly associated with subinvolution.

4. Assessment confirms normal involutional processes and facilitates early identification of infection.

5. Assessment assists in differentiating normal postpartum findings from breast infection.

6. Trend analysis in conjunction with physical examination assists in formulation of medical diagnosis.

7. Leukocytosis accompanies inflammation. However, normal postpartal levels are increased (15,000 to 30,000/mm^3) and diagnosis depends on complete integration of all pertinent suspect data.

8. These measures limit exposure to contaminants and facilitate healing.

9. Temperature increase may be a result of dehydration; fluid output reflects renal function.

10. Protein and vitamin C promote healing. Iron, whether from food sources or supplementation, may be necessary to correct anemia.

11. Pulmonary exercises facilitate oxygenation and prevent pooling or accumulation of secretions, minimizing risk of atelectasis and pneumonia.

12. Activity provides data base which assists in identification of thrombophlebitis.

Interventions

13. Encourage rest and uninterrupted sleep. Coordinate assessments and procedures for this purpose.

14. Additional individualized interventions: _____

Rationales

13. Rest promotes a decreased metabolic rate which garners physiologic and emotional resources needed for healing.

14. Rationales: _____

GOAL 2: Identify early signs of infection and intervene accordingly.

Interventions

1. Note temperature trends. Monitor for infection (see discussion of physical findings on page 119).

2. Administer the following medications as indicated: after culture and sensitivity tests, antibiotics such as penicillin, gentamicin (Gentacidin), clindamycin (Cleocin), tetracycline (Sumycin), cefoxitin (Cefoxin), chloramphenicol (Chloromycetin), or metronidazole (Metizol); oxytocics, such as ergonovine (Ergotrate) and methylergonovine (Methergine).

3. Discontinue breast-feeding with a diagnosis of suppurative mastitis.

4. Closey monitor fluid input and output; administer I.V. fluids with electrolytes; withhold food and fluids if the patient has persistent vomiting or paralytic ileus.

5. Insert a nasogastric tube, monitor continuous nasogastric suction, and assess bowel sounds.

6. Additional individualized interventions: _____

Rationales

1. Compilation of data assists in early identification and treatment of infection.

2. Various antibiotic drugs are used either alone or in combination to combat and resolve infection, whereas oxytocics assist in stimulating uterine contractions and expulsion of retained placental fragments.

3. With suppurative mastitis, breast milk becomes infected: The suckling infant's nose and throat usually harbor the organism, most frequently *S. aureus,* that causes the infection and, possibly, reinfection.

4. Dehydration secondary to pyrexia, vomiting, or diarrhea and fluid retention associated with peritonitis deplete resources, that is, water and electrolytes.

5. Paralytic ileus associated with peritonitis warrants mechanical decompression. Restoration of bowel function is gauged by cessation of symptoms and ability to expel flatus.

6. Rationales: _____

Nursing diagnosis: *Pain related to inflammatory processes and exudate entrapment*

GOAL: Reduce or minimize pain.

Interventions

1. Establish rapport with patient and significant others. Call patient by preferred name.

2. Assess for pain and its characteristics, including quality, frequency, location, and intensity.

3. Minimize distracting environmental stimuli.

4. Perform comfort measures, including position changes, relaxation techniques, rubdowns, and pharmacologic analgesia.

Rationales

1. A positive relationship facilitates trust and decreases anxiety; regressive behaviors, anger, resistance, and noncompliance may, thereby, decrease.

2. Pain profile may assist in formulation of medical diagnosis.

3. External stimuli may tend to increase perception of pain. Unwarranted interruptions of rest periods sap patient's emotional reserve.

4. Increased tissue perfusion and stimulation of large afferent, sensory fibers decrease sensation or perception of pain. Pharmacologic analgesia provides central control of pain.

POSTPARTUM

Interventions	Rationales
5. Additional individualized interventions: _____	5. Rationales: _____
_____	_____

ASSOCIATED PLANS AND APPENDICES
• Cesarean Section Birth
• Hemorrhage
• Normal Antepartum
• Premature Rupture of Membranes
• Puerperium
• Aspects of Psychological Care—Maternal (Appendix 4)

ADDITIONAL NURSING DIAGNOSES
• Fluid volume deficit related to dehydration secondary to pyrexia, decreased fluid intake, and emesis
• High risk for altered body temperature related to bacterial contamination and pathogenic invasion of genital tract
• Knowledge deficit related to source of infection, its course, outcome, and implications for the infant

POSTPARTUM
Thromboembolic Disease

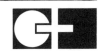

DEFINITION
Thromboembolic disease is a complication of the puerperium and includes deep-vein thrombosis (DVT) in the forms of thrombophlebitis and phlebothrombosis. Thrombophlebitis is thrombus or clot formation that is preceded by vein inflammation. It has been suggested that the inflammatory process more firmly attaches the thrombus to the vein, minimizing the opportunity for dislodgment and embolism. Phlebothrombosis is clot formation in the absence of inflammation. The possibility of dislodgment and subsequent pulmonary emboli is presumably more prevalent. All thrombi have the potential for dislodgment and sequelae of embolism.

Venous stasis is a major factor in thrombosis formation. Predominant sites of thrombi formation include legs, thighs, and pelvis. Management is directed primarily at prophylaxis and at early recognition of symptoms, prevention of further complications, and pain relief.

ETIOLOGY AND PRECIPITATING FACTORS
• Patient at risk: history of oral contraceptive use and of previous venous thrombosis; obesity; use of estrogens for lactation suppression; prolonged inactivity or sitting during pregnancy.

PHYSICAL FINDINGS
Cardiovascular
• DVT
  □ initial low-grade fever followed by pyrexia and chills; tachycardia
  □ marked pain and edema of affected extremity, more frequently left leg; abrupt in onset
  □ possible increased warmth of extremity or positive Homans' sign
• Superficial thrombophlebitis
  □ slight temperature elevation; possible normal temperature
  □ slight increase in pulse
  □ heat, redness, and tenderness at affected site

Subjective
• calf pain

DIAGNOSTIC STUDIES
• Accurate and complete history and physical examination may furnish enough data for a definitive diagnosis, possibly rendering diagnostic studies unnecessary.
• Doppler ultrasonography detects reduced or obstructed venous blood flow.
• Impedance plethysmography identifies amount of blood passing through affected vessel.
• Phlebography confirms thrombus and impeded venous flow.

Collaborative problem: *Altered peripheral tissue perfusion related to venous stasis (2 goals)*

GOAL 1: Identify early signs of peripheral dysfunction.

Interventions

1. Ascertain from delivery room personnel the patient's outstanding medical and obstetric histories; type, time, and length of delivery; anesthesia administered; and postdelivery reaction time.

2. Assess calves and thighs bilaterally for size, color, temperature, peripheral pulses, pain, paresthesia, paralysis, and Homans' sign.

3. Monitor vital signs, especially temperature.

4. Monitor for and refer to physician the signs of superficial venous thrombosis.

Rationales

1. Information assists in identification of high-risk patients: those with history of varicosities or thromboses, prolonged immobility associated with surgical delivery or with lithotomy position, and protracted anesthesia recovery time.

2. Assessment provides data base and facilitates early recognition of dysfunction.

3. Persistent low-grade fever may indicate inflammation.

4. Superficial venous thrombosis is considered less serious, because the possibility of embolism is low.

Interventions

5. Monitor for and refer immediately to physician signs of DVT, including:
• sudden onset of severe leg or thigh pain accompanied by edema
• possible positive Homans' sign
• increases in temperature and pulse, and chills.

6. Additional individualized interventions: _____

Rationales

5. Phlegmasia alba dolens, or "milk leg," is a serious postpartum complication that usually involves the deep venous system from groin to foot and has a real potential for generating life-threatening emboli.

6. Rationales: _____

GOAL 2: Maintain and improve peripheral circulation.

Interventions

1. Maintain bed rest. Fully elevate affected leg on pillow. Avoid compression on popliteal space.

2. Do not gatch bed.

3. Apply warm packs to affected leg; remove for 10 minutes every hour.

4. Administer broad-spectrum antibiotics if fever is present.

5. Administer heparin, 5,000 to 7,500 units S.C. every 4 to 6 hours or by continuous I.V. drip 1 unit/ml of estimated blood volume. Dosage depends on activated partial thromboplastin time (APTT).

6. After acute inflammation has subsided, ambulate progressively. Apply fitted elastic support hose.

7. Additional individualized interventions: _____

Rationales

1. Bed rest minimizes pressure on peripheral venous system. Elevation facilitates blood flow back to the heart.

2. Positioning may impede peripheral flow or cause pelvic pooling, thereby compromising an already weakened system.

3. Resulting vasodilation facilitates blood flow. Pain will decrease, although analgesics may also be indicated.

4. Fever indicates inflammation or infection.

5. An anticoagulant, heparin prevents further thrombus formation. APTT 1½ to 2½ times the control in seconds is consistent with effective anticoagulant effect.

6. The support hose compress superficial veins and facilitate deep venous flow.

7. Rationales: _____

Nursing diagnosis: *Altered cardiopulmonary tissue perfusion related to pulmonary embolism secondary to dislodgment of deep-vein thrombus*

GOAL: Identify early signs of cardiopulmonary dysfunction and intervene accordingly.

Interventions

1. Monitor and report immediately signs of impaired cardiopulmonary status, including:
• any nonspecific alteration after an uncomplicated postpartum course, such as vague chest pain, anxiety, or apprehension
• respiratory rate greater than 16 breaths/minute
• chest pain, shortness of breath, tachypnea, restlessness, pallor, or diaphoresis
• possible crackles, friction rub, or increased jugular pressure.

2. Additional individualized interventions: _____

Rationales

1. Anticoagulant pharmacotherapy is indicated in suspected or confirmed embolism to minimize risk of further and possibly fatal thrombus formation. Whereas the classic symptoms of pleuritic pain, hemoptysis, and dyspnea are infrequently presented clinically, increased respirations are the most common and telling signs of embolism.

2. Rationales: _____

Nursing diagnosis: *High risk for fluid volume deficit related to blood loss secondary to overheparinization*

GOAL: Identify signs of bleeding and intervene accordingly.

Interventions	**Rationales**
1. Monitor APTT and hematocrit (HCT) value.	1. APTT is the most accurate indicator of effective heparinization. Decreasing HCT values are consistent with blood loss.
2. Monitor for signs of bleeding, including epistaxis; hematemesis; dark, tarry stools; hematuria; ecchymosis; petechiae; prolonged bleeding from sites of invasive procedures; or oozing or bleeding from any orifice.	2. Small bleeds usually precede frank bleeding.
3. Have protamine sulfate 1% on hand.	3. Protamine sulfate inactivates heparin.
4. Additional individualized interventions: _____	4. Rationales: _____

ASSOCIATED PLANS AND APPENDICES
• Normal Antepartum
• Puerperium
• Aspects of Psychological Care—Maternal (Appendix 4)

ADDITIONAL NURSING DIAGNOSES
• High risk for trauma related to prolonged standing and sitting secondary to compromised peripheral vasculature
• Impaired gas exchange related to obstructed pulmonary tree secondary to emboli
• Knowledge deficit related to heparin or warfarin use, indications, adverse effects, and interactions

POSTPARTUM

SECTION IV
NEWBORN INFANT ASSESSMENT GUIDES

Ballard Gestational-Age Assessment Tool   **127**
Newborn Infant Postdelivery Assessment   **128**
Major Neonatal Reflexes   **129**
Newborn Infant Nursery Assessment   **130**

Ballard Gestational-Age Assessment Tool

To use this tool, the examiner evaluates and scores the neuromuscular and physical maturity criteria, totals the scores, and then plots the sum in the maturity rating box to determine gestational age.

	−1	0	1	2	3	4	5

NEUROMUSCULAR MATURITY

	−1	0	1	2	3	4	5
Posture	−						−
Square window (wrist)	>90°	90°	60°	45°	30°	0°	−
Arm recoil	−	180°	140° to 180°	110° to 140°	90° to 110°	<90°	
Popliteal angle	180°	160°	140°	120°	100°	90°	<90°
Scarf sign							−
Heel to ear							−

PHYSICAL MATURITY

	−1	0	1	2	3	4	5
Skin	Sticky, friable, transparent	Gelatinous, red, translucent	Smooth, pink; visible vessels	Superficial peeling or rash; few visible vessels	Cracking; pale areas; rare visible vessels	Parchment-like; deep cracking; no visible vessels	Leathery, cracked, wrinkled
Lanugo	None	Sparse	Abundant	Thinning	Bald areas	Mostly bald	−
Plantar surface	Heel-toe 40 to 50 mm: −1; <40 mm: −2	>50 mm; no crease	Faint red marks	Anterior transverse crease only	Creases over anterior two-thirds	Creases over entire sole	−
Breast	Imperceptible	Barely perceptible	Flat areola, no bud	Stippled areola; 1- to 2-mm bud	Raised areola; 3- to 4-mm bud	Full areola; 5- to 10-mm bud	−
Eye and ear	Lids fused, loosely: −1; tightly: −2	Lids open; pinna flat, stays folded	Slightly curved pinna; soft, slow recoil	Well-curved pinna; soft, ready recoil	Formed and firm; instant recoil	Thick cartilage; ear stiff	−
Genitalia, male	Scrotum flat, smooth	Scrotum empty; faint rugae	Testes in upper canal; rare rugae	Testes descending; few rugae	Testes down; good rugae	Testes pendulous; deep rugae	−
Genitalia, female	Clitoris prominent; labia flat	Prominent clitoris; small labia minora	Prominent clitoris; enlarging minora	Majora and minora equally prominent	Majora large; minora small	Majora cover clitoris and minora	−

MATURITY RATING

Score	−10	−5	0	5	10	15	20	25	30	35	40	45	50
Weeks	20	22	24	26	28	30	32	34	36	38	40	42	44

Adapted from Ballard, J.L., Khoury, J.C., Wedig, K. et al. (1991). New Ballard Score, expanded to include extremely premature infants. *Journal of Pediatrics*, 119(3), 417-423. Used with permission from Mosby, Inc.

NEWBORN INFANT ASSESSMENT GUIDES

Newborn Infant Postdelivery Assessment

The Apgar scoring system, shown here, provides a way to immediately evaluate an infant's cardiopulmonary and neurologic status. The assessment is performed at 1 and 5 minutes after birth and repeated every 5 minutes until the infant stabilizes.

APGAR SCORING SYSTEM

Sign	0	1	2
Heart rate	Absent	Slow (below 100 beats/minute)	Over 100 beats/minute
Respiratory effort	Absent	Slow or irregular	Good cry
Muscle tone	Flaccid; limp	Some flexion of arms and legs	Active motion with flexion
Reflex irritability: Response to catheter in nostril (tested before oropharynx is clear) or to slapping on soles of feet	No response	Grimace; some motion	Cough, sneeze, or cry
Color	Blue or pale	Body pink; arms and legs pale or blue	Completely pink

Totals indicate:
0 to 3—Severe distress
4 to 6—Moderate difficulty
7 to 10—No difficulty

The initial assessment

Concomitantly, as you measure the Apgar score, make sure the infant has a patent airway and no obvious problems. Make the following assessments (which may vary from hospital to hospital). To prevent heat loss in the infant, perform the assessment with speed and accuracy. (See *Newborn Infant Nursery Assessment*, page 130, for normal findings.)
• UMBILICAL CORD—Presence on cut surface of two arteries and one vein: the arteries are smaller-lumened, papular structures; the vein is larger with a thinner vessel wall. Note length and time of delivery and umbilical cord clamping.
GENERAL APPRAISAL—Total appearance, state of maturity, size and relation of body parts, presence of congenital anomalies or birth trauma, and spontaneity of movement.
• CRY—Quality.
• SKIN—Color and condition.
• TEMPERATURE—First, take rectal temperature to rule out imperforate anus; afterward, take axillary temperatures.
• LENGTH
• WEIGHT
• ABDOMEN—Palpate for masses. If necessary, pass gastric tube through mouth to rule out esophageal atresia. Aspirate stomach contents to rule out high intestinal obstruction.
• RESPIRATIONS—Observe whether infant can breath with closed mouth to rule out choanal atresia.
• MOUTH—Palpate integrity of palate to rule out cleft palate.

Major Neonatal Reflexes

This chart summarizes the neonatal reflexes that exist at birth or shortly thereafter. Some reflexes, such as the pupillary and blink reflexes, persist throughout life. Others, including the Babinski, doll's eye, grasp, Moro, sucking, tonic neck, and trunk incurvation reflexes, disappear within a few weeks or months after birth.

Reflex	How to Elicit	Normal Response
Babinski	Lightly stroke one side of neonate's foot upward from heel and across ball of foot.	Toes fan; great toe dorsiflexes.
Blink (corneal)	Momentarily shine bright light directly into neonate's eyes.	Neonate blinks.
Crossed extension	With neonate supine, extend one leg and stimulate sole with light pin prick or finger flick.	Neonate swiftly flexes and extends opposite leg as if trying to push stimulus away from other foot.
Doll's eye	With neonate supine, slowly turn neonate's head to left or right.	Eyes remain stationary.
Grasp □ Palmar □ Plantar	Press finger against neonate's palm. Press object against ball of neonate's foot.	Fingers momentarily close around object. Toes curl downward and around object.
Moro (startle)	Make loud noise or suddenly disturb neonate's equilibrium.	Neonate stiffens and then briskly abducts and extends arm with hands open and fingers extended in "C" shape. Legs flex and abduct, and arms return to embracing posture. Crying is usual.
Placing	Hold neonate so that top of foot or anterior portion of lower leg lightly touches underside of flat surface.	Hips and knees flex; foot rises onto surface.
Pupillary	Darken room and shine penlight directly into each eye for several seconds.	Pupils constrict equally bilaterally.
Rooting	Touch finger to neonate's cheek or to corner of mouth.	Neonate turns head toward stimulus, opens mouth, and searches for stimulus.
Stepping	Hold neonate so that sole touches flat surface. (Test this reflex when testing placing reflex.)	Neonate makes walking or stepping motion.
Sucking	Place finger (or nipple) in neonate's mouth.	Neonate sucks on finger (or nipple) forcefully and rhythmically.
Tonic neck (fencing)	With neonate supine, turn head over shoulder to one side.	Arm and leg partially or completely extend on side to which head is turned; opposite arm and leg flex.
Trunk incurvation (Galant)	With neonate prone, stroke one side of spine about 1 cm (½") from midline.	Trunk curves to stimulated side; shoulders and pelvis move in same direction.

Newborn Infant Nursery Assessment

Assessment determines the infant's initial condition, establishes a baseline for subsequent care, and identifies potential and existing problems. The physical assessment usually is completed within the infant's first 24 hours.

PHYSICAL ASSESSMENT
Conduct the assessment in a well-lighted, warm, draft-free room. For the general survey and measuring and weighing, undress the infant completely, but leave a diaper over the infant's genital area to avoid soiling. (Remove the diaper to weigh the infant and to assess the hips, lower spine, genitals, and rectum.) Although any organized, consistent, and complete assessment method is satisfactory, the most common way to proceed is from head to toe (cephalocaudal), assessing vital signs, auscultating the heart, lungs, and abdomen, and then palpating the abdomen. These assessments are performed when the infant is quiet. Continue the general survey by assessing the infant's color, size, proportion, symmetry, nutritional status, posture, positioning, activity, reflexes (see *Major Neonatal Reflexes,* page 129), and behavior. Note gross abnormalities and disproportionate sizes. Assess hip abduction last because it frequently evokes infant crying. The infant features described below are common findings for the full-term normal neonate.

INITIAL SIZE AND VITAL SIGNS

Size includes length and weight. Vital signs include temperature, heart rate, and respiratory rate (see Appendix 9: Assessing Vital Signs in the Infant for more information). Average ranges follow:

Length
   crown to rump: 12″ to 14″
   (approximately 31 to 35 cm)
   head to heel: 19″ to 21″ (approximately 48 to 53 cm)
Weight: 5 lb, 5 oz to 8 lb, 13 oz (2,500 to 4,000 g)
Temperature
   axillary (skin): 97.7° to 98.6° F (36.5° to 37° C)
   rectal (core): 96° to 99.5° F (35.5° to 37.5° C)
Heart rate: 110 to 160 beats/minute
Respiratory rate: 40 to 60 breaths/minute

Skin
The skin appears soft, with desquamation by the 2nd to 3rd day, smooth, nearly transparent, elastic, ruddy to pale pink. The nail beds and scrotum are more deeply pigmented in black infants, with possible mongolian spots in darker-skinned infants. Physiologic jaundice commonly appears after the first 24 hours. The neonate has lanugo, especially over the shoulders and back, and vernix caseosa, especially under fingernails and in labial folds. Skin may show transient harlequin-like color change, mottling with stress, acrocyanosis, milia, miliaria rubra, erythema toxicum, and telangiectatic nevi. Nails are formed and firm.

Head
About one-fourth the body length, the head measures about 13″ to 15″ about (33 to 37 cm) in circumference. The head is flexed onto the chest. The smooth skull, with flat, soft but firm fontanels, may be asymmetric from uterine position, molding during birth, or positional compression. The anterior diamond-shaped fontanel measures about 1″ to 2½″ (3 to 6 cm) at its widest diameter; the smaller posterior diamond-shaped fontanel measures about ½″ to 1″ (1 to 2 cm). Skull sutures feel like ridges. A 2-cm illumination ring is apparent during transillumination of the frontoparietal skull, 1 cm over the occiput.

Neck
Short and supple, the infant's neck is also mobile, with tonic neck, neck righting, and otolith righting reflexes. The prone infant can hold the neck in line with the back and turn the head from side to side. The infant in a sitting position shows momentary ability to hold head erect.

Eyes
Usually tightly closed and frequently with edema of the eyelids, the infant's eyes are slate gray, dark blue-gray, or brown. The infant has a tearless cry. Transient strabismus may be evident. The pupils, usually equal, are round, with direct and consensual constriction in response to light. Reflexes include the red reflex and the optical blink reflex. Doll's eye fixation is also evident.

Ears
The ear canal is patent. Tops of the firm, elastic pinna parallel the eye's inner and outer canthi. Earlobes may have preauricular tags. The infant responds to loud sound with the startle (acoustic blink) reflex.

Nose and throat
Broad and patent, the nostrils may contain a mucous discharge. The infant is an obligate nasal breather, can sneeze, and can cry lustily. The tongue lies midline in the mouth; the palate is intact; the infant is edentulous with minimal salivation. Rooting, sucking, swallowing, yawn, and gag reflexes are present.

Chest and lungs

The circumference of the rounded chest measures about 12″ to 13″ (30.5 to 33 cm). Anteroposterior and lateral diameters are equal. The xiphoid tip protrudes anteriorly at the apex of the costal angle. The infant has chiefly abdominal respirations (about 40 to 60 breaths/minute), intermittently slow and shallow, or deep and rapid, with apneic episodes lasting 6 to 15 seconds. Breath sounds are bilaterally clear, loud, bronchovesicular, and hyperresonant. Breath sounds commonly are diminished on the chest side opposite the head's direction, and fine crackles may be heard at the end of inspiration. Possibly enlarged, the breasts may secrete milky fluid.

Heart

Following respiratory trends, the heartbeat (110 to 160 beats/minute) sounds clear and regular and frequently is labile. The point of maximal intensity may be seen at the fourth intercostal space left of the midclavicular line. S_1 is louder than S_2 at the apex and S_2 is louder than in the pulmonic area. S_2 splitting is common; innocent systolic murmurs may be evident.

Abdomen

Soft, cylindrical, and protruding, the abdomen may show a superficial venous pattern. The umbilical stump is drying and darkening. The following can be palpated; the liver (soft with a smooth edge) about 1 to 2 cm below the right costal margin; the spleen tip along the lateral aspect of the left upper quadrant; kidneys, on deep palpation, with lower poles about 1 to 2 cm above the umbilius. Urine, if apparent, is clear; bowel sounds are present; and regurgitation may accompany feedings. Femoral pulses are equal. The crawling reflex is present.

Male genitalia

The penis is straight. Foreskin covers and adheres to glans penis, which has a midline urethral opening at the tip. Testes in the edematous scrotum (or in the inguinal canal from which they can be milked) measure about 1 cm.

Female genitalia

The labia majora covers the labia minora. The clitoris appears large. The infant may have a mucoid, occasionally blood-tinged vaginal discharge. The urethra is located anterior to the vaginal orifice.

Rectum

The infant has a patent anus. There is passage of meconium plug or meconium. The anal reflex is evident. Perianal skin tags may be present.

Arms and legs

Arms and legs are straight and symmetric in size, shape, and position. The body is flexed and the hands are clenched. No simian crease is present in the palms. Plantar creases cover the soles. The hips are stable and do not dislocate. Ortolani's maneuver and Barlow's sign are negative. The infant has good muscle tone, especially with resistance to opposing flexion, and full range of motion in each major joint. Hands have 10 fingers; feet have 10 toes. Hands and feet may show some edema. Feet are flat with creased soles. Deep tendon and plantar reflexes are highly variable. Brachial and radial pulses are strong and equal bilaterally. Femoral pulses are strong and equal and regular bilaterally.

Back

The spinal column is straight. The buttocks have a symmetric midline crease.

BEHAVIORAL ASSESSMENT

The neonate moves successively through behavioral states, or degrees of alertness. Behavioral assessment evaluates the neonate's ability to react to and integrate various stimuli during these states.

The most commonly used behavioral evaluation tool is the Brazelton neonatal behavioral assessment scale (BNBAS), developed by pediatrician T. Berry Brazelton in 1973. This tool evaluates the neonate's behavioral state and behavioral responses.

For best results, behavioral assessment should be conducted in a quiet, softly lit setting. Findings should be interpreted in light of the period of reactivity and the neonate's gestational age.

Behavioral states

During *deep sleep*, the neonate makes few or no spontaneous movements; any movements that occur are brief and jerky. Respirations are even and regular. No rapid eye movements (REMs) occur. The neonate can be aroused from this state only for a few moments at a time.

During *light sleep*, the neonate can be easily aroused and brought to wakefulness; REMs can be detected. The neonate may move the arms and legs occasionally; movements are smoother than during deep sleep. Breathing patterns vary as the neonate drifts from light sleep to drowsiness.

During the *drowsy state*, the neonate tries to become fully alert, moves more frequently and regularly, and opens the eyes periodically. Responses to auditory and tactile stimuli are sluggish.

During the *alert state*, the neonate seems to be transfixed by external stimuli.

During the *active state*, the neonate responds to external stimuli with regular eye and body movements.

During the *crying state*, the neonate responds to both internal and external stimuli, cries vigorously and without interruption, and makes thrusting movements.

Behavioral responses

The neonate's behavioral responses fall into six basic categories: habituation, orientation, motor maturity, variations, self-quieting ability, and social behaviors. The chart below describes these responses.

Neonatal Behavioral Responses

Behavioral response	Description	When to assess
Habituation	Process of becoming accustomed to environmental stimuli, such as light and noise	During deep sleep, light sleep, or drowsy state
Orientation	Responsiveness to visual and auditory stimuli. Normally, neonate moves both head and eyes when orienting to visual or auditory stimulus. Nystagmus and gaze aversion after direct eye contact are normal. Neonate typically stops activity in response to auditory stimulus; sudden or loud stimulus usually causes crying.	During alert or active state
Motor maturity	Posture, muscle tone, muscle coordination, and movements. These should all be within normal parameters; arm and leg movements should be smooth, symmetric, and equal. However, motor responses may vary greatly during first 24 hours after birth.	During alert state
Variations	Frequency of changes in activity level, behavioral state, and skin color	During each behavioral state
Self-quieting ability	Promptness and effectiveness with which neonate self-quiets when crying. Self-quieting behaviors include moving hands toward mouth, sucking on fist, changing position, and responding to auditory or visual stimuli when crying.	During crying state
Social behaviors	Reflexive cuddling, smiling, and other behaviors, such as crying to be fed followed by stopping sucking after hunger has been sated	During alert or active state

SECTION V
INFANT

Acquired Immunodeficiency Syndrome — Infant **134**

Air Leak Syndromes **139**

Anemia **142**

Birth Trauma **146**

Bowel Obstruction, Small or Large **150**

Bronchopulmonary Dysplasia **154**

Choanal Atresia **158**

Circumcision **160**

Cleft Lip and Cleft Palate **164**

Congenital Heart Disease **170**

Congestive Heart Failure **177**

Drug Addiction and Withdrawal **183**

Fetal Alcohol Syndrome **190**

Full-term Infant, 38 to 42 weeks **194**

Hip Dysplasia **201**

Hyaline Membrane Disease — Respiratory
Distress Syndrome (RDS I) **205**

Hyperbilirubinemia **213**

Hypocalcemia **221**

Hypoglycemia **225**

Hypothermia and Hyperthermia **229**

Inappropriate Size or Weight for Gestational
Age, Large **235**

Inappropriate Size or Weight for Gestational
Age, Small **239**

Intracranial Hemorrhage **243**

Meconium Aspiration Syndrome **247**

Necrotizing Enterocolitis **251**

Postoperative Care **257**

Preoperative Care **263**

Preterm Infant, Less Than 37 Weeks **268**

Sepsis Neonatorum and Infectious Disorders **276**

Skin Disorders **283**

Spinal Cord Defects and Hydrocephalus **287**

Talipes Deformity **293**

Tracheoesophageal Fistula or Esophageal
Atresia **297**

Transient Tachypnea (RDS II) **303**

Acquired Immunodeficiency Syndrome — Infant

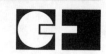

DEFINITION

Acquired immunodeficiency syndrome (AIDS) represents end-stage infection with the human immunodeficiency virus (HIV). It is characterized by T cell-mediated immune deficiency that is unexplained by congenital conditions or drug suppression. Because of profound immunosuppression, people with AIDS develop opportunistic infections from bacteria, fungi, protozoa, and viruses. See Appendix 13: 1993 CDC Revised Classification System for HIV Infection/AIDS Surveillance Case Definition for a diagnostic composite and the inclusive surveillance case definition for AIDS.

No other definition of AIDS has been developed for infants and children, and the classification system and surveillance definition may not apply. For this reason, two definitions have emerged: one for infants and children up to age 15 months who have been exposed to their infected mothers perinatally and the other for older children with perinatal infection and for infants and children who have acquired the virus through other means. AIDS in infants and children younger than 15 months who have perinatal infection and who were exposed to infected mothers in the perinatal period is defined by one or more of the following criteria:
• identification of HIV in the blood or tissues
• presence of HIV antibody (confirmed by repeatedly reactive screening test plus a positive Western blot analysis) and evidence of both cellular and humoral immune deficiency and a symptomatic infection
• signs and symptoms coinciding with those contained in Appendix 13.

This plan focuses on identifying infants at risk for HIV infection and on preventing HIV transmission to health care personnel and others who care for infants in the nursery. The maternal AIDS plan (see page 24) has prerequisite information and should be used with this plan.

Data included in the definition and plan are adapted from the Centers for Disease Control, "1993 Revised Classification System for HIV Infection and Expanded Case Definition for AIDS Among Adolescents and Adults," *Morbidity and Mortality Weekly Report,* December 18, 1992.

ETIOLOGY AND PRECIPITATING FACTORS
• presence of HIV, a retrovirus
• infant born to an HIV-seropositive mother (via perinatal transmission)
• infant receiving HIV-seropositive blood transfusion

PHYSICAL FINDINGS
Maternal history
• drug abuse or needle sharing
• sexual partner or partners with a positive HIV antibody test or AIDS-positive HIV, enzyme-linked immunosorbent assay (ELISA), and Western blot test as confirmation

Infant status at birth
• no obvious disease signs (HIV testing is not routinely performed unless the mother's blood is known to be seropositive)
• highly variable findings and symptoms, depending on the type of infection

BEHAVIORAL FINDINGS
• failure to achieve developmental milestones
• failure to thrive

DIAGNOSTIC STUDIES
Laboratory data
• ELISA—to detect HIV antibody, although seroconversion may take up to 6 months; in the neonate, HIV antibodies may appear from maternal infection, reflecting the placental transfer of maternal antibody.
• Western blot test—to confirm positive ELISA
• immunoglobulin level (antibody [IgM, IgA] detection—to identify antibodies that do not readily cross the placenta
• p24 HIV antigen testing—to identify the presence of antigen
• CD4 count—to help quantify the progression of HIV disease
• blood and tissue cultures—to identify HIV

Collaborative problem: *High risk for infection related to perinatal transmission of HIV and immunosuppression (3 goals)*

GOAL 1: Identify the infant at risk for HIV infection.

Interventions

1. Assess the infant's potential for developing HIV infection, including:

• maternal history of drug abuse, needle sharing, sexual partners with AIDS, positive HIV antibody test, or two positive ELISA tests on the same sample
• HIV antibody in the infant's blood or tissue

• tissue and blood cultures to identify infection with or without symptoms as well as abnormal immunoglobulin levels, CD4 and CD4:CD8 ratio, p24 antigen levels, and absolute cell count
• breast-feeding, if the mother is seropositive.

2. Additional individualized interventions: _____

Rationales

1. Assessment helps to identify the high-risk population and the infant's potential exposure and plan appropriate measures.
• Mother with this history is at high risk for developing AIDS and could transmit the disease to the infant.

• Early testing of the infant may reflect placental transfer of maternal antibody or infection, with the HIV antibody persisting for as long as 15 months.
• Testing reveals humoral and cellular immunodeficiency.

• Breast milk is thought to transmit the HIV antibody.

2. Rationales: _____

GOAL 2: Identify HIV-related illnesses in the perinatally exposed or seropositive infant.

Interventions

1. Assess the infant for signs that indicate infection, such as:
• failure to thrive
• weight loss over 10% at time symptoms appear
• elevated temperature
• diarrheal episodes (more than three times daily)
• lymph nodes measuring 0.5 cm (about ¼") at two or more sites
• hepatomegaly and splenomegaly
• rash.

2. Assess the infant for:
• cytomegalovirus disease
• herpes simplex virus infection with ulcer lasting longer more than 1 month
• lymphoid interstitial pneumonia
• toxoplasmosis of the brain
• HIV dementia
• HIV wasting syndrome
• bacterial sepsis
• coccidioidomycosis and histoplasmosis (disseminated)
• lymphoma
• other viral, fungal, or protozoal infections.

3. Additional individualized interventions: _____

Rationales

1. Infants may have signs and symptoms that persist for more than 1 month before a definitive AIDS diagnosis is made. In infants, signs and symptoms usually involve multiple organ systems and seldom occur as single entities.

2. Opportunistic infections occur because of a compromised and suppressed immune system.

3. Rationales: _____

GOAL 3: Minimize the effect of the infectious process.

Interventions	**Rationales**
1. Provide supportive care and treatment of potential and existing infections by preparing and administering anti-infective therapy.	1. This specific therapy treats opportunistic infections. Drugs of choice include penicillin G (Wycillin), ampicillin (Omnipen), methicillin (Staphcillin), carbenicillin (Geopen), cephalothin (Keflin), kanamycin (Kantrex), gentamicin (Garamycin), amikacin (Amikin), streptomycin, neomycin (Mycifradin), tobramycin (Kantrex), and amphotericin B (Fungizone).
2. Screen visitors for viral or other infections.	2. Because of immunosuppression, the infant is predisposed to infection from others.
3. Follow Centers for Disease Control and Prevention (CDC) recommendations for minimizing the risk of HIV transmission.	3. CDC studies show that these measures help to reduce HIV transmission.
4. Additional individualized interventions: _____	4. Rationales: _____

Nursing diagnosis: *High risk for injury related to transmission of HIV to personnel and other infants in the nursery*

GOAL: Prevent transmission of HIV by using universal precautions to protect caregivers and infants in nursery.

Interventions	**Rationales**
1. Wear gloves when examining or handling the potentially or known HIV-infected infant and when drawing blood or before potential contact with other body fluids, rashes, or skin breaks (for example, at I.V., catheter, dressing, or other exposure sites).	1. Gloves prevent the infant's body fluids from contact with skin breaks, which may permit transmission of the virus. *Note:* Neonates still have amniotic fluid and materials from the amniotic sac on their skin.
2. Wash hands with antiseptic solution before entering the nursery, before and after caring for the infant, and before and after touching contaminated articles.	2. Hands are considered contaminated unless washed properly.
3. Exclude the infant from the nursery, depending on whether the infant has enteritis, draining wounds, congenital syphilis, cytomegalovirus, herpes, rubella, or other viral infections. (Do not exclude the infant solely on the basis of HIV infection.)	3. Isolation of the infant with a positive culture for any infection helps to prevent transmission to other infants.
4. Wear a scrub or cover gown; change to a new gown for each infant.	4. A scrub gown permits easy handwashing. A new gown prevents cross-contamination.
5. Provide for proper disposal, decontamination, and sterilization of all equipment, supplies, or articles having infant contact (treat as hazardous waste), as follows: • Use disposable products if possible. • Dispose of used gowns, catheters, and other materials in clearly marked containers according to local, state, and federal regulations. • Follow standard sterilization, disinfection, cleaning, and housekeeping procedures according to hospital policy. • Double-bag nondisposable infectious material, using a water-soluble plastic inner liner, and color-code the bags.	5. Sequestering, disinfecting, and sterilizing infectious matter are methods of isolating and destroying the virus, helping to avoid self-inoculation as well as contamination of others and the environment.

Interventions

• Disinfect spills with a 1:10% solution of 5.25% sodium hypochlorite (household bleach) or approved chemical germicides.
• Clearly label laboratory specimens and secure in a plastic bag. Then notify the laboratory.

6. Follow the protocol in Appendix 14: CDC Guidelines for Preventing HIV Transmission in Health Care Settings.

7. Additional individualized interventions: _____

Rationales

6. These guidelines describe ways to prevent HIV transmission.

7. Rationales: _____

Nursing diagnosis: *Fear (parental) related to infant's future death as a result of HIV infection*

GOAL: Parents verbalize less fear.

Interventions

1. Assess level and cause of fear by:
• listening to expressions of fear
• determining what the parents know about AIDS
• observing nonverbal expressions of fear.

2. Provide information about AIDS based on what is known:
• cause of disease
• presence of HIV in infant
• possible implications of testing positive for HIV
• possible additional information and treatment as research efforts progress
• potential for positive future because disease may take 6 months or more to develop or may never develop
• importance of maintaining hope.

3. Maintain a calm, positive attitude when interacting with parents.

4. Encourage parents to use a support network, such as clergy, family, or others.

5. If the mother has AIDS or is positive for HIV, support her decision to seek abortion counseling (if she says she is considering this option) as well as counseling related to birth control and future pregnancies.

6. Refer the parents to community resources and home health care services.

7. Additional individualized interventions: _____

Rationales

1. Parents' fear level may increase with lack of information and distorted perceptions.

2. Increased knowledge will reduce anxiety and fear and give some reassurance that disease may not develop. Although AIDS currently results in death, research to develop effective identification, prevention, and treatment intensifies daily.

3. A calm, positive attitude conveys caring and concern.

4. A support system can help parents to cope with a potentially critically ill child.

5. Abortion is an option for pregnant women who test positive for HIV or who have AIDS.

6. These referrals provide parents and family with continued support before and after discharge.

7. Rationales: _____

ASSOCIATED PLANS AND APPENDICES
• Acquired Immunodeficiency Syndrome—Maternal
• Drug Addiction and Withdrawal
• Inappropriate Size or Weight for Gestational Age, Small
• Sepsis Neonatorum and Infectious Disorders
• 1993 CDC Revised Classificaton System for HIV Infection/AIDS Surveillance Case Definition (Appendix 13)
• CDC Guidelines for Preventing HIV Transmission in Health Care Settings (Appendix 14)

ADDITIONAL NURSING DIAGNOSES
• Altered nutrition: Less than body requirements related to immunosuppression and infectious processes
• Anticipatory grieving (parenting) related to potential loss of infant
• Anxiety (parental) related to interpersonal disease transmission and contagion and threat of future death of infant
• Ineffective individual coping related to situational crisis, inadequate support system, or unrealistic perceptions
• High risk for altered parenting related to reaction to HIV diagnosis
• High risk for caregiver role strain related to impact of HIV diagnosis and care
• High risk for infection related to immunosuppression

INFANT
Air Leak Syndromes

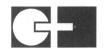

DEFINITION
Air leak syndromes are a group of clinical conditions characterized by air leakage from ruptured alveoli, with air escaping into tissue where it is not normally present. As the alveoli rupture, air escapes into the interstitium of the alveolar walls and then passes through the lung's perivascular and peribronchial tissues. The results are decreased pulmonary compliance and pulmonary interstitial emphysema. The air may subsequently enter the loose tissue of the mediastinum, causing pneumomediastinum. As pressure rises from the accumulation of large blebs at the hilum, the blebs rupture and air from the mediastinum enters the pleural space, causing pneumothorax. Further extension of air may involve other areas, such as the pneumopericardium and pneumoperitoneum.

Incidence of these disorders varies; type, severity, therapy, and gestational age are the deciding factors in management. Prognosis is good if the complication is managed and hypoxia is avoided to prevent cerebral damage.

This plan focuses on the recognition and immediate treatment of extraneous air syndromes as complications of other respiratory disorders. It does not include air embolus and air leaks at other sites.

ETIOLOGY AND PRECIPITATING FACTORS
• may occur spontaneously
• may occur after a difficult resuscitation
• lung immaturity
• complication of diseases, such as respiratory distress syndrome (RDS), lung infection, pulmonary anomalies, and meconium aspiration
• complication of vigorous use of continuous positive airway pressure, intermittent positive-pressure breathing, or positive end-expiratory pressure, in which inhalation, insufflation, or retention of large amounts of air causes the rupture

PHYSICAL FINDINGS
Infant status at birth
• prematurity, gestational age abnormality, or postmaturity
• resuscitation efforts
• meconium staining of amniotic fluid

Cardiovascular
• pneumothorax—hypotension, decreased pulse pressure and heart rate, and shift of apical pulse
• pneumomediastinum—possible muffled heart sounds or bulging sternum or both

Gastrointestinal
• pneumothorax—palpable liver or spleen because both organs are pushed down by the diaphragm; abdominal distention

Integumentary
• cyanosis when breathing room air

Neurologic
• pneumothorax—restlessness and irritability

Pulmonary
• pneumothorax—tachypnea (130 breaths/minute), grunting, nasal flaring, diminished breath sounds, and mediastinal shift to unaffected side
• pneumomediastinum—tachypnea

BEHAVIORAL FINDINGS
• restlessness
• irritability
• lethargy

DIAGNOSTIC STUDIES
• Chest X-ray to identify interstitial emphysema reveals cystlike or linear radiolucencies in the medial and peripheral lung fields in one or both lungs.
• Chest X-ray to identify pneumothorax reveals underexpanded lung and heart displacement away from affected side and free air in the pleural space. Transillumination of chest reveals air in pleural space in preterm infant.
• Chest X-ray (anteroposterior, lateral view) to identify pneumomediastinum reveals air behind sternum in the superior portion of the mediastinum between heart and chest wall.

Laboratory data
• arterial blood gas (ABG) measurements—show increased CO_2 retention ($PaCO_2$ above 50 mm Hg), decreased oxygen (PaO_2 below 70 mm Hg), decreased oxygen saturation (SaO_2 below 90%), and decreased pH (below 7.35)

Collaborative problem: *Interference with gas exchange related to respiratory insufficiency from ruptured alveoli, reduced lung compliance, and lung collapse (2 goals)*

GOAL 1: Identify respiratory distress and infant at risk for air leak.

Interventions

1. Assess for factors that indicate the infant is at risk for air leak syndromes, including:
• prematurity or postmaturity
• resuscitation at birth
• lung immaturity
• conditions such as RDS and meconium aspiration
• use of mechanical ventilation with high pressure.

2. Assess for changes in respiratory status, including:

• respiratory rate, depth, and ease, with tachypnea as high as 130 breaths/minute

• expiratory grunting

• nasal flaring

• cyanosis when breathing room air (infant may have dusky appearance)

• diminished breath sounds or muffled heart sounds

• hypotension, decreased heart rate, or both; restlessness or irritability
• serial ABG measurements

• serial X-rays and fiberoptic transillumination.

3. Additional individualized interventions: _____

Rationales

1. Assessment permits early intervention to prevent spread of air released to other areas from increased pressure.

2. Early recognition of an abnormality allows for immediate treatment and prevention of complications.
• Infant may have increased respiratory rate from an attempt to increase oxygen level.
• This is the sound of the closing glottis, stopping exhalation of air by forcing it against the vocal cords.
• Flaring is an attempt to reduce resistance to respirations caused by narrow nostrils.
• Cyanosis is the result of decreased oxygen.

• These symptoms are caused by decreased compliance and a bulging sternum.
• These are associated signs of air leak syndrome.

• ABG measurements reflect tissue oxygenation and the presence of acidosis.
• Changes in these diagnostic tests indicate the spread or location of air in tissues or spaces.

3. Rationales: _____

GOAL 2: Improve, maintain, and maximize pulmonary function.

Interventions

1. Assist with needle aspiration of chest until a chest tube can be inserted.

2. Administer warm and humidified oxygen, as ordered. Give enough oxygen to relieve cyanosis (even 100% if needed).

3. Assist with insertion of chest tube connected to closed underwater seal with continuous negative pressure section.

4. Monitor vital signs electronically for changes in heart rate, blood pressure, and pulse pressure.

5. Monitor serial ABG levels from umbilical artery catheter at least every hour.

Rationales

1. Needle aspiration removes air from the pleural space. This procedure is done only as an emergency because it may damage the myocardium.

2. Methods depend on oxygen need, infant acuity, and need for ventilatory assistance (see Hyaline Membrane Disease—Respiratory Distress Syndrome [RDS I], page 205, for methods and procedures).

3. Chest tube insertion attempts to remove air from the pleural space and reestablish lung expansion.

4. Changes in vital signs can indicate improvement or deterioration in the infant's status. By electronically monitoring vital signs, changes can be identified quickly without disturbing the infant and appropriate measures can be instituted rapidly.

5. ABG levels indicate tissue oxygenation and determine acid-base balance.

Interventions

6. Monitor serial chest X-rays and perform transillumination.

7. Check and calibrate all monitoring and measuring devices.

8. Additional individualized interventions: _____

_____

Rationales

6. These tests indicate improvement or deterioration in pulmonary pathology.

7. These practices assure safe functioning of all equipment and an accurate assessment of the infant's status.

8. Rationales: _____

_____

ASSOCIATED PLANS AND APPENDICES
• Bronchopulmonary Dysplasia
• Hyaline Membrane Disease—Respiratory Distress
Syndrome (RDS I)
• Meconium Aspiration Syndrome
• Assessing Vital Signs in the Infant (Appendix 9)
• Normal Lab Values for the Newborn Infant (Appendix 10)

ADDITIONAL NURSING DIAGNOSES
• Altered growth and development related to environmental and stimulation deficiencies
• Fear (parental) related to critical condition of infant
• High risk for injury related to complication from use of mechanical ventilation
• Ineffective individual coping (parental) related to situational crisis

Anemia

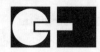

DEFINITION
Anemia is characterized by a decreased number of erythrocytes and a concentration of hemoglobin (Hb) below normal levels. At birth, the average red blood cell (RBC) count is 5,000,000/mm³. Levels fall to 3,000,000 to 4,000,000/mm³ during the next 8 weeks because new RBCs are not produced for replacement. Hb levels, normally between 16 and 20 g/dl (cord blood) at birth, fall to 10 to 11 g/dl during the next 8 weeks and as low as 7 to 9 g/dl in preterm infants. Physiologic anemia results from decreased Hb and RBC production, a 90-day survival rate for RBCs, increased blood volume, and hemodilution because of rapid growth. Preterm infants develop anemia earlier and with greater severity than full-term infants.

Blood volume at birth is about 90 ml/kg, with an average of 300 ml in full-term infants. Optimal blood volume is transferred to the infant at birth if the cord is clamped 30 seconds after delivery and if the infant is placed below the level of the placenta to allow gravity to enhance blood transfer.

This plan focuses on care of the infant at risk for anemia or with anemia, whether acute or chronic.

ETIOLOGY AND PRECIPITATING FACTORS
• hemolysis of RBCs in hemolytic disease (ABO and Rh erythroblastosis or other genetic conditions)
• lag in hematopoiesis while growth occurs
• defects in clotting mechanisms from vitamin K deficiency, causing deficiencies in coagulation factors
• platelet abnormality from infections
• iron deficiency from lack of iron intake and low iron stores
• blood loss before, during, or after parturition, as from the following situations:
    □ trauma, rupture, or tear of cord
    □ incision into placenta during cesarean delivery
    □ disorders such as placenta previa and abruptio placentae
    □ clamping of cord too soon with infant above level of placenta
    □ fetofetal bleeding (chronic transfer of blood from one twin to another) or fetomaternal hemorrhage
    □ trauma during labor, causing intracranial hemorrhage or hemorrhage into liver, spleen, or kidneys
    □ trauma after cardiac massage
    □ multiple blood sampling.

PHYSICAL FINDINGS
Maternal history
• blood type, Rh isoimmunization
• obstetric accident, traumatic delivery, tear in cord
• cesarean delivery
• iron deficiency, poor nutrition
• prenatal care
• intrauterine or intravenous transfusion

Infant status at birth
• prematurity and gestational age
• twin or multiple birth
• time cord was clamped and infant's level at birth in relation to placenta
• Apgar score, skin color

Cardiovascular
• tachycardia (over 160 beats/minute)
• feeble or absent pulses
• hypotension (30 to 50 mm Hg systolic)

Gastrointestinal
• palpable enlarged liver
• upper abdominal distention
• failure to gain weight and poor feeding

Integumentary
• pallor of skin and mucous membranes
• cyanosis despite oxygen therapy
• petechiae or ecchymoses with thrombocytopenia

Neurologic
• weak cry
• diminished activity or flaccidity
• listlessness
• temperature instability

Pulmonary
• tachypnea and dyspnea
• gasping and retractions
• episodes of apnea or bradycardia

BEHAVIORAL FINDINGS
• irritability
• lethary

DIAGNOSTIC STUDIES
Laboratory data
• complete blood count (CBC)—to detect decrease in RBC, Hb (less than 14 g/dl for term infant and less than 13 g/dl for preterm infant), and hematocrit (HCT) (less than 40 g/dl) values; mean corpuscular volume with smaller newly formed RBC and mean corpuscular hemoglobin with RBC less filled with Hb
• reticulocyte levels—to detect increases in response to decreases in RBCs (attempts to replace RBCs)
• bilirubin levels—increased as RBCs are destroyed
• iron levels—decreased to less than 100 mcg/dl
• blood type and Rh factor of mother and infant
• stool—for frank or occult blood

Collaborative problem: *Fluid imbalance related to blood loss before, during, or after birth (2 goals)*

GOAL 1: Identify infant at risk for anemia or one who is anemic.

Interventions	Rationales
1. Assess for risk of anemia; include the following considerations:	1. If risk is established, preparation can be made to offset life-threatening condition.
• indication in maternal history	• Maternal condition may predispose infant to anemia.
• prematurity or possibility of twins	• Anemia is more severe and occurs earlier in a preterm infant.
• Apgar score	• Apgar score indicates adequacy of circulation and oxygenation.
• traumatic birth	• Trauma causing hematoma results in blood loss into tissue.
• ABO type and Rh factor	• Assessment indicates possibility of hemolytic disorder and destruction of RBCs.
• bilirubin level	• Increased bilirubin level reveals amount of RBC destruction.
• RBC, HCT, and Hb values and decreased iron and serum-bound iron levels.	• Anemia is indicated by an HCT value of less than 40 g/dl (normal value at birth is 48 to 60 g/dl), a venous blood level of Hb of less than 13 g/dl, capillary blood level of less than 14.5 g/dl (normal level at birth is 16 to 20 g/dl cord blood), and a serum-bound iron level of less than 100 mcg/dl. Decreases greater than normally expected after birth may indicate anemia.
2. Assess for signs of anemia from blood loss, including: • pallor • tachypnea (over 60 breaths/minute) • tachycardia (over 160 beats/minute) • arterial hypotension (less than 30 mm Hg).	2. These signs indicate hemorrhage caused by accident or great blood loss with possible shock and decrease in oxygen-carrying capacity of the blood.
3. Assess for signs and symptoms of anemia that indicate hemorrhage, including: • abdominal distention • periumbilical ecchymoses • shifting dullness • apnea • seizure activity.	3. These signs and symptoms indicate internal hemorrhage from trauma during labor or bleeding into the central nervous system.
4. Assess for signs and symptoms of anemia from hemolysis, including: • jaundice • lethargy or diminished activity • poor feeding • increased bilirubin level and decreased RBC count.	4. These signs and symptoms indicate hemolysis of RBCs.
5. Assess for signs and symptoms of anemia from iron deficiency, including: • pallor • irritability • decreased Hb, HCT, and iron values • occult blood in stool.	5. These signs and symptoms indicate iron deficiency anemia.
6. Assess for symptoms of anemia from a platelet disorder, including: • petechiae • ecchymoses.	6. These symptoms indicate anemia from thrombocytopenia.

Interventions	**Rationales**
7. Assess for signs and symptoms of anemia from a clotting disorder, including: • pallor • lethargy • bleeding from umbilical cord • bloody or black stools • hematuria • decreased Hb and HCT values and platelet count.	7. These signs and symptoms indicate anemia from poor response to vitamin K or from low levels of clotting factors (usually factors I and V).
8. Additional individualized interventions: _____	8. Rationales: _____

GOAL 2: Prevent or minimize anemia and its complications.

Interventions	**Rationales**
1. Record HCT and Hb values initially and every 4 hours, as ordered.	1. Monitoring HCT and Hb values reveals changes indicating improving or deteriorating status. Decreasing values may signal blood loss.
2. If HCT and Hb values decrease below 40 g/dl and 13 g/dl, respectively, notify physician; check CBC and reticulocyte values, as ordered.	2. Decreased values indicate that the infant may need iron or an exchange transfusion if RBCs are not being produced.
3. Calculate or measure blood volume according to agency techniques, and closely monitor amount of blood drawn.	3. Monitoring blood volume allows for quick detection of imbalances. Blood volume may be calculated by using an average volume of 90 ml/kg and estimating the loss based on decreases in HCT and Hb values after birth (method varies among agencies).
4. Administer warmed and humidified oxygen, as needed.	4. This treats tachypnea and dyspnea and prevents hypoxia with a decreased oxygen-carrying capacity of blood.
5. Maintain a thermoneutral environment.	5. A thermoneutral environment reduces the metabolic demands for additional oxgyen.
6. Monitor arterial blood pressure and central venous pressure via umbilical artery catheter (UAC); measure other vital signs continuously.	6. Monitoring provides ongoing assessment of the infant's condition and the effects of treatment.
7. Prepare for transfusion of packed RBCs; if infant is symptomatic, give whole blood.	7. Transfusion may be needed to relieve hypoxia by increasing RBC count and Hb level (see Hyperbilirubinemia plan, page 213, for transfusion procedure).
8. Carry out gavage feedings by gastric tube.	8. Feedings provide nutrition if poor feeding is a problem. Oral feedings are not given with UAC in place.
9. Prepare and administer vitamin K I.M. or I.V. after birth.	9. Administration of vitamin K protects against prolonged prothrombin time.
10. Prepare and administer oral liquid iron preparation daily as supplement; provide iron-fortified formula or vitamins with iron as alternatives.	10. These measures treat iron deficiency and prevent anemia based on reticulocyte level. If situation is acute and infant is bleeding, give blood. If patient is a growing preterm infant, give vitamins plus iron.
11. Additional individualized interventions: _____	11. Rationales: _____

Nursing diagnosis: *Knowledge deficit related to need for transfusion or medication administration after discharge*

GOAL: Provide appropriate information about treatment and continuing drug therapy

Interventions

1. Inform parents about:
• infant's condition
• reason for transfusion
• screen of blood products and selection of donors according to blood bank standards
• their opportunity to select a donor if the donor fits bank guidelines
• infant's improved condition after the transfusion.

2. Instruct parents in administration of oral iron supplement as follows:
• how to measure correct amount in dropper and administer
• time of day to give iron
• how to store drug
• what drug does and possible adverse effects.

3. Instruct parents in appropriate nutritional sources of iron, such as iron-fortified formulas and cereals.

4. Encourage questions and clarify information as requested. Allow for a return demonstration of preparing and giving medication.

5. Refer parents and family for possible community and home health care follow-up.

6. Additional individualized interventions: _____

Rationales

1. Information helps relieve parents' fears that the transfused blood may transmit acquired immunodeficiency syndrome, hepatitis, or other diseases to the infant.

2. Thorough instruction regarding administration and drug therapy promotes compliance. Treatment may continue for 3 months or longer to maintain normal iron level.

3. Adequate nutrition provides sufficient calories plus additional sources of iron to combat any deficiency.

4. Explanations and demonstrations reinforce understanding.

5. Referral to community and home health care services helps to support parents and ensure compliance with medical regimen.

6. Rationales: _____

ASSOCIATED PLANS AND APPENDICES
• Birth Trauma
• Hyperbilirubinemia
• Intracranial Hemorrhage
• Preterm Infant, Less Than 37 Weeks
• Normal Lab Values for the Newborn Infant (Appendix 10)

ADDITIONAL NURSING DIAGNOSES
• Altered peripheral tissue perfusion related to decreased oxygen-carrying capacity of blood
• Anxiety (parental) related to possible life-threatening illness of infant
• Fear (parental) related to transmission of disease to infant via transfusion or to belief that allowing transfusion will violate religious convictions

Birth Trauma

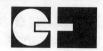

DEFINITION
Birth trauma, in this plan, refers to all traumatic conditions caused by labor and delivery. The term encompasses mechanical and asphyxial events. Most cases of traumatic birth are mild and transient, but some cause permanent disability. The trauma may affect the infant's skin, skull, bones, brain, spinal cord, eyes, peripheral nerves, or abdominal organs, and it may result in hemorrhage, hematoma, fractures, abrasions, or paralysis.

Birth trauma occurs in approximately 2 to 7 of every 1,000 live births. Its incidence has declined with better monitoring of labor and the fetus, with careful mid- or high-forceps use with difficult presentations, and with cesarean delivery for abnormal presentations.

This plan focuses on the identification of birth trauma and care of the affected infant.

ETIOLOGY AND PRECIPITATING FACTORS
• dystocia and severe contractions during labor
• small maternal pelvis size
• breech or abnormal vertex presentations
• pressure produced by forceps or against bony pelvis
• inaccurate application of forceps
• large baby 8 lb, 13 oz (4,000 g), or baby too large for pelvic outlet
• stretching of body parts or crushing of organs that may be enlarged, such as the liver
• blood clotting disorders

PHYSICAL FINDINGS
Maternal history
• difficulty during delivery and use of forceps
• mother's size
• type of delivery: vaginal or cesarean

Infant status at birth
• presentation at birth
• weight, especially if large for gestational age

Integumentary
• edema of scalp (caput succedaneum)
• edema and cyanosis of buttocks, arms, or legs
• bluish color to scalp (cephalohematoma)
• firm blue or red lesions on face, shoulders, back, arms, and thighs (subcutaneous fat necrosis)
• scalp abrasions
• molding of head with gradual rise to apex of posterior half
• petechiae or ecchymoses of purplish color, from pinpoint size to large bruises
• pallor with anemia associated with liver injury

Musculoskeletal
• fracture of skull or long bones (clavicle or humerus) with diminished motion of arm or leg and pain with movement

Neurologic
• hypotonia, bulging anterior fontanel, (subdural hemorrhage)
• paralysis of arm, including shoulder and arm muscles, with absent Moro's reflex on affected side (Erb's paralysis)
• paralysis involving hand and forearm (Klumpke's paralysis)
• paralysis of the side of the face (cranial nerve VII) or asymmetry indicating that the nerve is stretched but not permanently damaged

Pulmonary
• possible apneic episodes

BEHAVIORAL FINDINGS
• lethargy
• shrill cry
• irritability

DIAGNOSTIC STUDIES
• X-rays of bones and chest—to detect fractures and diaphragm paralysis
• lumbar puncture with cerebrospinal fluid (CSF) specimen—to detect red blood cells (RBCs)
• Computed tomography (CT) scan—to determine whether blood appears in brain or ventricles
• Electroencephalogram—to determine damage and prognosis if infant is recovering from bleeding

Laboratory data
• Hematocrit (HCT) value and platelet count—to detect decreased values with hemorrhage
• bilirubin levels—to detect increases with hematomas because of increased load of RBCs to liver for destruction
• coagulation studies—to determine clotting disorders

Nursing diagnosis: *High risk for injury related to difficult labor and delivery (2 goals)*

GOAL 1: Identify infant with birth trauma or at risk for birth trauma.

Interventions

1. Assess infant for predisposing factors and presence of trauma, including:

• large size, use of forceps, presentation at birth

• edema, color, lesions, abrasions, hematoma, and petechiae of skin

• X-rays of bones and chest

• movement of arms and legs

• apneic episodes, respiratory distress, shrill cry, poor feeding, lethargy, irritability, and bulging and widening fontanels

• straight, limp arm with fist closed and absent Moro's reflex

• loss of grasp reflex with wrist drop and relaxed fingers

• immobility on side of face when crying, with eye closing and lips deviating toward normal side

• edema, hematoma, and shape of the head

2. Additional individualized interventions: _____

Rationales

1. Forces and pressures from labor and delivery may cause trauma to infant's bones, soft tissue, and nervous system.

• These are the most common factors that predispose the infant to trauma.

• These skin changes reflect injury, hemorrhage, breaks, or clotting disorders.

• X-rays indicate fractures, diaphragm paralysis, or both.

• Abnormal movement indicates fracture, paralysis or palsy, or intracranial hemorrhage.

• These signs indicate intracranial hemorrhage, causing pressure against the respiratory center.

• Erb's paralysis is caused by injury to cervical nerve V or VI, causing brachial plexus injury.

• Klumpke's paralysis is caused by injury to cervical nerve VII or VIII, causing brachial plexus injury.

• Facial paralysis is caused by injury to cranial nerve VII.

• Edema may occur within 24 hours after birth; hematoma, within 24 to 48 hours after birth; and subdural hematoma, from hours to a few days after birth, with bleeding between periosteum and skull bone or in space between dura and arachnoid lining (tentorial tears). Molding of head with some elongation may follow birth.

2. Rationales: _____

GOAL 2: Support recovery from injury.

Interventions

1. Provide for special needs of infant with facial paralysis:

• Assist with feeding (sucking) by using soft nipple with large hole for bottle-fed infant and compressing areolar area for breast-fed infant.

• Instill artificial tears every 2 to 4 hours.

• Perform gavage feedings.

2. Provide for special needs of infant with brachial palsy:

• Position arm in abducted and external rotation.

• Perform passive range-of-motion exercises on arm daily.

• Dress and undress infant carefully; start with unaffected arm when undressing and affected arm when dressing.

Rationales

1. Facial paralysis may impede feeding and prevent appropriate nutrition.

• Because part of mouth droops, the infant may not be able to close lips around nipple.

• Eyelid may not close on affected side; medication prevents drying.

• These feedings may be indicated to prevent aspiration if infant has difficulty with normal feeding.

2. Brachial palsy requires special care to prevent permanent complications.

• This position maintains humeral head in glenoid fossa of scapula and prevents contracture of paralyzed muscle.

• This ensures muscle tone and function.

• This prevents unnecessary stress on the affected muscle.

Interventions

• Maintain desired position of arm by pinning shirt sleeve to the mattress or placing arm in a sling and pinning the sling to the mattress.

• Prepare for and assist with splint or cast application.

3. Provide for special needs of infant with a fracture:

• Maintain proper body alignment.

• Handle and pick up the infant carefully, supporting injured part. Carefully dress and undress the infant.

• Pin shirt or clothing to sheet.

• Prepare for and assist with cast.

4. Provide for special needs of infant with intracranial hemorrhage:

• Monitor intracranial pressure.

• Position infant with head slightly elevated (30 to 45 degrees).

• Monitor I.V. fluids if given.

• Perform gavage feedings if infant's sucking reflex is affected.

• Review CSF analysis, CT scan, HCT value, platelet count, bilirubin level, and coagulation studies.

• Prepare and assist with blood transfusion if needed.

5. Additional individualized interventions: _____

Rationales

• This immobilizes arm in desired position.

• Splinting or casting may be used to maintain desired position.

3. Special care prevents fracture complications.

• Proper body alignment prevents contractures.

• This technique prevents pain or further injury.

• This immobilizes injured part, when necessary, while decreasing discomfort.

• A cast may be indicated for immobilization.

4. For needs associated with intracranial hemorrhage, see Intracranial Hemorrhage plan, page 243.

• Intracranial pressure increases if infant's condition worsens, indicating increased bleeding.

• This position relieves pressure on the brain by allowing fluid to flow downward.

• I.V. monitoring prevents fluid overload.

• Alternate feeding methods provide nourishment.

• These tests can indicate bleeding from hematoma, petechiae, liver damage, and cranial injury.

• Transfusion replaces blood loss.

5. Rationales: _____

Nursing diagnosis: *Knowledge deficit (parental) related to infant's condition, treatment, and progress*

GOAL: Provide appropriate information regarding infant's condition and expected progress.

Interventions

1. Inform parents about the following:
• cause of injury
• infant's condition
• progress toward resolution of trauma
• treatment being given
• effects of trauma usually being temporary
• time usually needed for effects of trauma to disappear.

2. For cranial injury:

• Keep parents informed of the seriousness of the injury and of changes in the infant's condition.

• Explain all tests and procedures to the parents.

• Inform parents that scalp abrasions or hematoma will disappear but that cranial hemorrhage will take longer to resolve.

Rationales

1. This information reduces parents' anxiety and concerns about the infant's appearance, effects of the injury, and whether these effects will be permanent.

2. Cranial injury at birth may involve intracranial or intraventricular hemorrhage.

• Ongoing information about infant's condition assists in allaying parental anxiety.

• Potential for anemia or hyperbilirubinemia requires several tests. A lumbar puncture may be ordered to detect intraventricular bleeding.

• Different types of trauma require different healing times.

Interventions

• Inform parents that infant will need transfusion and that blood is first tested for safety.

• Discuss risks and benefits of transfusion.

3. Allow for the parents' questions and clarify information as requested.

4. Encourage parental contact with infant and participation in infant's care.

5. Additional individualized interventions: ⎯⎯⎯⎯⎯⎯

Rationales

• Acquired immunodeficiency syndrome is a common fear of parents when blood transfusion is mentioned.

• No one can be 100% certain that blood is safe because some blood donors may have undetected human immunodeficiency virus antibodies (in rare instances). This risk must be weighed against benefit of transfusion.

3. This reinforces parental understanding.

4. This promotes bonding and increases parental confidence and comfort regarding infant care.

5. Rationales: ⎯⎯⎯⎯⎯⎯⎯⎯⎯⎯⎯⎯⎯⎯⎯⎯⎯

ASSOCIATED PLANS
• Anemia
• Hyperbilirubinemia
• Inappropriate Size or Weight for Gestational Age, Large
• Intracranial Hemorrhage

ADDITIONAL NURSING DIAGNOSES
• Anxiety (parental) related to threat of change in infant's health status
• High risk for fluid volume deficit related to excessive blood loss
• Ineffective family coping: compromised related to fear, guilt
• Pain related to injury

Bowel Obstruction, Small or Large

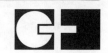

DEFINITION

Bowel obstructions are congenital abnormalities of the gastrointestinal (GI) system that occur in the intestinal tract. They may obstruct the intestinal tract partially or completely. Intestinal atresia of the duodenum, jejunum, or ileum is an interruption in the continuity of the bowel; it causes total obstruction. Intestinal stenosis, which may affect any segment of the intestine, is a narrowing, or constriction, in the bowel; it causes an incomplete or partial obstruction. Single or multiple areas of stenosis or atresia may exist.

Another abnormality causing obstruction is malrotation, in which the cecum fails to assume its correct anatomic position. The duodenum is pulled out of position, and duodenal bands maintain the abnormal position of the cecum. The loosely connected mesentery allows the small intestine to twist around it. This twisted loop of bowel (volvulus) causes obstruction and, possibly, strangulation of the superior mesenteric artery.

Such conditions as imperforate anus and strangulated inguinal hernia may cause obstruction. Imperforate anus, an imperfect fusion of the anal area, may be a high or low type, depending on whether or not the rectum passes through the puborectalis muscle. It may be associated with a fistula leading to the vagina in girls or to the urethra in boys. In inguinal hernia, a portion of the intestine prolapses through the inguinal ring because of weakness or incomplete closure of the inguinal ring at 32 weeks' gestation or later. This prolapsed portion of the bowel may become incarcerated or strangulated, causing complete obstruction.

This plan focuses on care of the infant who displays signs and symptoms of GI obstruction and on the prevention of complications before surgical intervention.

ETIOLOGY AND PRECIPITATING FACTORS

• failure of the gut to recanalize in utero because of ischemic injury to the bowel below the duodenum or from abnormality where the common bile duct and the pancreatic duct enter into the upper duodenum; either condition may cause atresia or stenoses

• duplications of any length or segment of the GI tube, with or without continuity with the normal segment
• functional obstructions caused by such conditions as achalasia, pyloric stenosis, megacolon, and meconium plug syndrome
• incomplete closure of inguinal ring, allowing intestine to protrude through it

PHYSICAL FINDINGS
Maternal history
• polyhydramnios
• ultrasound results

Infant status at birth
• usually appears normal at birth
• closed anal area or only a small aperture, making insertion of rectal thermometer impossible; anal dimple possible (imperforate anus)

Gastrointestinal
• bile-stained vomitus (early occurrence coincides with higher obstruction; later occurrence, with lower obstruction)
• abdominal distention (intermittent with duodenal obstruction; persistent with jejunal or ileal obstructions and with imperforate anus or inguinal hernia strangulation)
• failure to pass meconium or diminished stools
• weight loss

DIAGNOSTIC STUDIES
• X-ray studies of bowel—upper GI, barium series results indicating pattern of double bubble from distended duodenum or dilated loops of bowel
• X-ray contrast studies of upper GI tract—to determine malrotation; barium enema studies to determine obstruction by inguinal hernia strangulation
• X-ray studies of infant in upside down position—allows gas in colon to rise and outline blind rectal pouch and position in relation to the anal opening (in imperforate anus)

Collaborative problem: *Bowel obstruction related to congenital GI abnormality* (2 goals)

GOAL 1: Identify infant at risk for or with bowel obstruction.

Interventions

1. Assess for signs and symptoms of partial or complete bowel obstruction, including:

Rationales

1. Prompt reporting of GI abnormalities allows for immediate interventions to treat an acute condition and prevent complications.

Interventions

- bile-stained vomitus (also noting amount of vomitus and time vomiting occurred)

- diminished or absent stools

- abdominal distention and tense abdomen

- results of upper and lower GI tract X-ray studies.

2. Assess for other congenital conditions, such as Down syndrome, herniation, and absence of anus.

3. Additional individualized interventions: _____

Rationales

- Greenish vomitus indicates bowel obstruction; earlier vomiting indicates that the obstruction is located higher in the GI tract.
- Diminished stools indicate partial or evolving obstruction; absent stools indicate complete obstruction.
- These signs indicate failure of GI tract to rid itself of gas and secretions because of obstruction.
- Study results identify location and extent of obstruction.

2. These conditions commonly accompany GI anomalies.

3. Rationales: _____

GOAL 2: Reduce risk of physical complications associated with bowel obstruction.

Interventions

1. Maintain fluid and electrolyte balance and caloric needs by:
- administering and monitoring I.V. solution (dextrose 10% in water calculated individually for infant in ml/kg/day as ordered by physician) with added electrolytes, if needed
- weighing infant daily if condition permits
- monitoring fluid intake and output hourly (with output including gastric drainage of at least 2 to 3 ml/kg/hour) and comparing output with I.V. intake.

2. Provide gastric decompression and monitor its effect by:
- measuring abdominal girth
- ensuring patency of gastric tubing by noting drainage and carefully aspirating it without exerting pressure
- noting vomiting
- auscultating bowel sounds.

3. Prevent pulmonary aspiration of vomitus by positioning infant on abdomen or side and administering oxygen if needed.

4. Maintain thermoneutral environment by:

- taking infant's axillary temperature every 2 hours

- placing infant in Isolette or incubator or using radiant warmer.

5. Prepare infant for surgical intervention after diagnosis has been made.

6. Additional individualized interventions: _____

Rationales

1. Fluid and electrolyte balance and caloric needs must be maintained to prevent dehydration and hypoglycemia and their complications.

2. Gastric decompression prevents abdominal distention by removing contents.
- Increases in girth indicate distention.
- This action ensures properly functioning suction apparatus for decompression.
- Vomiting indicates ineffective decompression.
- Bowel sounds indicate that air and fluid are moving through the bowel.

3. The infant's pulmonary system is compromised if aspiration occurs.

4. Maintaining appropriate environment prevents cold stress, which would further compromise sick infant and increase oxygen needs.
- Temperature readings reveal decreases in body temperature.
- Depending on infant needs, thermoregulation will maintain optimal temperature (see Hypothermia and Hyperthermia plan, page 229).

5. Adequate physical and psychological preoperative preparation aids postoperation recovery. Bowel obstruction is corrected by surgical removal or repair of affected part (see Preoperative Care plan, page 263).

6. Rationales: _____

Nursing diagnosis: *Parental anxiety related to uncertain outcome of surgical intervention*

GOAL: Minimize parental anxiety, and support parents through crisis situation.

Interventions

1. Maintain calm and accepting environment.

2. Encourage parents to ask questions. Give honest and accurate answers or obtain information for them. For example, they may need to know that:
• small-bowel surgery involves resection and anastomosis of the intestinal segments
• malrotation involves releasing bands across small bowel and releasing cecum
• anal deformity involves removing anal membrane, or if deformity is in high position, colostomy may be performed until correction can be completed.
• inguinal hernia repair is needed if the mass cannot be reduced or bowel becomes strangulated
• temporary gastrostomy may be performed or total parenteral nutrition administered after surgery.

3. Use pamphlets and drawings to reinforce and clarify physician's information about surgical procedure, prognosis, and postsurgical care.

4. Spend as much time as possible with parents. Keep them informed of infant's care and progress. Explain procedures and their rationales.

5. Additional individualized interventions: _____

Rationales

1. A calm, accepting environment allows parents to feel comfortable expressing feelings and asking questions.

2. Encouragement promotes trust and decreases anxiety; information alleviates fear of the unknown.

3. Information may need to be repeated or reinforced because the parents may be too anxious to absorb it all at once; this action also provides for a better-informed consent before surgery.

4. These actions show your caring and supportive attitude.

5. Rationales: _____

Nursing diagnosis: *Ineffective family coping: compromised related to emotional crisis of infant with a congenital defect and potential for long-term care after surgery*

GOAL: Support parents in coping with parenting changes required to deal with sick infant needing surgery.

Interventions

1. Help parents to appraise the crisis in terms of their needs and their infant's needs.

2. Involve parents in care, as appropriate, encouraging as much contact with infant as possible.

3. Help parents verbalize their feelings about loss of the "perfect child," the intensive care nursery, change in child's appearance if colostomy or gastrostomy must be performed, as well as other feelings, such as their guilt during possible long-term treatment.

4. Reassure parents of their ability to care for their infant after surgery.

5. Refer parents to social services and community resources for additional help.

Rationales

1. This will identify needed changes and possible coping strategies necessary because of the crisis.

2. Involvement of parents encourages the bonding process.

3. By reassuring parents that their feelings are normal, you show your acceptance of their concerns and fears.

4. Reassuring the parents creates feelings of self-confidence and ability in parenting.

5. Referral to other services ensures continuing support as infant progresses and is ready to leave the hospital.

Interventions	Rationales
6. Additional individualized interventions: _____	6. Rationales: _____

ASSOCIATED PLANS AND APPENDICES
• Hypoglycemia
• Hypothermia and Hyperthermia
• Postoperative Care
• Preoperative Care
• Transporting an Infant to Another Hospital
(Appendix 11)

ADDITIONAL NURSING DIAGNOSES
• Altered family processes related to situational crisis
• Altered nutrition: less than body requirements related to feeding status and gastric decompression
• Fear (parental) related to possible loss of child as result of surgery
• High risk for altered body temperature related to extremes of age and weight, dehydration
• High risk for fluid volume deficit related to nutritional status and gastric decompression
• Knowledge deficit (parental) related to lack of exposure to information

INFANT
Bronchopulmonary Dysplasia

DEFINITION

Bronchopulmonary dysplasia (BPD) is a respiratory disorder of infants, with or without hyaline membrane disease, who need supplemental oxygen to prevent cyanosis. Also called respirator lung disease, this disorder is characterized by mucosal dysplasia, fibrosis, and bronchovascular muscle hypertrophy, causing thickening and necrosis of alveolar walls, basement membranes, and bronchiolar epithelial lining layers and leading to impaired oxygen diffusion from alveoli to capillaries.

BPD does not seem to have a single discrete cause; it results from a combination of iatrogenic factors and patient characteristics. Two common respiratory treatments—oxygen therapy and mechanical ventilation—have been strongly implicated in BPD.

The onset of oxygen toxicity is noted by the infant's need for increased oxygen and ventilatory pressure after recovery from respiratory distress syndrome (RDS) or by a continued need for support for 5 to 10 days after recovery should have occurred. BPD occurs in 20% to 30% of neonates with RDS requiring ventilation with oxygen; two-thirds recover within 6 to 12 months, but some suffer persistent respiratory system abnormalities throughout childhood. Complications include right heart failure, right ventricular hypertrophy, and, later in life, susceptibility to pulmonary infections.

This plan focuses on care of the infant at risk for BPD from ventilation therapy and on appropriate preventive and supportive measures.

ETIOLOGY AND PRECIPITATING FACTORS

• related to fraction of oxygen in inspired air (FIO_2) levels greater than 70% for more than 5 days, but condition may also occur in those with lower FIO_2 levels
• related to trauma from mechanical ventilation with use of an endotracheal tube
• lung immaturity
• surfactant deficiency
• pulmonary edema, air leak
• family history of reactive airway disease
• systemic-to-pulmonary shunt through a patent ductus arteriosus

PHYSICAL FINDINGS
Infant status at birth
• RDS
• prematurity

Integumentary
• cyanosis, pallor, poor capillary filling time

Pulmonary
• increased respiratory distress with subcostal and intercostal retractions, tachypnea
• diminished breath sounds, bilateral crepitant crackles

BEHAVIORAL FINDINGS
• decreased interaction with environment
• activity intolerance
• feeding difficulties

DIAGNOSTIC STUDIES
• chest X-ray—reveals areas of irregularly shaped density in lungs, with atelectasis resulting from obstruction of small bronchioles. This is followed by air cysts among dense patches, indicating multifocal emphysema with collapsed alveoli, edema, and fibrosis. This is followed by bubbly appearance to lungs from enlarging air cysts, progressive emphysema with hyperinflation, flattened diaphragm, and cardiomegaly.

Laboratory data
• arterial blood gas (ABG) measurements—indicate increased carbon dioxide (CO_2) level and decreased oxygen (O_2) level, with acidosis.

Collaborative problem: *Respiratory deficiency and impaired gas exchange related to alveolar impairment caused by continued use of mechanical ventilation and by increased concentrations of oxygen (2 goals)*

GOAL 1: Identify signs and symptoms of respiratory distress and deviations from desired functioning with oxygen administration.

Interventions

1. Assess for changes in respiratory status and need for continued oxygen and ventilatory support after recovery from RDS or other pulmonary condition, noting:

• tachypnea or retractions with rate taken for 1 full minute

Rationales

1. Need for continued oxygen and ventilatory support may indicate that lung damage has occurred, so allow time for treatment to prevent complications.

• Respiratory rate over 60 breaths/minute is considered tachypneic.

Interventions

- diminished breath sounds

- cyanosis
- X-ray findings

- serial capillary blood gas (CBG) measurements or ABG measurements
- need for tracheal aspirate culture and sensitivity (C and S) tests and Gram stain (if patient is intubated)
- oxygen concentration administered by mechanical ventilation with endotracheal tube and duration of ventilation

2. Additional individualized interventions: _____

Rationales

- Diminished breath sounds indicate ventilatory impairment.
- Cyanosis indicates low oxygen level and hypoxemia.
- X-rays may indicate that such changes as atelectasis with lung densities are progressing to hyperinflation and fibrosis.
- Increased CO_2 and decreased O_2 levels may lead to acidosis; CBG or ABG measurements will detect this.
- Pulmonary infection may occur if infant is on ventilator.

- This method of oxygen administration and length of therapy is considered a predisposing factor for the condition. C and S tests identify causative organism and appropriate drug therapy.

2. Rationales: _____

GOAL 2: Minimize oxygen toxicity while supporting respiratory efforts.

Interventions

1. Administer warm, humidified oxygen in amount and method ordered.

2. Monitor amount and duration of oxygen administered by continuous positive airway pressure, positive end-expiratory pressure, and continuous positive pressure ventilation via endotracheal tube.

3. Apply a transcutaneous PO_2 monitor and check and record hourly while lowering O_2 levels, including FIO_2; or apply a pulse oximeter as ordered.

4. Verify changes in FIO_2 concentration with O_2 analyzer or pulse oximeter; calibrate analyzer each shift.

5. Perform serial CBG or ABG measurements to determine FIO_2 concentrations.

6. Prepare and assist with tracheostomy if needed.

7. Prepare furosemide (Lasix) I.V. to be given if pulmonary edema is present.

8. Perform chest physiotherapy, as ordered.

9. Additional individualized interventions: _____

Rationales

1. Oxygen must be administered in smallest doses for shortest time to maintain normal PO_2 (50 to 70 mm Hg usually sufficient) level, but amount must be adequate to treat infant.

2. Monitoring maintains optimal oxygen level for treatment (see Hyaline Membrane Disease—Respiratory Distress Syndrome [RDS I] plan, page 205, for procedures and precautions for various mechanical ventilation methods).

3. These actions allow the infant to be slowly weaned from dependence on increased oxygen administration; sensor site rotation every 3 to 4 hours is required to prevent skin burns. Using pulse oximeter to monitor oxygen level is safer because it does not produce heat that can cause burns.

4. Verifying changes assures adequate FIO_2 concentrations and accuracy of readings.

5. Serial measurements help detect changes in levels quickly. Long-term therapy requires monitoring of O_2 and CO_2 levels. CO_2 is more important in evaluating chronic condition; O_2 is more important when infant is sick because O_2 requirements will rise.

6. This procedure may be indicated in long-term, chronic cases for continued treatment and weaning.

7. Furosemide is the diuretic of choice in conditions associated with congestive heart failure.

8. Chest physiotherapy helps to drain and clear copious tenacious secretions (commonly seen in infants with BPD).

9. Rationales: _____

Nursing diagnosis: *Ineffective family coping: compromised related to crisis of sick infant and long-term implications*

GOAL: Increase family understanding and comfort with infant's condition and long-term needs.

Interventions

1. Provide accurate information, including:
• infant's condition and progress
• hospital routines and use of equipment on infant
• procedures done on infant
• rationales for care being given.

2. Reinforce information given by physician regarding length of hospitalization, long-term use of ventilator, and future use of O_2 at home after discharge.

3. Offer privacy and opportunity to express feelings about crisis and concern about infant's welfare. Look for clues of readiness to talk. Help parents obtain counseling as needed.

4. Encourage family communication about infant status.

5. Discuss with parents expectations for themselves and for infant, including BPD spells and other complications.

6. Inform infant's family that in time and with growth, pulmonary function may become normal.

7. Allow parents as much contact with infant as possible. Offer open visitation and participation in infant care.

8. Refer family to community and home health care resources.

9. Additional individualized interventions: _____

Rationales

1. Information reduces parental anxiety.

2. The family may be facing a difficult hospitalization of infant for 6 months or longer and years of predisposition to pulmonary problems.

3. Expressing feelings gives parents an opportunity to identify ways of coping with crisis.

4. Communication strengthens family relationships.

5. Unrealistic expectations may cause frustration.

6. Long-term or lasting effects of BPD are unknown, but new lung parenchymal growth is believed to occur until about age 6.

7. These actions encourage bonding and comfort with infant care.

8. Referral promotes parental adjustment and provides continuing emotional and physical support.

9. Rationales: _____

Nursing diagnosis: *Knowledge deficit (parental) related to long-term care of sick infant at home*

GOAL: Provide information about the disease and follow-up care.

Interventions

1. Inform parents about:
• disease process
• treatments and procedures
• signs and symptoms of respiratory problems
• follow-up care and therapy.

2. Instruct parents about ordered treatments, including:
• home oxygen therapy
• mechanical ventilation
• chest physiotherapy
• drug therapy
• nutritional therapy.

Rationales

1. Providing parents with information alleviates their anxiety and helps them prepare for the infant's discharge.

2. Proper instruction promotes compliance and helps dispel fears about equipment and procedures.

Interventions

3. Encourage family to participate in infant's care.

4. Teach parents and family how to balance infant's activities with rest and how to evaluate infant's tolerance for activities.

5. Arrange for home health care follow-up.

6. Additional individualized interventions: ⎯⎯⎯⎯⎯⎯

⎯⎯⎯⎯⎯⎯⎯⎯⎯⎯⎯⎯⎯⎯⎯⎯⎯⎯⎯⎯⎯⎯⎯⎯⎯⎯⎯⎯⎯⎯

Rationales

3. Participating in care helps alleviate parents' feelings of inadequacy and prepares them to care for infant at home.

4. Stimulation of activity is necessary to promote normal growth and development, which may be delayed from prolonged hospitalization. Activity tolerance varies from one infant to the next.

5. Home health care referral offers parents and family continued support outside the hospital.

6. Rationales: ⎯⎯⎯⎯⎯⎯⎯⎯⎯⎯⎯⎯⎯⎯⎯⎯⎯⎯⎯⎯

⎯⎯⎯⎯⎯⎯⎯⎯⎯⎯⎯⎯⎯⎯⎯⎯⎯⎯⎯⎯⎯⎯⎯⎯⎯⎯⎯⎯⎯⎯

ASSOCIATED PLANS AND APPENDICES
• Congestive Heart Failure
• Hyaline Membrane Disease—Respiratory Distress Syndrome (RDS I)
• Preterm Infant, Less Than 37 Weeks
• Normal Lab Values for the Newborn Infant (Appendix 10)

ADDITIONAL NURSING DIAGNOSES
• Altered growth and development related to prolonged hypoxia and environmental stress
• Altered parenting related to interruption in bonding process, chronic condition of infant, prolonged hospitalization, lack of family support, unrealistic expectations of self, infant
• Dysfunctional ventilatory weaning response related to inability to maintain adequate oxygen saturation level
• Fear (parental) related to eventual outcome of disorder, care of infant on ventilator at home
• Fluid volume excess related to compromised regulatory mechanism
• Impaired gas exchange related to disease process

INFANT

Choanal Atresia

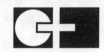

DEFINITION

Choanal atresia is a congenital malformation of the respiratory tract in which the choanae (posterior nares opening into the nasopharynx) are obstructed by a membranous or bony structure covering the openings. One or both nares may be affected, with partial or complete obstruction.

Because the neonate is an obligate nose breather, this malformation causes severe respiratory distress by preventing the infant from inspiring air.

This plan focuses on the identification and immediate care of the infant before surgical correction.

ETIOLOGY AND PRECIPITATING FACTORS
• cause unknown

PHYSICAL FINDINGS
Infant status at birth
• able to take first breath through mouth, with further attempts at breathing difficult or impossible

• experiences severe retractions and cyanosis from air hunger when not crying; symptoms disappear when infant cries because he can then breathe through mouth

Integumentary
• pink color when crying, blue color when not crying

Pulmonary
• thick, mucus-filled nose
• catheter cannot be passed through nose
• suprasternal and substernal retractions
• snorting respirations

DIAGNOSTIC STUDIES
• X-ray of head or neck—to determine abnormality

Collaborative problem: *Ventilatory insufficiency related to obstruction from congenital defect*

GOAL: Establish and maintain airway patency and support respiratory efforts.

Interventions

1. Insert size 0 or 00 oral airway.

2. Perform endotracheal intubation if airway is not maintained by oral airway.

3. Assess respiratory efficiency, including:
• continued crying since delivery
• pink color when crying and cyanotic when not crying
• accumulation of nasal secretions.
• arching of head and neck on attempt to breathe
• retractions on inspiration.

4. Position infant with head of the bed elevated.

5. Prepare and assist with examination by otolaryngologist.

6. Prepare infant for surgery to correct defect.

7. Additional individualized interventions: _____

Rationales

1. This immediate intervention allows for mouth breathing when nares are obstructed.

2. Intubation is necessary to accommodate breathing and to prepare infant for surgery.

3. Neonatal unit nurse may be first to differentiate choanal atresia from other respiratory distress problems.

4. Elevating the head of the bed improves air exchange.

5. In rare cases, examination and puncture of the obstruction, if it is caused by a membrane only, may be done.

6. Surgery is necessary to achieve airway patency (see Preoperative Care plan, page 263).

7. Rationales: _____

Nursing diagnosis: *Ineffective family coping: compromised related to anxiety, guilt, and emotional conflict as a result of infant's defect*

GOAL: Promote understanding and a comfortable adjustment to infant's condition and needs in crisis situation.

Interventions

1. Allow and encourage parental expression of feelings and fears about loss of the "perfect child."

2. Reinforce the infant's normal and healthy aspects and the possibility that surgery will correct the defect, leaving no visible effects.

3. Encourage parents to hold and cuddle the infant and to give care as appropriate. Support their efforts to do so.

4. Provide accurate information regarding:
• condition of infant and symptoms that must be observed
• etiology, prevalence, and nature of defect
• equipment used and procedures performed on infant
• rationales for care being given
• preparation for surgery and care after surgery, if anticipated.

5. Allow time for questions about and discussion of the prognosis and the infant's needs.

6. Additional individualized interventions: _____

_____

Rationales

1. Expression of feelings helps promote trust and decrease parental anxiety.

2. Positive reinforcement helps reduce sadness and increase positive feelings about possible correction of the problem.

3. Involving parents in care promotes bonding and development of parent-child relationship.

4. Accurate information reduces parental anxiety and maximizes understanding.

5. Open discussion reinforces information given and parents' ability to cope with crisis.

6. Rationales: _____

_____

ASSOCIATED PLANS
• Postoperative Care
• Preoperative Care

ADDITIONAL NURSING DIAGNOSES
• Altered nutrition: less than body requirements related to inability to ingest feedings while breathing through mouth
• Altered parenting related to interruption in bonding process
• Dysfunctional grieving (parental) related to loss of the perfect child
• Fear (parental) related to impending surgery and possible loss of child
• Knowledge deficit (parental) related to lack of information

Circumcision

DEFINITION

Circumcision is the surgical removal of the prepuce— commonly known as the foreskin—from the glans penis. The procedure is done within the first few days after birth (usually after 24 hours), and after the infant's physiologic status stabilizes. The procedure may be postponed because of neonatal illnesses, congenital anomalies, or prematurity. In the Jewish faith, circumcision is performed as a religious custom on the 8th day after birth during a ceremony called a bris; it is performed by a specially trained individual called a mohel.

Controversy exists about the medical value of circumcision. Those favoring it argue that it enhances hygiene, reduces the risk of urinary tract infections, and decreases the risk of phimosis, cancer of the penis, and cancer of the cervix in partners. Some believe circumcision also reduces the risk of sexually transmitted diseases. Those opposing circumcision argue that it presents an unnecessary risk to the infant and reduces sexual gratification later in life. The American Academy of Pediatrics states that there is no absolute medical indication for the procedure based on current research findings. The procedure is done at the parents' request and requires a signed consent form that includes information about advantages and disadvantages of the procedure.

This plan focuses on infant care after a circumcision and on prevention of complications during the healing process.

ETIOLOGY AND PRECIPITATING FACTORS

• a common practice in the United States associated with social pressure, cosmetic purposes, custom, or cultural beliefs
• a religious ritual for those practicing Judaism

PHYSICAL FINDINGS
Family and maternal history
• religious affiliation
• no bleeding disorders, such as hemophilia
• no maternal medications, such as aspirin or anticoagulants

Infant status at birth
• prematurity and gestational age (infant should be full term)
• birth weight of 5 lb, 8 oz (2,500 g) or more
• vital signs within normal ranges
• administration of vitamin K to enhance blood coagulation

Genitourinary
• normal genitalia with testes in scrotal sac
• absence of congenital abnormalities, such as epispadias, hypospadias, ambiguous genitalia, hydrocele, inguinal hernia

DIAGNOSTIC STUDIES
Laboratory data
• hematocrit (HCT) and hemoglobin (Hb)—levels must be within normal range (48% to 60% for HCT; 16 to 20 g/dl for Hb) for procedure to be done
• clotting time—5 to 8 minutes (normal) unless coagulation abnormality is present
• blood testing—not needed for normal neonate unless a problem existed during birth or signs and symptoms that warrant investigation are present.

Nursing diagnosis: *Pain related to trauma of surgical incision and irritation to incision from urine or diaper*

GOAL: Minimize or reduce pain.

Interventions

1. Assess infant for pain characteristics, including:
• total body movement
• loud crying.

2. Remove infant from restraining apparatus (Circumstraint) immediately after completion of the procedure, and hold and cuddle him. Dress and feed infant, speaking in soft, calm voice. Allow parents to hold and caress infant.

Rationales

1. Although controversy exists over how mature the infant's neurologic system is, pain perception seems to exist based on reactions to painful stimuli.

2. Reactions to pain usually stop when caregiver or parent provides distractions.

Interventions

3. Perform comfort measures, including:

• applying diapers loosely and changing them frequently after each voiding or soiling.
• applying petrolatum dressing around surgical site for first 24 hours and replacing dressing as needed at diaper change
• applying oxidizing cellulose (Oxycel).
• placing infant on his side, not abdomen, for the first 24 hours.
• avoiding contact of incision with soaps, alcohol, or lotions.

4. Assess for continued reactions of infant after procedure, including:
• altered crying and irritability
• feeding pattern changes
• sleeping pattern changes
• urinary pattern changes.

5. Additional individualized interventions: _____

Rationales

3. Such noninvasive measures usually promote comfort in the infant.
• Burning and irritation result when incision comes in contact with urine or stool or rubs against diaper.
• Petrolatum dressings protect incision from urine and prevent diaper from sticking to incision.

• Oxycel enhances clotting when bleeding persists.
• Positioning infant on his side prevents pressure on and irritation to the site.
• Using soap or other cleaning agents or alcohol causes burning and irritation.

4. Circumcision, considered a stressful procedure for infants, may result in behavior changes because of discomfort for up to 12 hours. Identifying changes allows for interventions to prevent complications.

5. Rationales: _____

Nursing diagnosis: *High risk for infection related to break in primary defense (skin) because of invasive procedure (2 goals)*

GOAL 1: Recognize early signs and symptoms of infection.

Interventions

1. Assess for possible infection of surgical site.

• Observe for redness, purulent drainage, and edema with each diaper change after removal of petrolatum dressing.
• Check for foul odor.
• Take axillary temperature every 4 hours.

• Review platelet count and white blood cell (WBC) count for decrease and differential for changes, especially in neutrophils, which indicate infection.

2. Additional individualized interventions: _____

Rationales

1. Because of infant's underdeveloped immune systems, they are susceptible to infection. Early recognition of signs and symptoms allows for early treatment and prevention of complications.

• Redness or purulent drainage indicates infectious process. Yellowish exudate around site is normal healing by granulation and should not be disturbed.
• Odor indicates possible infection at circumcision site.
• An unstable temperature, even a low temperature of 96° to 97° F (35.5° to 36.1° C), may indicate infection. An elevated temperature may be the result of infection or of excess blankets, clothing, or hats (an infant cannot get rid of excess heat because sweating capability is poorly developed). Thus, elevated temperature may be from infection or other causes.
• Deviations from normal may indicate infection. Normal levels for a full-term infant are:
    □ platelets—100,000 to 300,000/mm³
    □ WBC count—15,000/mm³
    □ neutrophils—45%
    □ basophils and eosinophils—3%
    □ lymphocytes—30%
    □ monocytes—5%.

2. Rationales: _____

GOAL 2: Prevent infection at circumcision site and promote healing.

Interventions	**Rationales**
1. Assess incision for healing and cleanliness; make sure that plastic bell is in place, if used.	1. Complete healing usually takes 7 to 10 days with proper care. If plastic bell method is used, prepuce and bell will drop off in 1 to 2 weeks.
2. Carry out proper handwashing before attending infant. Wash hands with a povidone-iodine preparation before entering nursery.	2. Proper handwashing prevents cross-contamination, which may transmit infectious organisms to infant.
3. Wear gown in nursery when caring for infant.	3. By wearing a gown, caregiver protects infant from exposure to infectious agents.
4. Clean penis with clear, warm water and soft sponge as needed.	4. Careful cleaning removes contaminants, such as urine and feces. Antiseptics usually are not needed.
5. Monitor urinary pattern for return of urination within 8 hours after procedure.	5. Edema or inflammation from the procedure may cause inability to void.
6. Additional individualized interventions: _____	6. Rationales: _____

Nursing diagnosis: *High risk for fluid volume deficit related to blood loss secondary to hemorrhage from incisional area*

GOAL: Prevent hemorrhage from circumcision site.

Interventions	**Rationales**
1. Assess circumcision for amount of bleeding, hourly for first 12 hours, then every 2 hours.	1. Some bleeding and oozing are normal for a new circumcision. Excess bleeding may indicate a decrease in clotting factors, a possible clotting disorder, or another condition that requires prompt attention.
2. Report continued oozing of blood or failure to form clot.	2. Continued bleeding may require suturing to stop bleeding or local hemostatic material to enhance clotting.
3. Take blood pressure and pulse rate if bleeding continues. Note decreases. Base estimate of blood loss on weight and blood pressure changes.	3. Blood volume averages 90 ml/kg in a full-term infant, an estimated 25% in volume is reduced with each 50% decline in blood pressure. Acute blood loss of more than 10% volume must be replaced, so careful monitoring and correction of bleeding are essential to prevent complications.
4. Cover site with petrolatum dressing. Avoid using a dry dressing.	4. Petrolatum dressings prevent dried blood from sticking to diaper, which may cause bleeding when diaper is removed and changed.
5. If dressing or diaper is stuck, loosen with warm sterile water to soften before attempting to remove it.	5. This technique prevents disturbance of clot by pulling, which causes subsequent bleeding.
6. Additional individualized interventions: _____	6. Rationales: _____

Nursing diagnosis: *Knowledge deficit (parental) related to care of circumcision and prevention of complications*

GOAL: Provide information to parents about the care of circumcised infant, with emphasis on preventing complications and on the healing process.

Interventions

1. Demonstrate the following procedures and allow for return demonstration by parents:

• Gently clean infant with warm water to remove feces and urine, wiping from front to back or away from circumcision.

• Apply petrolatum dressing as needed during diaper change, unless plastic bell is used.

• Change diaper after each voiding, and apply loosely.

• If dressing becomes stuck or dry, moisten it with warm sterile water before attempting removal.

• Position infant on his side for 24 hours after procedure.

2. Inform parents about possible complications to report, such as:
• excessive bleeding, foul odor, pus, or drainage at circumcision site
• failure to heal completely in 7 to 10 days regardless of method used.

3. Additional individualized interventions: _____

_____

Rationales

1. Hands-on experience by parents will increase their comfort level and feeling of competence in caring for the circumcised infant.

• Some parents may have fears about handling the penis during cleaning; practice will help reassure them that they will not harm the infant.

• Petrolatum dressing promotes comfort and cleanliness by preventing irritation or pain from contact with urine or feces.

• Applying diaper loosely avoids irritation and pressure on circumcision site.

• Moistening prevents discomfort or possible bleeding when diaper is removed.

• Side-lying position prevents discomfort and irritation because of pressure from diaper.

2. Awareness of potential complications associated with infection or hemorrhage provides for prompt reporting and for immediate intervention. Most circumcisions heal in 4 to 7 days; if a plastic bell is used, the foreskin and the bell covering the glans penis will fall away when healing is completed.

3. Rationales: _____

_____

ASSOCIATED PLANS
All plans have applications for the care of the infant who may develop abnormal conditions. For specific information, refer to the appropriate plans.

ADDITIONAL NURSING DIAGNOSES
• Altered urinary elimination related to meatal inflammation and edema resulting from trauma of surgical procedure
• Fear (parental) related to care of circumcised infant

Cleft Lip and Cleft Palate

DEFINITION

Cleft lip and cleft palate are the two most common forms of facial malformations. Cleft lip occurs in 1 of every 700 to 800 births and cleft palate, in 1 of every 2,500 births. Both malformations may accompany other birth defects, such as spina bifida, heart defects, extra fingers or toes, fusing together of fingers or toes, or talipes deformity. The abnormality may involve clefts of the lip and the palate, cleft of the lip only, cleft of the hard or soft palate only, or bilateral deformities.

Cleft lip with or without cleft palate — cosmetically the most distressing of the two abnormalities — develops when the maxillary prominence fails to fuse with the nasal elevations, causing failure of nostril and upper lip formation. Cleft lip develops during the 6th to 8th week of gestation and may be unilateral, involving one nasal cavity, or bilateral, involving both. It may involve the lip only or extend to the nose.

Cleft palate occurs during formation of the fetal neck and jaws and develops when downward movement of the tongue is delayed, causing a failure of the palate, to fuse above the tongue to form the roof of the mouth. Cleft palate develops during the 7th to 12th week of gestation and may be partial or complete. It may affect only the soft palate and uvula or may extend to the hard palate. The malformation interferes with feeding and speech development.

Cleft lip with or without cleft palate is more common in boys; cleft palate is more common in girls. Treatment is accomplished by team approach with nurse, pediatrician, orthodontist, speech therapist, plastic surgeon, and psychologist contributing to care.

This plan focuses on care of the infant with one or both of these defects before surgical intervention. Surgical correction of cleft lip usually occurs from 6 weeks to 8 months after birth; sometimes it is performed immediately. Correction of cleft palate occurs between ages 1 and 2; time of correction depends on the infant's condition, parental acceptance, and surgeon's preference.

ETIOLOGY AND PRECIPITATING FACTORS

• actual cause unknown; believed to be the result of inherited factors, mutant genes, or chromosomal abnormalities
• environmental factors — such as medications or teratogens ingested during a critical period of pregnancy or maternal exposure to radiation or infection — may play a role

PHYSICAL FINDINGS
Family history
• family member or relative with cleft lip or cleft palate

Infant status at birth
• visible unilateral or bilateral cleft lip
• mouth examination reveals visible cleft palate involving soft or hard palate with opening between mouth and nasal cavity

Gastrointestinal
• difficulty sucking (with cleft lip and cleft palate)

Nursing diagnosis: *Altered nutrition: less than body requirements related to inability to ingest food because of difficulty sucking (2 goals)*

GOAL 1: Recognize early signs of inadequate nutrition.

Interventions

1. Assess nutritional status and needs, including:

• sucking or swallowing ability

• daily caloric and fluid intake

• daily weight gain or loss.

Rationales

1. Infant's appetite is not affected by defect, but the ability to suck properly is impaired, so intake may be reduced.

• Infant may be unable to form adequate seal for sucking.

• Documented daily intake helps determine whether infant is meeting nutritional needs or whether feeding method needs to be changed, possibly to gastric gavage.

• Monitoring weight daily evaluates success of feeding pattern and reveals optimal weight gain desired or need for change in feeding method to minimize weight loss.

Interventions

2. Additional individualized interventions: _____

Rationales

2. Rationales: _____

GOAL 2: Facilitate and maintain nutritional status.

Interventions

1. Based on assessment, calculate minimum calories per kilogram per day and milliliters per kilogram per day of feeding needed.

2. Facilitate breast-feeding as follows:

• Instruct mother to massage breast and nipples before nursing.

• Apply pressure to areola with fingers, guide nipple to side of infant's mouth, and hold it there during feeding.

• Allow extra feeding time.

• Burp infant frequently during feeding.

• Hold infant in upright or sitting position while feeding.

• If infant cannot breast-feed, encourage mother to pump breasts and feed infant with bottle.

3. Facilitate bottle-feeding as follows:

• Hold infant in upright or near-sitting position during feeding.

• Select a nipple with a flange, Lamb's nipple (big and soft with large holes), regular preterm nipple with large holes, Breck feeder (rubber-tipped Asepto syringe), or soft plastic bottle to squeeze formula into infant's mouth.

• Place nipple at side or back of infant's tongue.

• Thicken milk with small amount of cereal.

• Feed infant small amounts slowly, and burp infant after each 10 to 15 ml of milk.

• Refrain from removing nipple from infant's mouth if not necessary.

• Give some water after feeding.

• Gently wipe milk away from face and nose with damp cloth, and pat dry.

4. Additional individualized interventions: _____

Rationales

1. This provides nutritional requirements for infant (see Appendix 8: Fluid and Nutritional Needs in Infancy).

2. Infant with cleft palate may or may be able to breast-feed; infant with cleft lip may be able to breast-feed if cleft doesn't affect sucking.

• Massaging breast and nipples brings milk near surface for ease in sucking and hardens breast, helping infant to hold nipple in mouth.

• Holding nipple in infant's mouth allows infant to nurse with gums rather than by sucking if sucking is difficult.

• Feeding may take up to 1½ hours.

• Infant swallows more air during feedings.

• Holding infant in upright or sitting position enhances swallowing and prevents milk from coming through defect and out of nose, thus decreasing risk of aspiration.

• Pumping breast milk satisfies mother's desire to breast-feed and provides an excellent source of nourishment.

3. Safe bottle-feeding maintains infant's nutritional status.

• Holding infant in upright or near-sitting position reduces risk of aspiration and of swallowing air.

• Various feeding devices may be used; mother may have to experiment to find the most suitable for infant, depending on defect.

• Placing nipple at side or back of infant's tongue avoids cleft and enhances swallowing.

• Thicker milk allows for easier swallowing because of increased gravity flow.

• Feeding slowly and burping infant regularly prevent regurgitation or vomiting by expelling air that is swallowed when feeding.

• Removing nipple may cause infant to cry, making feeding more difficult.

• Water rinses milk away from mouth and defect.

• Wiping removes milk that may have entered and drained from nose.

4. Rationales: _____

SPECIAL FEEDING DEVICES

Various devices, shown below, may be used to feed an infant with cleft lip or cleft palate.

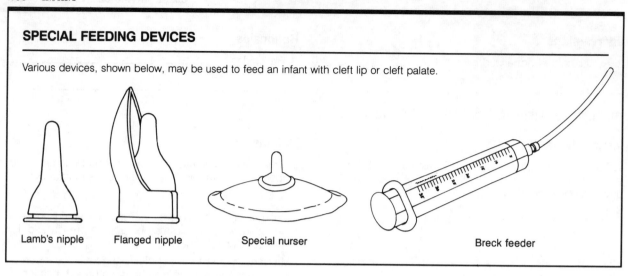

Lamb's nipple   Flanged nipple   Special nurser   Breck feeder

Nursing diagnosis: *Ineffective airway clearance related to possible aspiration of secretions or milk as result of defect*

GOAL: Promote and maintain airway clearance.

Interventions

1. Assess respiratory status, including:
• rate, depth, and effort
• dyspnea and cyanosis
• nasal flaring and chest retractions
• breath sounds
• skin color
• capillary refill.

2. Observe for abdominal distention.

3. Carefully suction oropharynx and nasopharynx when needed.

4. Position infant on abdomen or side.

5. Feed infant in upright position, and elevate head of crib 30 degrees after feedings.

6. Place infant in mist tent with cool air.

7. Additional individualized interventions: _____

_____

Rationales

1. Assessment provides data about respiratory status and function. Aspiration of secretions or milk can cause tachypnea, abnormal breath sounds, bluish skin, or delayed capillary filling from decreased oxygenation.

2. Distention, resulting from swallowed air, will compromise respirations.

3. Suctioning removes excess liquids and secretions in hypopharynx.

4. These positions prevent infant's tongue from falling back and obstructing airway.

5. This positioning prevents aspiration of milk.

6. Mist tent keeps secretions loose.

7. Rationales: _____

_____

Nursing diagnosis: *Altered oral mucous membrane related to defect and retention of formula in oral cavity*

GOAL: Protect and maintain tissue integrity of oral mucous membrane.

Interventions

1. Assess for impairment, by observing:
• reddened, tender areas on lip or palate
• formula in oral cavity or crust formation.

Rationales

1. Impairment may cause irritation or inflammation of mucous membrane.

Interventions

2. Clean cleft lip with small amount of water (or 0.45% sodium chloride and hydrogen peroxide) after each feeding.

3. Apply small amount of cream or baby oil to infant's lips.

4. Report persistent irritation for further treatment.

5. Additional individualized interventions: _____

_____

Rationales

2. Cleaning rinses away milk after feeding. Hydrogen peroxide solution has bactericidal cleaning action.

3. Cream or oil prevents drying and cracking.

4. Persistent irritation may lead to infection if mucosa breaks down.

5. Rationales: _____

_____

Nursing diagnosis: *Ineffective family coping: compromised related to anxiety, guilt, or emotional conflict as a result of infant's defect (2 goals)*

GOAL 1: Promote trusting relationship so that adaptation process can begin.

Interventions

1. Encourage and allow parental expression of feelings and fears about caring for infant, what others might say, or loss of the "perfect child."

2. Allow parents to see and hold infant as soon after birth as possible, after obstetrician has informed them of the defect.

3. Allow parents to grieve the loss of the perfect child.

4. Reinforce infant's normal and healthy aspects when interacting with parents.

5. Handle infant in caring manner, and encourage parents to hold and cuddle infant.

6. Allow for open visitation with infant when desired, encouraging parents' active role in giving care.

7. Encourage participation in support groups for parents of infants with congenital defects.

8. Additional individualized interventions: _____

_____

Rationales

1. Society places great importance on physical appearance; impairment causes parental shock, guilt, and disappointment.

2. Delay in seeing infant may heighten parents' anxiety and sadness.

3. Grieving may help parents to accept the child with a defect.

4. Reinforcement helps to reduce parents' sadness and anger and to begin their adaptation to the crisis.

5. Careful handling promotes bonding process and infant's normal social and emotional development.

6. Visits promote flexible, secure environment for development of parent-child relationship.

7. Group members offer support and a positive view of the treatment outcome.

8. Rationales: _____

_____

GOAL 2: Promote parental understanding of infant's defect.

Interventions

1. Assess parents' (or family's) understanding of cleft lip and cleft palate.

2. Assure parents in a positive way that the defect can be repaired with surgery.

3. Provide information regarding:

• infant's condition, its causes and prevalence, and the nature of the defect

Rationales

1. Assessment reveals their need for information, the kind of information, and past misinformation.

2. Providing this information in a calm, positive way reassures the parents that the defect can be corrected and assists in the grieving process.

3. Information maximizes parents' understanding of defect.

• Explaining infant's condition helps resolve parents' guilt feelings about defect.

Interventions

• infant's short-term needs, such as feeding

• infant's long-term problems, such as impaired speech, dental problems, upper respiratory tract and ear infections, and possible need for surgery.

4. Allow parents to ask as many questions as they would like.

5. Additional individualized interventions: _____

Rationales

• This reduces anxiety about the most difficult problem in caring for infant.

• This prepares parents for long-term health needs. The palate is essential to speech formation, and changes in structure—even after surgery—may permanently affect speech. Mouth breathing may cause changes in shape of the mouth and dental problems, with need to straighten teeth and correct shape of jaw. Middle ear infections from failure of eustachian tube to drain may contribute to hearing loss. Upper respiratory tract infections are common. Depending on deformity, subsequent surgeries may be needed for additional revisions.

4. The more questions parents ask, the better able they will be to adapt.

5. Rationales: _____

Nursing diagnosis: *Knowledge deficit (parental) related to feeding of infant and surgical procedure to correct defect*

GOAL: Provide appropriate information regarding feeding and defect repair.

Interventions

1. Inform parents of general timing of surgical repair and what to expect from infant. Show them before and after photographs of surgically repaired cleft lips.

2. Instruct parents in breast- or bottle-feeding techniques, whichever method is applicable.

3. Instruct parents in procedures to perform before surgery, including:

• avoiding nipple feeding unless specifically ordered by plastic surgeon. Instead, feed by syringe with 1" to 2" of latex tubing attached, or feed with Breck feeder.

• using restraints, such as jackets with pockets for tongue-depressor splints, to hold arms straight and away from mouth, or applying commercially available restraints, until suture line heals.

• periodically positioning infant on back (using infant seat) so he can be closely observed for excessive secretions.

4. Instruct parents in postoperative care measures, including:

• incision care

Rationales

1. If weight is optimal and other neonatal anomalies are ruled out, cleft lip may be repaired shortly after birth to minimize parents' shame or embarrassment; or it may be repaired in 2 to 3 months or as late as 8 months to allow for bonding and to rule out other congenital anomalies. Cleft palate may be repaired in two steps by 12 to 16 months; or repair of soft palate may proceed in 6 to 18 months and repair of hard palate, as late as age 5. Timing of procedures is related to normal growth changes and repair before speech development.

2. Proper feeding technique helps maintain infant's nutritional status without complications.

3. A few days before surgery, introduction of care techniques will help infant adapt to restrictions.

• Teaching parents how to feed infant by non-nipple devices prevents injury to surgical site.

• Restrictive positioning prevents disturbance of suture line.

• Back position is position of choice to maintain respiratory function after surgery.

4. Providing information helps dispel parents' anxiety and promotes their compliance in aiding infant's recovery.

• Cleaning the incision aids healing of the suture line.

Interventions	Rationales
• dietary modifications	• Dietary modifications help meet infant's nutritional needs while maintaining integrity of the suture line.
• avoidance of sucking and blowing	• Sucking and blowing put stress on the suture line.
• avoidance of placing silverware or straws into infant's mouth	• Inserting objects into the mouth could traumatize the suture line.
• rinsing of oral cavity with sterile water after feeding.	• Rinsing the oral cavity removes residual food or fluids, which could irritate the incisional area and lead to infection.
5. Refer parents to community and home health care resources.	5. Referrals help the parents and family with continued physical and emotional support outside the hospital.
6. Use pamphlets to illustrate procedure, suture lines, fading scar, and appliance used (Logan bow).	6. Illustrations show what to expect and possible outcomes.
7. Additional individualized interventions: _____	7. Rationales: _____

ASSOCIATED PLANS AND APPENDICES
• Postoperative Care
• Preoperative Care
• Skin Disorders
• Fluid and Nutritional Needs in Infancy (Appendix 8)
• Parent Teaching Guides (Appendix 12)

ADDITIONAL NURSING DIAGNOSES
• Altered home maintenance related to care of infant with defect
• Dysfunctional grieving (parental) related to loss of the perfect child
• High risk for altered parenting related to crisis of having infant with defect or interruption in parental bonding process
• High risk for infection related to trauma to oral mucosa as result of improper feeding technique
• Ineffective infant feeding pattern related to physical defect

Congenital Heart Disease

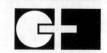

DEFINITION

Congenital heart disease (cardiovascular malformation at birth) is found in 8 to 10 of every 1,000 neonates. One-third also have noncardiac anomalies. In infants with a birth weight of less than 5 lb, 8 oz (2,500 g), incidence of congenital heart disease is as high as 16%.

Cardiac defects most commonly identified during the first weeks of an infant's life are transposition of the great vessels, hypoplastic left heart syndrome, tetralogy of Fallot, pulmonary atresia, patent ductus arteriosus (PDA), coarctation of the aorta, ventricular septal defect (VSD), and combined defects. Noncardiac anomalies associated with cardiac defects include chromosomal syndromes, such as trisomy 13, 18, or 21; Turner's, Hunter's, DiGeorge's, Marfan's, Williams, or Laurence-Moon-Biedl syndrome; abnormalities of the skeleton, skin, muscles, gastrointestinal tract, or renal system; and visceral malformations and malpositions.

Heart defects are classified as cyanotic (high-risk infant) and acyanotic (low-risk infant). Cyanotic defects cause an interference or shunting in the pulmonary blood flow, producing desaturation of hemoglobin because insufficient blood is moving through the lungs to oxygenate it. This, rather than a lack of circulation to peripheral tissue, causes the infant's blue appearance. (For descriptions, see *Cyanotic heart defects*.)

Acyanotic defects allow for a flow of oxygenated blood to the body with no cyanosis because shunting either does not occur or occurs from a high-pressured left side to a low-pressured right side. Acyanotic defects are more common than cyanotic defects. When using this classification, note that lesions that may potentially cause cyanosis do not always do so. In acyanotic defects, signs and symptoms may be absent if the defect is small and the heart can compensate for the increased workload. If the defect is more severe, the infant may become cyanotic if pulmonary vascular changes take place or if he has secondary defects. (For descriptions, see *Acyanotic heart defects*, page 172.)

Cyanosis in the first hours or days of life usually results from transposition of the great vessels, tricuspid atresia, tetralogy of Fallot, truncus arteriosus, or congestive heart failure occurring because of hypoplastic left heart syndrome, severe coarctation of the aorta, interrupted aortic arch, severe aortic stenosis, or a combination of shunt lesions.

This plan focuses on care of the infant with congenital heart disease and clinical manifestations specific to the particular defect before surgical correction or palliative intervention.

ETIOLOGY AND PRECIPITATING FACTORS

• thought to be caused by multifactorial inheritance, which is a combination of genetic, environmental, and intrauterine factors, accounting for higher risk among infants who have a parent or sibling with a congenital heart defect
• associated with maternal diseases, such as rubella during first 8 weeks of pregnancy, diabetes mellitus, and alcoholism
• associated with drugs taken by mother during pregnancy, such as hydantoin, alcohol, and trimethadione

PHYSICAL FINDINGS
Maternal history
• high-altitude birth
• congenital heart disease or previous child with congenital heart defect
• drugs taken during pregnancy

Infant status at birth
• preterm or full-term, low birth weight, or small for gestational age
• visible anomaly or deformity
• cyanosis
• heart murmur
• possibly asymptomatic at birth

BEHAVIORAL FINDINGS
• irritability
• agitation
(For assessment findings, see *Cyanotic heart defects* and *Acyanotic heart defects*, page 172.)

DIAGNOSTIC STUDIES
• chest X-ray—to reveal small ventricle
• electrocardiography (ECG)—to detect abnormal changes
• cardiac catheterization—to determine abnormal communication between chambers, obstructions in vessels, chamber pressures, and oxygen saturation
• Doppler flow in color—to evaluate ductus
• M-mode echocardiography—to determine anatomy and function of the circulation, including valve motion, great vessel size and location, location and size of chambers, and left ventricle function
• contrast echocardiography—to determine location of right-to-left shunting in the heart
• two-dimensional or real-time ultrasound echocardiography—reproduces intracavitary angiograms

Laboratory data
• hyperoxygenation test—to rule out heart disease; PO_2 must exceed 100
• arterial blood gas (ABG) measurements—to determine levels of pH, $PaCO_2$, PaO_2, and HCO_3 and changes resulting from cardiac or pulmonary disease
• electrolyte analysis (of potassium, sodium, and chloride)—to detect changes in congestive heart failure

CYANOTIC HEART DEFECTS

The chart below describes the major cyanotic heart defects and associated assessment findings.

Defect	Description	Assessment findings
Tetralogy of Fallot	• Defect is a combination of four defects: ventricular septal defect (VSD), overriding aorta, pulmonic stenosis, and right ventricular hypertrophy. • Unoxygenated blood shunts through VSD, mixing with oxygenated blood in left ventricle. Cyanosis results. • Pulmonary blood flow is restricted by pulmonic stenosis, causing increased pressure in and hypertrophy of right ventricle as it attempts to shunt blood through restricted pulmonary valve.	*If severe:* • Cyanosis with hypoxic spells (increases after patent ductus arteriosus [PDA] closes) • Murmur associated with blood flow through pulmonary valve • Aortic ejection click with larger aorta • Dyspnea on exertion • Limpness or seizures *Later:* • Dyspnea • Clubbing of fingers and toes • Tachypnea • Fatigue • Squatting position (to relieve respiratory distress) • Growth retardation • Systolic murmur • Single second heart sound on auscultation • Thrill palpated in lower left region of sternal border
Truncus arteriosus	• Single vessel overriding ventricles (caused by failure of aorta and pulmonary artery to separate) carries blood for pulmonary and systemic circulations. • Both ventricles pump oxygenated and unoxygenated blood into common artery, causing cyanosis. • VSD also may occur.	• Cyanosis with ashen appearance • Fatigue • Dyspnea *Later:* • Systolic murmur at lower left sternal border • Single second heart sound • Tachypnea • Crackles • Growth retardation • Congestive heart failure
Tricuspid atresia	• Tricuspid valve is absent. • Blood flow is diverted from right atrium to left atrium, resulting in mixing of arterial and venous blood in left ventricle. Entry of mixed blood into circulation causes cyanosis. • Pulmonary blood flows through PDA (if present).	• Cyanosis • Dyspnea • Anoxic spells • Fatigue • Single first and second heart sounds • Absence of murmur • Pansystolic murmur with VSD • Congestive heart failure
Transposition of the great vessels	• Aorta leaves right ventricle; pulmonary artery leaves left ventricle. • Systemic circulation bypasses lungs for oxygenation; pulmonary blood flows through heart and back to lungs without entering systemic circulation.	• Cyanosis, especially during or after feeding or crying • Tachypnea • Systolic murmur or congestive heart failure with VSD • Metabolic acidosis from hypoxia • Abnormal heart sounds, depending on type of defect
Hypoplastic left heart syndrome	• Left ventricle is nonfunctional. • Pulmonary blood returns to left atrium through atrial septum to right atrium. Systemic output, carried by right-to-left flow of blood through PDA, is restricted by normal PDA closure after birth.	• Marked cyanosis • Respiratory distress with grunting • Worsening of symptoms as PDA narrows • Congestive heart failure • Death within 1 week unless wide-open PDA and atrial septal defect are present

ACYANOTIC HEART DEFECTS

The chart below describes the major acyanotic heart defects and associated assessment findings.

Defect	Description	Assessment findings
Ventricular septal defect	• Ventricular septum has abnormal opening. • Oxygenated blood from left ventricle shunts through abnormal opening and then mixes with unoxygenated blood in right atrium.	*If small:* • Murmur *If large:* • Tachypnea • Irritability • Tachycardia • Difficulty feeding • Slight cyanosis from heart failure • Dyspnea with feeding • Growth retardation
Atrial septal defect	• Atrial septum has abnormal opening (caused by improper closure of foramen ovale or atrial septal wall). • Blood passes from left atrium to right atrium through abnormal opening. • Defect occurs in three types: ostium secundum, ostium primum, and sinus venosus.	• May be asymptomatic • Dyspnea on exertion • Fatigue • Orthopnea • Transient cyanosis *Later:* • Soft, pulmonic midsystolic murmur • Growth retardation
Patent ductus arteriosus	• Defect represents failure of vascular conduit between descending aorta and pulmonary artery to close after birth. • Blood shunts from aorta to pulmonary artery.	• Continuous murmur at second and third left intercostal spaces • Widening pulse pressure • Tachycardia • Difficulty feeding • Fatigue • Weak cry *Later:* • Dyspnea
Coarctation of the aorta	• Aorta is narrowed. • Defect may be preductal (in front of area of ductus arteriosus) or postductal (behind area of ductus arteriosus).	• Increased blood pressure and bounding pulse proximal to defect • Decreased blood pressure and weak pulse distal to defect • Dizziness • Headache • Fainting • Epistaxis • Discoloration of legs • Cold feet *If severe:* • Poor weight gain • Difficulty feeding • Congestive heart failure • Possible murmur at sternal border
Pulmonic stenosis	• Blood flow from right ventricle to lungs is obstructed. • Obstruction may be above or below pulmonic valve, or defect may occur as stenosis of valve. • Resistance to blood flow, (caused by stenosis) leads to right ventricular hypertrophy.	• Dyspnea • Fatigue • Cold arms and legs • Peripheral cyanosis • Systolic ejection murmur over second left intercostal space, accompanied by systolic thrill with murmur radiating over precordium and back • Less distinct second heart sound (may disappear)
Aortic stenosis	• Aortic valve is narrowed, causing obstruction of blood flow from left ventricle and persistent fetal circulation.	*If severe:* • Faint peripheral pulses • Tachycardia • Fatigue on exertion • Pale skin • Irritability • Syncope • Angina pectoris • Diaphoresis • Epistaxis

Collaborative problem: *High risk for complications related to congenital heart disease (2 goals)*

GOAL 1: Identify the low-risk and high-risk infant with cardiac condition for signs and symptoms and complications.

Interventions

1. Assess for infant at risk for congenital heart disease by checking for the following factors:
• maternal history of congenital heart defects and such conditions as diabetes, rubella, and infections early in pregnancy; maternal drugs taken
• birth at high altitude
• presence of other congenital abnormalities.

2. Assess infant at low risk for cardiac conditions; include the following considerations:
• review of X-ray and echocardiography results
• identification of murmur and its location
• difficulty feeding (lack of energy and pauses to rest)
• pale or mottled skin
• dyspnea
• developing congestive heart failure (if defect is severe).

3. Assess infant at high risk for cardiac conditions, including:
• review of X-ray, ECG, echocardiography, cardiac catheterization, and hyperoxygenation test results
• generalized cyanosis
• respiratory distress and tachypnea
• skin mottling
• poor pulse rate and blood pressure changes
• hypotonia
• congestive heart failure with weight gain and increased central venous pressure (CVP); cool, cyanotic arms and legs; periorbital edema; and hepatomegaly
• soft murmur with single second heart sound
• ABG measurements, with hypoxemia and, possibly, mild hypercapnia generally indicating primary heart disease.

4. Additional individualized interventions: _____

Rationales

1. Assessment provides information about possible defect, if infant appears asymptomatic, or about risk for developing congenital heart disease.

2. Of infants with congenital heart diseases, 30% to 40% have ventricular septal defect. Less common, but important within the low-risk group, are atrial septal defect and patent ductus arteriosus. Pulmonic and aortic stenoses and simple coarctation of the aorta usually are not symptomatic in the first months of life; signs and symptoms depend on the severity of the defect.

3. Presenting signs and symptoms of severe cardiac disease in infant depend on the defects. Cyanosis results from intracardiac or intrapulmonary shunting of blood from right to left and indicates low arterial oxygen saturation. Respiratory distress results from pulmonary hypertension and congestion; tachypnea will result with hypoxemia and acidosis. Congestive heart failure may occur with either right- or left-ventricular failure in the infant with hepatosplenomegaly and in the infant with systemic venous congestion. Low cardiac output causes skin mottling, poor pulse rate, hypotonia even when infant is asleep, and cyanosis because of increased oxygen extraction in peripheral tissues.

4. Rationales: _____

GOAL 2: Maintain and support cardiac function and prevent congestive heart failure.

Interventions

1. Prepare and provide continued support for infant undergoing cardiac tests and procedures.

2. Prepare and administer I.V. glycoside and diuretic as appropriate and prescribed, and accurately monitor fluid intake and output.

3. Provide continuous mechanical monitoring of heart and rhythm by oscilloscope and ECG; discuss changes with physician.

Rationales

1. The caregiver's presence and continued physical support of cardiac status during diagnostic procedures decreases potential for complications.

2. These drugs are given to improve myocardial function and decrease fluid retention (see Congestive Heart Failure plan, page 177, for complete care of this complication).

3. Hemodynamic changes in CVP, pulse rate, blood pressure, and cardiac dysrhythmias must be noted continuously to prevent complications in severe cases and in infants needing surgery.

Interventions	Rationales
4. Monitor CVP and maintain it at 3 to 8 cm H_2O, unless otherwise ordered.	4. Evaluation of CVP helps assess changes in fluid volume status. CVP monitoring is not a standard procedure because of difficulty in obtaining reliable readings; an umbilical venous catheter is needed in addition to the umbilical artery catheter.
5. Monitor arterial blood pressure; note changes and discuss them with physician.	5. Blood pressure changes must be noted for indications of heart failure.
6. Monitor ABG levels, and discuss changes in PaO_2 and $PaCO_2$ levels with physician.	6. Changes indicate potential for hypoxemia and acidosis and whether problem is cardiac or pulmonary.
7. Administer oxygen by hood, nasal continuous positive airway pressure, or endotracheal tube.	7. Oxygen may be necessary to relieve respiratory distress and improve ventilation and perfusion.
8. Place infant in semi-Fowler's position.	8. Semi-Fowler's position is more comfortable and promotes diaphragmatic movement and lung expansion.
9. Maintain infant's temperature at 98.6° F (37° C).	9. Maintaining a neutral thermal environment prevents excessive oxygen consumption.
10. Prepare infant for surgery if emergency procedure for duct-dependent lesions is indicated.	10. In life-threatening conditions related to heart defects, immediate surgery may be performed (see Preoperative Care plan, page 263).
11. Additional individualized interventions: _____	11. Rationales: _____

Nursing diagnosis: *Altered nutrition: less than body requirements related to poor feeding as result of lack of energy*

GOAL: Improve and maintain nutritional requirements.

Interventions	Rationales
1. Use soft nipple with larger holes.	1. Soft nipple facilitates flow and reduces need for infant to suck harder to feed (causing fatigue).
2. Allow infant to feed for short time in the upright position; pause, continue to feed, and then pause again for short periods.	2. Shortened feeding periods allow infant to rest between sucking and expending energy. Upright positioning promotes lung expansion.
3. Feed for 30 minutes; if infant cannot finish, discontinue bottle feedings and initiate gavage feedings.	3. Gavage feedings assure adequate nutrition for infant whose long-term outcome may be growth retardation.
4. Additional individualized interventions: _____	4. Rationales: _____

Nursing diagnosis: *High risk for activity intolerance related to fatigue and dyspnea on exertion*

GOAL: Promote activity and rest according to limitations.

Interventions	Rationales
1. Take measures to minimize infant's energy expenditure.	1. Energy expenditure affects cardiac output and increases the metabolic demand for oxygen.

Interventions

• Refrain from handling infant more than required.
• Do not wake infant for feedings or care procedures.
• Anticipate infant needs to minimize crying.
• Allow rest periods during feeding or other essential care.

2. Additional individualized interventions: _____

Rationales

2. Rationales: _____

Nursing diagnosis: *Anticipatory grieving (parental) related to potential loss of infant*

GOAL: Assist parents with constructive grieving process for sick infant.

Interventions

1. Allow for parental expression of feelings, concerns, fears, anger, and guilt; allow for shock, denial, and feeling of loss of the "perfect child" envisioned during pregnancy.

2. Identify signs and symptoms of anticipatory grieving, including:
• feelings of sadness
• irritability
• crying or depression
• inability to eat or sleep
• constant thinking about infant
• withdrawal.

3. Provide a quiet, accepting environment, using listening and touch techniques when appropriate.

4. Offer open visiting privileges and participation in care, if feasible.

5. Provide information about infant's condition, care, progress, and potential outcomes.

6. Provide support from clergy or others with similar problem, as acceptable to parents.

7. Avoid judgmental attitudes when interacting with parents who are angry, critical, or sad.

8. Additional individualized interventions: _____

Rationales

1. Expression of feelings helps acknowledge shock and normal grieving process for potential loss of infant or for long-term care and responsibilities.

2. These signs and symptoms indicate that the grief process is taking place.

3. A quiet, attentive atmosphere shows caring and fosters trust.

4. Open visitation promotes bonding and infant-parent relationship and offers needed time with infant.

5. This helps allay parental fears of unknown and reinforces hope for recovery.

6. Empathetic support assists parents in the grieving process.

7. Nonjudgmental attitudes assure parents that their behaviors are normal.

8. Rationales: _____

Nursing diagnosis: *Knowledge deficit (parental) related to lack of information regarding infant's condition, long-term care, and treatment*

GOAL: Provide appropriate information to ensure safe short-term and long-term infant care.

Interventions

1. Identify parents' knowledge needs, interest in learning, and readiness and capability to learn

Rationales

1. Learning assessment provides the basis for developing a teaching plan commensurate with parents' abilities and needs.

Interventions

2. Provide information regarding:
• infant's condition and progress
• possibility of immediate surgery
• possible surgery at later date, depending on defect and infant's condition (noting that plans may change)
• infant's need for rest and sleep
• need to minimize infant's fatigue and exertion, including directives to feed slowly and frequently with rest periods
• need to observe for cyanosis and dyspnea
• need to avoid exposing infant to respiratory infections.

3. Impart accurate and complete information about defect and what is and is not known about its cause.

4. Instruct parents in oral administration of glycoside and diuretic, including:

• name of medication, how to measure it, and amount to give

• how to add drug to formula or what formula to purchase and how to prepare it

• withholding of glycoside if infant's heart rate is less than 90 to 100 beats/minute

• need to record infant's input and output and weight daily

• need to report adverse effects of nausea, vomiting, diarrhea, and dermatitis and to discontinue medication if these reactions occur.

5. Use visual aids and pamphlets to assist in teaching; write information in language appropriate to parents.

6. Allow for questions and clarifications, including opportunities to prepare medications and to plan care.

7. Arrange for social services, community services, and home health care follow-up.

8. Additional individualized interventions: _____

_____

Rationales

2. Information makes parents feel more secure in caring for infant and reduces their anxiety about infant's future. Long-term care may place parents in chronic crisis situation.

3. Parents may feel responsible for infant's cardiac defect.

4. Instruction provides for safe administration of medications and timely reporting of effects to physician.
• Knowing drug name, dosage, and form is fundamental to safe administration.
• Infant medications should be given in liquid form.

• Lowered heart rate is sign of drug toxicity.

• These actions help monitor diuretic effect and fluid balance status.
• These are common responses to diuretic therapy, and physician should be made aware of them.

5. These teaching methods reinforce learning.

6. Repeating information may be necessary while parents are in crisis state.

7. These referrals provide parents and family with continued support before and after discharge.

8. Rationales: _____

_____

ASSOCIATED PLANS AND APPENDICES
• Congestive Heart Failure
• Postoperative Care
• Preoperative Care
• Sexually Transmitted Diseases/TORCH

ADDITIONAL NURSING DIAGNOSES
• Altered peripheral tissue perfusion related to unoxygenated blood supply reaching arms and legs
• Decreased cardiac output related to malfunction of heart and impaired blood flow as result of defect
• High risk for altered parenting related to interruption in bonding process
• High risk for injury related to invasive diagnostic procedures
• Ineffective infant breathing pattern related to dyspnea or tachypnea as result of fluid accumulation in lungs

• Ineffective individual coping (parental) related to chronic situational crisis
• Ineffective infant feeding pattern related to lack of energy and fatigue

Congestive Heart Failure

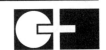

DEFINITION

Congestive heart failure (CHF) is the heart's inability to pump and circulate the oxygen and nutrients needed to maintain the metabolic requirements that sustain life. In the infant, this condition usually results from congenital defects causing fluid overload, left-to-right shunt through ductus, or surgical correction of these heart defects. The onset may occur soon after birth (in the 1st month or year, depending on the cause). A weak myocardium that can't meet normal demands as a result of asphyxia is the usual cause of CHF in the first few days after birth. Such defects as a narrowed passage or an obstruction, a fistula, or a shunt lesion hinder blood flow and increase the heart's workload, causing CHF in the first few weeks after birth.

Cardiac dysfunction activates sympathetic nervous system compensatory mechanisms, producing peripheral vasoconstriction, which diverts blood from the skin and renal circulation to the heart and brain. The decreased renal perfusion activates the angiotensin-aldosterone mechanism, causing hyperaldosteronism. The results are sodium and water retention and increased blood volume.

Ventricular dysfunction increases end-diastolic pressure and produces systemic venous or pulmonary venous engorgement, depending on which ventricle is affected. The ventricles dilate and hypertrophy. Because the infant's myocardium is less compliant and contains less contractile mass, a small increase in ventricular volume will increase the pressure, but the ventricles may be unable to hypertrophy in response to the increased pressure. This produces signs and symptoms of CHF (most often both left and right ventricular failure) with both systemic and venous engorgement resulting. Deterioration occurs more rapidly in the preterm infant than in the full-term infant because the preterm infant has even less compliance (ability to comply with changes in volume and pressure) and smaller contractile mass than the full-term infant.

Prompt treatment of CHF is necessary to maintain systemic perfusion. This plan focuses on early identification, prevention, and treatment.

ETIOLOGY AND PRECIPITATING FACTORS

• congenital heart defects, such as transposition of the great vessels, severe coarctation of the aorta, hypoplastic left or right heart syndromes, severe aortic stenosis, interrupted aortic arch, and combined defects that cause increased pressure
• such conditions as anemia, hypoglycemia, hypocalcemia, hypomagnesemia, and hypokalemia, which affect cardiac muscle fiber contractility, or respiratory distress syndrome (RDS) with hypoxia because lungs cannot keep up with tissue demands for oxygen

• handling and repair of the heart (for correction of tetralogy of Fallot or truncus arteriosus) in the older infant; temporary surgeries, such as creative shunts and pulmonary artery banding, performed on the neonate

PHYSICAL FINDINGS
Infant status at birth
• prematurity
• low Apgar score (1 to 4) with hypoxia and bluish skin
• congenital heart defect

Cardiovascular
• tachycardia with rates as high as 200 beats/minute
• peripheral vasoconstriction with cool arms and legs
• increased central venous pressure
• distended neck and, occasionally, superficial veins

Gastrointestinal
• poor feeding with prolonged feeding time and poor sucking
• propensity to fall asleep during feedings because of exhaustion
• vomiting after feedings
• gastric distention
• hepatomegaly or splenomegaly with palpable liver in severe instances

Integumentary
• pale or mottled skin and nail beds
• cyanosis
• periorbital edema and possibly peripheral edema on backs of hands and feet; dependent edema on flank and scalp

Neurologic
• restlessness and irritability
• lethargy

Pulmonary
• tachypnea and dyspnea with rates as high as 100 breaths/minute
• intercostal muscle retractions
• rhonchi and crackles on auscultation
• possible carbon dioxide retention in preterm infant receiving ventilation therapy

Renal
• oliguria or reduced urine output despite adequate fluid intake

BEHAVIORAL FINDINGS
• irritability
• agitation
• lethargy
• difficulty bonding and interacting with parent

DIAGNOSTIC STUDIES

• echocardiography, phonocardiography, and vectorcardiography—to identify heart abnormalities
• electrocardiography (ECG)—to identify dysrhythmias (after controlling CHF)
• cardiac catheterization—to determine heart abnormalities
• chest X-ray—to show heart enlargement in response to increased workload

Laboratory data

• hematocrit and hemoglobin values—to detect decreases suggesting anemia
• serum glucose analysis and Chemstrip testing—for blood glucose levels; decreases suggest hypoglycemia
• cardiac glycoside serum levels—to determine therapeutic levels of digitalis
• white blood cell count, platelet count, and neutrophil studies—to indicate possible infection
• arterial blood gas (ABG) studies—for possible acidosis
• electrolyte analysis—to identify serum sodium and potassium levels

---

Collaborative problem: *Decreased cardiac output related to decreased cardiac muscle contractility, causing CHF (3 goals)*

GOAL 1: Identify the infant at risk for or with CHF.

Interventions

1. Assess risk factors related to developing CHF:
• prematurity
• RDS and hypoxia
• congenital heart defects (note type and severity)
• surgery for heart defect
• hypoglycemia, hypocalcemia, hypokalemia, anemia, and hypomagnesemia.

2. Assess for signs and symptoms of CHF, including:

• tachycardia as high as 200 beats/minute with gallop rhythm

• oliguria (urine output range less than 0.5 to 1 ml/kg)

• pale or mottled skin and nail beds; cool arms and legs
• tachypnea and dyspnea (60 to 100 breaths/minute or more)

• intercostal muscle retractions
• crackles and rhonchi on auscultation

• cyanosis

• frothy sputum

• hepatomegaly (palpable liver below right costal margin)

• periorbital edema and edema on backs of hands and feet
• restlessness, irritability, and lethargy

Rationales

1. Risk factors and subtle signs of impending abnormal conditions, such as decreased serum glucose, calcium, hematocrit, and hemoglobin values, are a warning of CHF.

2. Assessment and identification of impending CHF allow for immediate interventions.
• Tachycardia results from sympathetic nervous system stimulation and renal compensatory mechanisms (impaired cardiac output [CO] and renal perfusion); CO varies with infant's weight but normally is about 200 ml/kg/minute.
• Renal perfusion is impaired because of decreased CO, causing reduced urine output.
• These signs result from peripheral vasoconstriction and the diversion of blood to vital organs.
• These changes result from pulmonary venous engorgement, causing decreased lung compliance. Tachypnea results from decreased oxygenation; dyspnea results from decreased ability of the lungs to distend, creating the need for additional effort in respiration (retractions).
• Retractions occur from increased effort to take in oxygen.
• Abnormal breath sounds indicate fluid accumulation in the lungs, indicating pulmonary edema.
• Cyanosis results from low oxygen saturation and decreased blood volume.
• Frothy sputum results from pulmonary effusion of fluid in alveoli.
• Hepatomegaly results from systemic venous engorgement, which increases central venous pressure and causes liver congestion.
• Edema results from fluid retained in tissues as renal perfusion is affected by decreased CO.
• Restlessness and irritability are caused by oxygen and nutrient deprivation of the tissues and organs.

Interventions

- tiring during feeding, causing prolonged feeding time and low intake
- gastric distention or vomiting after feedings.

3. Additional individualized interventions: _____

Rationales

- Sucking and breathing efforts increase metabolic demands for oxygen and exhaust the infant.
- Distention or vomiting results from air swallowed during feeding and from rapid breathing.

3. Rationales: _____

GOAL 2: Improve and maintain cardiac contractility while reducing excess intravascular fluid.

Interventions

1. Prepare and administer cardiac glycosides, such as digoxin or digitoxin, I.V.

2. Assess serum digoxin levels for evidence of toxicity and ECG changes for bradycardia. Withhold the dose and report infant heart rates ranging less than 90 to 100 beats/minute.

3. Prepare and administer a diuretic, such as furosemide (Lasix), to promote diuresis in infants with CHF.

4. Assess for effect of diuretic and for electrolyte losses. Note:

- administration time and degree of response
- serum sodium, chloride, and potassium values for decreases

- ABG or venous blood gas analysis for increased carbon dioxide levels.

5. Have sodium chloride or potassium chloride on hand to prevent hypochloremia.

6. Prepare and administer a sympathomimetic drug, such as dopamine or dobutamine, to treat low CO.

7. Prepare and administer sodium nitroprusside or nitroglycerin I.V. Either may be given with dopamine.

8. Assess patient response and prevent adverse reactions to sympathomimetic and vasodilation therapy.
- Continuously monitor heart rate and rhythm electronically.

Rationales

1. Cardiac glycosides increase the force of contractions; decrease heart rate; slow conduction of impulses via the atrioventricular node; increase renal perfusion and urine output; all of which decrease heart size, venous pressure, and edema. Their use is controversial, however, in preterm infants and may be reserved for infants age 1 month to 12 months rather than neonates.

2. The therapeutic serum digoxin level ranges from 1.1 to 2.2 ng/ml (SI: 1.1 to 2.2 nmol/liter). Toxicity is more common in preterm infants because digoxin has a longer half-life in preterm infants than in full-term infants.

3. Diuretic therapy helps reduce fluid retention. Treatment of CHF with diuretics may be preferred in the 1st week because digoxin use in preterm infants may cause toxicity.

4. The assessment data identify the patient's response to therapy, indicate whether the dosage needs to be adjusted, reveal deteriorating patient condition, and suggest whether I.V. administration of drugs is needed.
- This information reveals the effect of the drug.
- Electrolyte balance must be maintained; electrolytes are lost with water excretion resulting from diuretic effect of such drugs as furosemide.
- Changes in electrolyte levels may predispose the infant to acid-base imbalances. Hypochloremia causes an increase in base bicarbonate, and hypokalemia causes increased renal excretion of hydrogen ion; together they may cause metabolic acidosis.

5. These medications are used to prevent metabolic alkalosis and replace electrolytes. *Warning: Do not administer I.V. potassium chloride rapidly because rapid administration may cause death.*

6. An inotropic agent is used to improve urine output (in a lower dose) or to increase heart rate and contractility (in a higher dose).

7. A vasodilator treats severe heart failure by decreasing the heart's workload, thereby improving myocardial performance.

8. Continual assessment prevents adverse effects of drugs and treatment.
- Inotropic agents and vasodilators may cause tachycardia or dysrhythmias.

Interventions

• Monitor blood pressure by umbilical artery catheter and transducer with continuous readings on a screen. Keep alarm on at all times.

• Administer nitroprusside through a volume-control set with tubing covered and solution changed every 4 to 6 hours. Do not mix with other drugs. Change tubing without interrupting administration.

• Make dosage changes one drug at a time.

• Have volume expanders on hand to be given I.V. during vasodilation therapy.

• Monitor serum thiocyanate levels every 2 days for nitroprusside toxicity. Also review platelet and clotting factors.

9. Additional individualized interventions: _____

Rationales

• Accurate monitoring helps prevent hypotension from excessive vasodilation.

• Volume-control set provides safe drug administration according to agency policy.

• This action allows assessment of patient's response to each drug.

• Volume expanders treat hypovolemia.

• Nitroprusside breakdown produces thiocyanate and cyanide, decreasing the platelet count and, thus, the blood's clotting ability. The toxic level for thiocyanate is 10 mg/dl.

9. Rationales: _____

GOAL 3: Decrease cardiac and respiratory demands.

Interventions

1. Limit the infant's physical activity by minimizing handling and performing as few procedures as safely possible.

2. Maintain a thermoneutral environment by:
• monitoring temperature radially or electronically
• providing a radiant warmer or an incubator.

3. Maintain optimal respiratory function by:
• elevating the infant's head to semi-Fowler's position or using an infant seat if appropriate
• providing supplemental warmed and humidified oxygen by mask, with nasal prongs for adequate fraction of oxygen in inspired air
• placing a padded roll under the infant's shoulders for support.

4. Additional individualized interventions: _____

Rationales

1. Limited handling preserves the infant's energy (needed for feeding), minimizes metabolic oxygen demands, and prevents dyspnea, which occurs with exertion.

2. Because the infant has little subcutaneous fat to maintain its body temperature, a thermoneutral environment reduces the infant's need to consume more oxygen to maintain body temperature.

3. Semi-Fowler's position decreases the infant's breathing effort by allowing greater chest expansion. Oxygen relieves cyanosis and respiratory distress, and padding beneath the infant's shoulders extends the airway to ease breathing.

4. Rationales: _____

Nursing diagnosis: *Fluid volume excess related to compromised cardiac function*

GOAL: Promote fluid balance.

Interventions

1. Assist in promoting and assessing fluid loss by:
• weighing the infant once or twice daily at the same time and on the same scale
• measuring and recording fluid intake and output (including weighing diapers)
• including all methods of fluid intake and output in comparisons

Rationales

1. Daily weights are a good indicator of fluid balance. Note a weight gain or loss of 50 g or more. Include insensible losses, I.V. fluids given, and urine output in the calculation. Evaluating all aspects together produces an accurate picture of the infant's fluid status.

Interventions	Rationales
• assessing the infant's response to the diuretic. Note time and amount of diuresis.	
2. Limit fluid intake, if appropriate, scheduling amounts to be given.	2. CHF may result in fluid retention. Limits on oral and I.V. fluid intake may be required to prevent additional fluid retention.
3. Additional individualized interventions: _____	3. Rationales: _____

Nursing diagnosis: *Altered nutrition: less than body requirements related to inability to ingest feedings because of dyspnea or exhaustion*

GOAL: Maintain nutritional intake.

Interventions	Rationales
1. Offer small feedings when the infant appears hungry or after rest periods.	1. Sucking requires exertion, which causes dyspnea, making feeding more difficult. Small feedings require less energy.
2. Limit feeding to 30 minutes. Use a soft nipple with larger holes.	2. Shorter feeding times and a soft nipple allow sucking with less effort; lengthy feeding sessions stress and exhaust the infant.
3. If the infant on fluid restriction is stable enough to eat, a low-sodium formula may be indicated.	3. Low-sodium formulas are used to reduce sodium and fluid retention, although urine output and sodium excretion should be occurring.
4. According to the infant's condition, provide caloric additives in oral feedings if fluid intake is restricted.	4. Providing adequate caloric intake when fluids are restricted is difficult; high-calorie formulas are given to restrict feeding volume and provide additional calories for growth and repair.
5. Prepare and administer gavage feedings if oral feedings are impossible. Gavage is a better alternative until the infant's condition is stable enough to permit oral feedings.	5. The infant's respiratory rate may be increased or the infant may be exhausted from trying to suck, so another method might be used to meet the infant's caloric demands (see Hyaline Membrane Disease—Respiratory Distress Syndrome [RDS I] plan, page 205, for gavage procedure).
6. Provide a pacifier during gavage if the infant tolerates the pacifier.	6. A pacifier enhances digestion, thus promoting nutrition.
7. Additional individualized interventions: _____	7. Rationales: _____

Nursing diagnosis: *Ineffective family coping: compromised related to guilt and emotional crisis associated with infant's illness*

GOAL: Promote and support parents' coping behaviors.

Interventions	Rationales
1. Assess the parents' verbal and nonverbal expression of their anxieties and fears as well as their use of coping mechanisms.	1. This assessment helps all parties identify coping strategies and develop more constructive ones.

Interventions

2. Help the parents to express their feelings about the intensive care nursery, neonatal care, the treatments, and the acuity of their infant's condition.

3. Encourage the parents to have contact with their infant, touching it and providing care as appropriate.

4. Continually inform the parents of the infant's condition and progress.

5. Additional individualized interventions: _____

Rationales

2. Helping parents express feelings promotes trust in the caring environment. By helping the parents express their concerns, you demonstrate acceptance of their concerns and fears.

3. Parental participation in care promotes bonding.

4. Knowledge about what is happening to their infant may help decrease the parents' anxiety.

5. Rationales: _____

Nursing diagnosis: *Knowledge deficit (parental) related to the infant's condition, treatment, and progress*

GOAL: Provide appropriate information regarding infant's condition, progress, and long-term care.

Interventions

1. Inform parents of the following:
• CHF's possible cause, stressing how little is known about its actual cause
• infant's condition
• current treatment and its effect
• condition's seriousness
• infant's progress.

2. Tell the parents the following about the infant's medication regimen:
• drug name and action
• dose and times to give drug
• how to give drug
• adverse reactions to watch for
• what to do if infant vomits drug
• where and how to store drug safely.

3. Allow time for questions; clarify information given.

4. Refer parents to community and home health care services.

5. Additional individualized interventions: _____

Rationales

1. This information may relieve possible parental guilt, anxiety, and concern that they caused the infant's illness.

2. The infant may remain on maintenance dosages of a cardiac glycoside and a diuretic. The parents need a knowledge base for administering and monitoring drug therapy when the infant goes home.

3. Explanations and clarification reinforce the learning process, thereby enhancing understanding.

4. Referals provide continued support for the parents and family before and after discharge.

5. Rationales: _____

ASSOCIATED PLANS
• Congenital Heart Disease
• Hypothermia and Hyperthermia
• Preterm Infant, Less Than 37 Weeks

ADDITIONAL NURSING DIAGNOSES
• Activity intolerance related to exertional dyspnea
• Anticipatory grieving (parental) related to potential loss of infant

• Fear (parental) related to possible death of infant
• High risk for altered parenting related to interruption of bonding process
• Ineffective breathing pattern related to tachypnea, dyspnea
• Ineffective infant feeding pattern related to exertional dyspnea

INFANT
Drug Addiction and Withdrawal

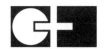

DEFINITION
Mothers addicted to such drugs as heroin, morphine, methadone, and barbiturates deliver infants who are passively addicted to the same drug and who display withdrawal symptoms. Depending on the type and quality of the drug used, symptoms may appear as early as 12 to 24 hours after birth or as late as 2 to 4 weeks after birth. Symptoms may last for 6 to 8 weeks (hyperirritability, 3 to 4 months) with the most pronounced symptoms occurring between 48 and 72 hours after birth. Most symptoms appear in the first 24 hours of life.

Long-term effects on the infant suffering from drug withdrawal are not known. Ongoing concerns focus on the importance of safe care in the home after discharge by a mother who can function, who is dependable, and who is following a treatment program. Supervision by social services and home visits by Visiting Nurses' Association personnel are necessary when an infant is discharged in the mother's care. If this is not possible, foster care must be obtained until the parent or family achieves stability.

This plan focuses on care of the infant who displays signs and symptoms of drug withdrawal and on recognition of the potential for inappropriate care or neglect by the mother after discharge.

ETIOLOGY AND PRECIPITATING FACTORS
• maternal addiction to drug (heroin, methadone, amphetamine, cocaine, or other substance)
• maternal treatment for seizure condition with phenobarbital

PHYSICAL FINDINGS
Maternal history
• drug addiction or dependence: name of drug used, time of last dose, length of time addicted, and route; names of drugs given in intrapartal phase
• type and length of prenatal care (if any)
• prenatal conditions associated with pregnancy, such as placenta previa and hypertension
• prenatal disorders, such as bacterial and TORCH infections, sexually transmitted diseases, human immunodeficiency virus (HIV) seropositivity, and poor nutrition
• participation in drug treatment or rehabilitation program
• previous addiction to narcotics because effect on infant (growth deficiency) may extend beyond addiction
• alcohol abuse
(*Note:* Because an addicted mother may be an unreliable information source, you may need to interview another family member to confirm history.)

Infant status at birth
• Apgar score, indicating possible asphyxia in utero
• infant small for gestational age (SGA) if maternal nutrition is poor or if mother uses heroin, cocaine, or morphine
• infant large for gestational age (LGA) with maternal use of methadone
• preterm birth
• cardiovascular disorders
• cleft lip or cleft palate

Gastrointestinal
• low birth weight, with difficulty in gaining weight or weight loss
• poor feeding resulting from uncoordinated sucking and swallowing
• vomiting or regurgitation after feeding caused by hyperactivity; overfeeding from constant need for sucking
• abdominal cramps, diarrhea caused by GI hyperactivity

Integumentary
• redness; abrasion marks on knees, elbows, or face caused by constant restlessness, kicking, and hyperactive movements associated with rubbing against sheets or clothing
• jaundice with maternal use of methadone
• slight to excessive sweating and flushed appearance
• sudden circumoral pallor
• excoriated buttocks
• facial scratches

Neurologic
• restlessness, hyperactivity from drug effect on central nervous system (CNS) functioning
• hypertonicity, hyperactive reflexes, hyperflexic arms and legs, kicking at times when mother would be due for drugs
• seizures

Pulmonary
• excessive mucus, stuffy nose, sneezing
• tachypnea, chest retractions
• periods of apnea

Cardiovascular
• tachycardia

BEHAVIORAL FINDINGS
• decreased sleep periods and lengthened awake periods
• dislike for cuddling and close contact
• frequent or prolonged sneezing or yawning
• high-pitched or weak cry, inconsolability
• irritability

DIAGNOSTIC STUDIES
Laboratory data
• toxicology screen—to identify drug and drug levels in mother's and infant's blood and urine
• serum electrolyte levels—to detect losses associated with vomiting and diarrhea; also used to determine other causes of neurologic symptoms or seizures, such as hypocalcemia
• serum glucose test—to determine decreases, if cause of neurologic symptoms or seizures is hypoglycemia
• capillary blood gases (serial) studies—to identify PO_2 and pH changes, increased PCO_2 from hypoxia, and metabolic acidosis as need for oxygen increases during withdrawal because of irritability, crying, and tachypnea
• complete blood count—to detect decreased white blood count, changes in ratio of immature to mature neutrophils, and decreased platelet count (with sepsis); decreased hematocrit and hemoglobin values and red blood cell count if the infant has anemia (these abnormal measurements result from conditions acquired in utero or intrapartally)
• blood culture—to identify sepsis
• HIV antigen test—to identify HIV exposure (especially if mother used I.V. drugs)

Collaborative problem: Neurologic and respiratory instability related to withdrawal from drug addiction (2 goals)

GOAL 1: Recognize and facilitate withdrawal.

Interventions

1. Assess for withdrawal symptoms, including:
• restlessness or wakefulness
• irritability; excessive yawning; high-pitched, shrill cry; hyperpyrexia
• hyperactivity, hypertonicity, poor coordination, tremors
• seizure activity or twitching
• vomiting or diarrhea.

2. Ask about maternal use of drug during pregnancy— names, time, route, and amount of last intake—and review serum and urine toxicology screen for drug identity.

3. Provide calming techniques, including:

• holding, rocking, and cuddling infant

• touching, patting, smiling, and talking to infant. Use infant carrier for closeness.

• limiting or increasing contact, depending on response

• tightly swaddling infant in prone or side-lying position and supporting back with small pillow

• providing quiet, dim environment for sleep

• planning care around rest periods and limiting procedures whenever possible.

4. Prepare to give medications ordered for withdrawal symptoms and to evaluate their side effects.

• Paregoric may be given P.O. with formula or in water. Drug dosage is decreased over 2 to 4 weeks.

• Chlorpromazine may be given P.O. with formula or I.M. in vastus lateralis.

• In the unstable infant, phenobarbital may be given I.V. initially until oral drugs can be introduced.

Rationales

1. About 90% of infants of addicted mothers display signs and symptoms of withdrawal as early as 12 hours after birth. Early recognition allows for early interventions and prevention of complications. Early signs of withdrawal include irritability and hyperactivity. Later manifestations of withdrawal include seizures, GI responses.

2. Severity of drug effect on infant depends on degree of abuse, time of last dose, and possible use of more than one drug. Because history taken from mother may be unreliable, more objective data are necessary to assess neonatal involvement.

3. Calming techniques help soothe infant and reduce irritability and hyperactivity.

• Cuddling quiets and comforts infant.

• These actions provide contact.

• Close contact may increase or decrease infant irritability.

• Positioning provides restful environment to discourage hyperactivity and increase comfort while reducing stimuli.

• Quiet environment reduces external stimuli that may increase infant's irritability.

• Planning care allows for needed rest and reduces external stimuli.

4. Pharmacologic agents alleviate withdrawal symptoms.

• By increasing smooth muscle tone of GI tract (thereby decreasing digestive secretions), paregoric acts to decrease GI tract motility and peristalsis.

• Chlorpromazine controls vomiting, producing sedation by acting on the hypothalamus and reticular formation.

• Give phenobarbital to control hyperactivity, irritability, and seizures. It acts to interfere with impulse transmission of cerebral cortex by inhibiting reticular activating system.

Interventions

• Phenytoin may be given I.V. if phenobarbital fails to stop seizures; then give I.V. or P.O. for maintenance.

• Diazepam may be given I.V., but it is not the drug of choice because it displaces bilirubin from its albumin binding sites.

5. Monitor serum glucose and calcium levels for decreases.

6. Additional individualized interventions: _____

Rationales

• Phenytoin acts to reduce voltage, frequency, and speed of electrical discharges in the motor cortex.

• Diazepam is given if respiratory status is controlled and infant is not preterm or jaundiced. It acts at limbic and subcortical levels of CNS, with shorter duration than chlorpromazine.

5. This can rule out hypoglycemia and hypocalcemia, which may manifest symptoms similar to those of withdrawal, such as tremors, irritability, tachypnea, and seizures.

6. Rationales: _____

GOAL 2: Minimize risk of injury and complications.

Interventions

1. Assess respiratory status and airway clearance; include the following considerations:

• respiratory rate, depth, and effort location and severity of chest contractions and nasal flaring

• increased secretions, stuffy nose

• bluish tint to face, trunk, nail beds, arms and legs, and mucous membranes

• crackles heard by auscultation

• Apgar score or apneic periods.
Note: Infant may be placed on apnea monitor or cardiopulmonary monitor.

2. Carefully suction mucus from infant's nose and mouth, as needed.

3. Position infant with head slightly elevated or use infant seat.

4. Assess for signs and symptoms of seizures, including:
• twitching movements (as opposed to tremors)
• uncoordinated movements of mouth or tongue, such as thrusting tongue, sucking, or chewing
• muscular rigidity, with arching of back
• nystagmus, blinking, and staring.

5. Identify potential HIV seropositivity. Use universal precautions in caring for infant. Carry out other protective procedures for infant and personnel according to agency protocols or those recommended by the Centers for Disease Control and Prevention.

6. Additional individualized interventions: _____

Rationales

1. Assessment provides data related to respiratory function and airway patency.

• Respirations often are depressed with narcotic addiction. Tachypnea of 60 breaths/minute or more indicates distress. Normal respiratory rate for infant is 30 to 50 breaths/minute.

• Secretions cause respiratory difficulty because infant can breathe only through nose.

• Cyanosis is a sign of hypoxia and requires immediate attention.

• Auscultation allows for comparison of breath sounds to identify abnormalities.

• Apgar score indicates infant status at birth regarding asphyxia and hypoxia. Cause of apnea must be established because withdrawal may be complicated by sepsis or birth-related respiratory condition or preterm status. Monitoring infant allows for continuous monitoring of vital signs if potential for severe respiratory distress exists.

2. Suctioning clears nose and allows for ease of breathing, especially during feedings.

3. This position facilitates breathing by promoting lung expansion.

4. Infant undergoing withdrawal is at risk for seizures because of CNS involvement. Tonic seizures are more common in preterm infants; clonic seizures, in full-term infants. Carefully observing infant for these signs and symptoms of seizures allows for immediate treatment to prevent injury.

5. I.V. drug users are high-risk candidates for acquired immunodeficiency syndrome, which can be passed on to the infant.

6. Rationales: _____

Nursing diagnosis: *Altered nutrition: less than body requirements related to poor or low intake because of lack of coordination in sucking or swallowing and because of vomiting*

GOAL: Improve nutritional status of neonate.

Interventions

1. Assess nutritional status and needs, including:

• gestational age and weight

• uncoordinated sucking and swallowing

• handling of secretions and gag reflex

• vomiting, regurgitation, and diarrhea (compare output with intake if infant is on oral feedings)

• daily intake (I.V., oral, or gastric lavage), including calorie count

• serum glucose review.

2. Provide appropriate nutrition as follows:

• If infant is unstable, assure proper administration of the I.V. infusion and delay feedings.
• When infant is stable, start feedings at half-strength, 10 ml every 3 hours.
• Check for residuals after oral feedings; reduce feeding amounts if residuals are high. Then, increase feedings as tolerated to 5 to 10 ml hourly if hyperactivity is decreasing.
• Place infant on right side, supporting back with small pillow or towel, or place infant on abdomen after feedings, once they have been started.
• If gastric gavage (intermittent or continuous) is given:

☐ Insert tube through mouth and confirm placement.

☐ Administer measured amount as ordered or by gravity or volumetric pump.

☐ Position infant on right side with head slightly elevated for 1 hour or as tolerated.
☐ Evaluate tolerance of feedings and record any emesis.

Rationales

1. Infant's nutrition in utero may reflect poor maternal nutrition.
• Infants of drug-addicted mothers often are SGA with low birth weight, or they may be preterm from poor nutrition during prenatal period, causing reduced number of organ cells.
• CNS stimulation causes hyperactivity, which leads to poor feeding.
• In preterm infants, gag reflex may not be complete.
• CNS stimulation causes GI hypermotility and irritation, which may result in inability to retain or absorb nutrients, a later manifestation of withdrawal.
• I.V. fluids should probably be given until infant is stable because feeding an irritable infant with possible seizures might foster aspiration. Infant may not tolerate full-strength feeding and may need to increase strength gradually when fed orally or by gastric gavage.
• Serum glucose test identifies hypoglycemia caused by inadequate reserve or maternal malnutrition.

2. A full-term infant needs 100 to 200 calories/kg daily. An SGA infant needs more, based on age and projected daily weight gain.
• These actions avoid aggravating the GI problem if infant cannot tolerate feedings.
• Smaller feedings facilitate nutritional intake if GI tract can accept feeding.
• This action prevents vomiting from overfeeding while still providing I.V. fluids according to infant's tolerance.

• This action prevents vomiting or aspiration after feedings and may prevent residuals and distention.

• Gastric gavage is an alternate feeding route when infant cannot tolerate oral feedings.
☐ Mouth route is used because infant breathes through nose, which may be stuffy.
☐ Gravity administration permits slow instillation, minimizing gastric distention; use of volumetric pump allows the feeding to be given at a controlled rate over a specified time, eliminating the risk of overfeeding.
☐ Positioning prevents vomiting or aspiration.

☐ Evaluating how the infant tolerates the feedings helps to determine if changes in feeding are required. Feedings are increased to provide calculated caloric needs; infant may have emesis of 1 to 2 ml.

Interventions

□ Evaluate residual content before feedings and hold feedings if amount exceeds infant's acceptable quantity.

3. Measure abdominal girth every 2 hours and compare with past measurements.

4. Weigh infant daily and record weight on flow sheet for comparison; monitor fluid intake and output.

5. Provide quiet environment and reduce light and noise.

6. Provide pacifier for sucking when infant is not feeding.

7. Allow mother to feed infant and help her offer food slowly and calmly while holding infant.

8. Additional individualized interventions: _____

_____

Rationales

□ Residual feedings may indicate infant's failure to digest or tolerate feedings and may lead to abdominal distention. With a 10-ml feeding, a residual of 2 ml or more after 3 hours is significant.

3. Widening girth indicates distention. This test may be done with oral feedings, too.

4. Weighing reveals gains or losses and need for feeding changes; monitoring fluid intake and output helps evaluate fluid balance.

5. Quiet environment reduces external stimuli, which may increase hyperactivity and irritability, thus increasing caloric and metabolic needs.

6. Pacifier helps to quiet infant by satisfying sucking need.

7. Mother's participation encourages bonding process, giving support and confidence to mother while preventing overfeeding.

8. Rationales: _____

_____

Nursing diagnosis: *High risk for fluid volume deficit related to diarrhea or vomiting*

GOAL: Maintain fluid and electrolyte balance.

Interventions

1. Assess for possible signs and symptoms of fluid or electrolyte imbalance; include the following:
• intake (oral and I.V.)
• urine output (weigh diapers: 1 g = 1 ml)

• fluid loss from phototherapy for bilirubin increases or radiant warmer
• vomiting or diarrhea

• urine specific gravity

• dry skin and mucous membranes, sunken fontanels, weight loss
• serum electrolyte levels.

2. Monitor and evaluate administration of I.V. fluids.

3. Additional individualized interventions: _____

_____

Rationales

1. Imbalances may occur from inadequate fluid or nutritional intake.
• Comparisons determine whether an imbalance exists.
• Normal urine output for a neonate is 2 to 3 ml/kg hourly; first voiding may occur as late as 24 hours after birth.
• Heat sources may promote fluid losses.

• Vomiting and diarrhea—later symptoms of withdrawal related to GI hypermotility—subject the infant to fluid loss as well as loss of such electrolytes as potassium and chloride.
• Normal specific gravity is 1.001 to 1.020 with increases being an indication of concentrated urine as a result of decreased output caused by fluid loss. Increases could be an indication of dehydration.
• Dryness indicates dehydration from fluid or electrolyte loss.
• GI fluid losses may cause hypokalemia.

2. Fluids and electrolytes are replaced by I.V. infusion with 10% to 20% increase based on severity of fluid loss

3. Rationales: _____

_____

Nursing diagnosis: *High risk for impaired skin integrity related to perianal irritation from diarrhea and rubbing against sheets because of hyperactivity*

GOAL: Preserve skin integrity.

Interventions

1. Inspect skin frequently for areas of redness or irritation.

2. Clean perianal area gently and apply soothing lotion with each diaper change, or leave area exposed to air to dry.

3. Pad infant's knees and elbows, cover hands with mittens, and place soft sheepskin under face.

4. Provide infant with a waterbed mattress.

5. Additional individualized interventions: _____

_____

Rationales

1. Frequent inspection promotes early detection and prevention of skin breakdown.

2. Cleaning and lotion application prevent irritation and possible skin breakdown from frequent diarrhea.

3. Padding prevents skin contact with linens and, thus, possible irritation; covering the hands with mittens prevents the infant from scratching the skin.

4. Waterbed mattress reduces pressure on skin surfaces.

5. Rationales: _____

_____

Nursing diagnosis: *Ineffective individual coping (maternal) related to drug abuse or inability to care for infant*

GOAL: Support development of coping skills and change in life-style.

Interventions

1. Assess mother's mental state; include the following:

• individual and family stressors; use of coping mechanisms, both constructive and destructive; mother's behavior and comments regarding infant; and mother's reaction to and willingness to participate in infant's treatment
• feelings of vulnerability

• mother's anxieties and fears regarding infant care, and her need to participate in drug rehabilitation program.

2. Help mother identify coping skills she needs and available support systems: family, church groups, drug assistance groups such as Born Free, and parenting classes.

3. Assess need for protected environment, such as halfway house, supportive follow-up at home with social service, Visiting Nurses' Association visits, foster home for infant, or hospital-based boarder infant program. Make appropriate referrals.

4. Additional individualized interventions: _____

_____

Rationales

1. Assessment provides information regarding mother's ability to care for infant and to pursue drug rehabilitation.
• Assessment offers clues to potential problems leading to infant neglect.

• Assessment allows for expression of concerns and reveals mother's ability to assume responsibility for infant.
• Assessment allows mother to understand own needs to change life-style.

2. This assists mother in determining need for help with drug addiction and infant care.

3. Follow-up care offers support and help to mother undergoing treatment and provides safe infant care.

4. Rationales: _____

_____

Nursing diagnosis: *Knowledge deficit (parental) related to emotional inadequacy and lack of exposure to information about infant care*

GOAL: Provide appropriate information for safe infant care.

Interventions

1. Identify parental knowledge needs, interest in learning, and readiness and capability for learning.

2. Provide information regarding:

• infant's condition and signs and symptoms of infant withdrawal and rationale for treatment
• need for infant stimulation as well as rest periods, depending on responses

• fact that drug is passed to infant if mother is breast-feeding while taking drugs; encourages bottle-feeding unless abstinence is assured.
• physical care of infant (feeding, bathing, clothing, and holding).

3. Determine need for social services and assistance at home after infant's discharge.

4. Advise mother of possibility of foster care for infant during drug treatment and rehabilitation.

5. Advise about medication administration with feedings, including times, amounts, and adverse effects.

6. Additional individualized interventions: _____

Rationales

1. This provides a basis for developing a teaching plan commensurate with parents' abilities and needs.

2. Information is needed if parent is to care for infant safely.
• Assessment determines maternal understanding of infant behavior and how to care for infant with symptoms.
• Diversity provides infant with needed rest and activity and promotes maternal-infant bonding without overtaxing the infant.
• Breast-feeding prolongs infant's addiction.

• This knowledge helps mother provide for safe infant care and increases her feeling of competence in parenting.

3. Social services' participation ensures ongoing follow-up and safety of the infant while in the mother's care.

4. Foster care may be an alternative until stability is achieved.

5. This ensures safe administration of medications given for withdrawal if they are needed after discharge.

6. Rationales: _____

ASSOCIATED PLANS AND APPENDICES
• Acquired Immunodeficiency Syndrome—Infant
• Cleft Lip and Cleft Palate
• Congenital Heart Disease
• Fetal Alcohol Syndrome
• Inappropriate Size or Weight for Gestational Age, Small
• Intracranial Hemorrhage
• Preterm Infant, Less Than 37 Weeks
• Sexually Transmitted Diseases/TORCH
• Selected Substances and Fetal Abnormalities (Appendix 3)
• Aspects of Psychological Care—Maternal (Appendix 4)
• Parent Teaching Guides (Appendix 12)
• 1993 CDC Revised Classification System for HIV Infection/AIDS Surveillance Case Definition (Appendix 13)

ADDITIONAL NURSING DIAGNOSES
• Activity intolerance related to neurologic irritability
• Diarrhea related to GI hypermotility

• High risk for altered parenting related to previous lifestyle associated with drug abuse and unrealistic expectations of self and infant
• High risk for aspiration related to diminished gag reflex and poor swallowing and sucking
• Impaired home maintenance management related to inadequate support system, insufficient financial resources, and continuation of drug abuse patterns
• Ineffective breathing pattern related to decreased lung expansion, depressed respirations, apnea associated with prematurity, respiratory disorders, and nasal stuffiness affecting airway clearance
• Ineffective family coping (disabled) related to intolerance, rejection, and ambivalent family relationships
• Sleep pattern disturbance related to neurologic irritability

INFANT

Fetal Alcohol Syndrome

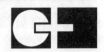

DEFINITION

Fetal alcohol syndrome (FAS) in the neonate results from the mother's chronic or periodic ethanol intake during pregnancy. Severity of effects on the infant depends on the degree and timing of alcohol consumption. For this reason and because it is not known what a safe limit of alcohol intake should be or when alcohol intake is most harmful to the fetus, pregnant women are advised to abstain from alcohol intake.

Neonates damaged from alcohol abuse may be physically and mentally deficient and may display multiple congenital abnormalities. Diagnosis is based on a cluster of findings rather than one isolated finding. Perinatal mortality is about 20%.

This plan focuses on care of the neonate displaying signs and symptoms of withdrawal and on maternal preparation for infant care after discharge.

ETIOLOGY AND PRECIPITATING FACTORS

• maternal chronic alcoholism
• social drinking
• binge drinking (taking large amounts periodically)

PHYSICAL FINDINGS
Maternal history

• alcohol consumption or use of street, scheduled, or prescription drugs
• participation in Alcoholics Anonymous or other treatment program or support group
• possible high risk for human immunodeficiency virus (HIV) seropositivity
• TORCH risk

Infant status at birth

• small for gestational age (SGA) with low birth weight and height
• congenital cardiac defects, joint contractures or malformations
• facial abnormalities, such as microcephaly, short eye slits, and midfacial hypoplasia

Neurologic

• abnormal reflexes, including hyperactive rooting and increased sucking
• irritability, poor coordination, hyperactivity from effect of drug on central nervous system (CNS) functioning, and maternal history of cross abuse, neonatal abstinence syndrome
• tremors, seizures

BEHAVIORAL FINDINGS

• sleeplessness
• inconsolability
• easily hyperstimulated by noise, light, and touch
• activeness with little inability to remain alert and attentive to environment

DIAGNOSTIC STUDIES
Laboratory data

• HIV seropositivity test—if indicated by history
• toxicology screen—for alcohol or other drugs in maternal or infant blood
• serum glucose levels—to determine hypoglycemia in infant who is SGA

Collaborative problem: *High risk for neurologic instability (short-term) and mental deficiency (long-term) related to alcohol addiction*

GOAL: Recognize and facilitate withdrawal.

Interventions

1. Assess for withdrawal symptoms, including:

• maternal use of alcohol during pregnancy, time and amount of last intake, and other drugs taken

• irritability, hyperactivity, tremors, restlessness, or poor coordination of infant

• results of toxicology screen to identify alcohol or other drugs.

2. Provide calming techniques as follows:
• Hold, rock, and cuddle infant. If possible, have volunteers perform these activities.

Rationales

1. Signs and symptoms of alcohol withdrawal usually appear within 12 hours after birth, although some infants do not display withdrawal patterns.

• Severity of effect on neonate depends on degree of abuse; withdrawal may be delayed if intake occurs just before birth.

• Monitoring degree of these symptoms helps determine whether treatment is reducing withdrawal responses.

• Mother may be an unreliable source of information about drug habit.

2. These techniques soothe the infant
• Holding assists in soothing infant and reducing irritability and hyperactivity.

Interventions

• Touch, pat, smile, and talk to infant; use infant carrier for closeness.

• Swaddle infant in prone or side-lying position, supporting back with small pillow. Provide quiet, dim environment for sleep.

• Plan care around rest periods and limit procedures if possible.

• Do not disturb infant if he is quiet.

3. Prepare to give medications ordered for withdrawal symptoms and to evaluate their side effects.

• Give paregoric with formula or water P.O. adjusted according to symptoms.

• Give I.V. phenobarbital initially to the unstable infant until P.O. drug can be introduced.

4. Recognize long-term effects of alcohol addiction.

• Assess for congenital anomalies, including microcephaly, cardiac defects, and musculoskeletal abnormalities.

5. Additional individualized interventions: _____

Rationales

• Touching quiets and comforts infant while providing personal contact.

• A restful, restricted environment reduces hyperactivity and provides comfort while reducing external stimuli.

• Careful scheduling reduces external stimuli, which increase irritability.

• This allows for needed rest and sleep.

3. Pharmacologic agents help reduce withdrawal symptoms.

• Paregoric treats withdrawal symptoms (see Drug Addiction and Withdrawal plan, page 183, for actions and adverse effects).

• Phenobarbital controls hyperactivity, irritability, and seizures (see Drug Addiction and Withdrawal plan, page 183, for actions and adverse effects).

4. Infants with FAS continue to have difficulties with growth and development throughout childhood.

• Neonates affected by FAS may have anomalies; 50% are estimated to have mental deficiencies.

5. Rationales: _____

Nursing diagnosis: *Altered nutrition: less than body requirements related to lack of nutritional reserves and to poor or low intake*

GOAL: Improve infant's nutritional status.

Interventions

1. Assess nutritional status and needs; include the following:

• gestational age and weight

• sucking or swallowing incoordination, handling (swallowing) of secretions

• daily intake (by I.V. or oral route or gastric gavage), including calorie count

• review of serum glucose levels.

2. Provide appropriate nutrition, as follows:

• Assure proper administration of I.V. infusion; delay feedings if infant is unstable.

• Start oral feedings at half-strength: 10 ml every 3 hours.

Rationales

1. Baseline nutritional status helps identify how best to meet infant's needs.

• Infants of alcoholic mothers are commonly SGA with low birth weight and length.

• Hyperactivity from CNS stimulation causes poor feeding.

• I.V. fluids should probably be given until infant is in stable condition; infant may not be able to tolerate full-strength feeding initially, so increase may have to be gradual.

• This determines hypoglycemia in SGA infant with low nutritional reserve. Ethanol intake causes hypoglycemia, which is passed on to infant because ethanol is metabolized like sugars.

2. Full-term infant needs 100 to 200 calories/kg daily; SGA infant needs more, based on age and projected daily weight gain.

• I.V. fluid administration ensures nutrient infusion; delayed feedings prevent complications when infant cannot tolerate feedings.

• Half-strength feedings facilitate nutritional intake if infant cannot tolerate full-strength feeding.

Interventions	Rationales
• Check for residuals after oral or gavage feedings and reduce amount of feeding if residuals are high, or increase feedings gradually, as tolerated, to 5 to 10 ml hourly while increasing strength of feedings.	• Monitoring residuals prevents overfeeding or vomiting after feedings.
• Place infant on right side, supporting back with small pillow, or place on abdomen when feedings are started.	• This positioning prevents overfeeding and vomiting.
• Monitor gastric gavage (intermittent or continuous).	• Gavage feeding provides an alternate feeding route when infant cannot tolerate oral feedings (see Interventions for gastric gavage in the Drug Addiction and Withdrawal plan, page 183.)
• Have suction equipment on hand and ready for use.	• Suction may be needed for aspiration.
3. Weigh infant daily and record weight on flow sheet for comparison.	3. Weighing reveals gains or losses and need for changes in feedings.
4. Provide pacifier for sucking when infant is not feeding.	4. Pacifier helps to quiet infant by providing means of satisfying need for sucking.
5. Provide quiet environment and reduce light and noise.	5. Quiet environment reduces external stimuli, which may increase hyperactivity and irritability, thus increasing caloric and metabolic needs.
6. Allow mother to feed infant; help her feed slowly and calmly, holding infant while feeding.	6. Mother's participation encourages bonding process; it also gives support to her while preventing overfeeding.
7. Additional individualized interventions: _____	7. Rationales: _____

Nursing diagnosis: *High risk for altered parenting related to previous life-style associated with alcohol abuse or to unrealistic expectations of self and infant (2 goals)*

GOAL 1: Support need for change in life-style.

Interventions	Rationales
1. Assess mental status of mother, including: • individual and family stressors • mother's behavior and comments regarding infant • mother's reaction to infant's possibly long-term treatment • developmental stage • use of coping mechanisms.	1. Assessment provides information about mother's ability to pursue treatment for alcohol abuse while offering clues to potential problems that may lead to infant neglect.
2. Offer information about parenting classes and alcohol rehabilitation programs; encourage attendance.	2. To change life-style successfully, support groups and rehabilitation are needed.
3. Assist mother to identify support systems, including family, spouse, church, or others, such as Born Free, Alcoholics Anonymous, and Al-Anon.	3. These support groups provide additional long-term assistance and decrease maternal fear or guilt.
4. Additional individualized interventions: _____	4. Rationales: _____

GOAL 2: Help mother acquire realistic expectations of self and infant.

Interventions	Rationales
1. Encourage mother to verbalize expectations, both realistic and unrealistic, and feelings about infant and her own capabilities.	1. This provides information about the mother's expectations, coping skills, fears, and anxieties.

Interventions

2. Assist mother to identify realistic expectations and develop strategies to fulfill them.

3. Allow for discussion of alcohol abuse and rehabilitation needs.

4. Refer mother to social services for community and home health care resources.

5. Additional individualized interventions: _____

Rationales

2. Success is more likely if mother is involved in decisions.

3. Self-assessment of alcohol abuse and need to change may influence realistic decisions about infant care.

4. Referrals to community and home health care resources provide continued support before and after discharge and promote compliance with follow-up regimen.

5. Rationales: _____

Nursing diagnosis: *Knowledge deficit (parental) related to lack of information about infant care*

GOAL: Provide appropriate information for safe infant care.

Interventions

1. Identify parents' knowledge needs, interest in learning, and readiness and capability to learn.

2. Provide information regarding infant's condition, signs and symptoms of infant withdrawal, and rationale for treatment as well as the following information:
• need for increased or decreased stimulation, depending on infant's reactions
• alcohol consumption during breast-feeding passes drug to infant
• mental effects of alcohol abuse on infant and possible behavioral difficulties
• physical care—including feeding, bathing, clothing, and holding infant.

3. Refer parents to social services for community resources and home health care.

4. Additional individualized interventions: _____

Rationales

1. This provides the basis of a teaching plan commensurate with parent abilities and needs.

2. Information will help mother understand infant behavior and how to care for the infant who has prolonged symptoms.
• Infant's responses to stimuli may be increased or decreased during withdrawal
• Alcohol is found in breast milk; continued alcohol intake will prolong infant's addiction if he is breast-fed.
• Alcohol addiction is known to cause mental and growth retardation in infants.
• This information will provide for safe care of infant and mother's increased feeling of competence in parenting.

3. Referrals provide emotional and physical support, promoting compliance with follow-up regimen.

4. Rationales: _____

ASSOCIATED PLANS AND APPENDICES
• Acquired Immunodeficiency Syndrome—Infant
• Congenital Heart Disease
• Drug Addiction and Withdrawal
• Hypoglycemia
• Inappropriate Size or Weight for Gestational Age, Small
• Intracranial Hemorrhage
• Parent Teaching Guides (Appendix 12)

ADDITIONAL NURSING DIAGNOSES
• Activity intolerance related to neurologic hyperirritability
• Altered growth and development related to maternal alcohol use and FAS

• High risk for aspiration related to uncoordinated sucking and swallowing
• Impaired home maintenance management related to continued alcohol abuse
• Ineffective family coping: disabled related to intolerance, rejection, ambivalent family relationships
• Ineffective individual coping (maternal) related to anxiety, fear, guilt; inadequate support systems; excessive drinking (alcohol); and unrealistic expectations, and perceptions
• Sleep pattern disturbance related to neurologic irritability

Full-term Infant, 38 to 42 Weeks

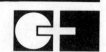

DEFINITION

An infant born after 38 to 42 weeks' gestation is considered full-term. At birth, it must leave the life-sustaining in utero environment and adapt to one that requires profound physiologic changes. Any interference with the infant's transition to extrauterine life affects its well-being. Some physiologic factors that can affect the transition include initiation of extrauterine cardiopulmonary function, thermoregulation, defenses against infection, neurologic impairment, fluid and nutritional deficits, congenital defects, and skin impairment.

The first 4 weeks, or 28 days, of life present the greatest risk to the infant. The incidence of death is highest during the 1st day, and two-thirds of all deaths during the 1st year of life occur within the 1st month.

In the first 24 hours are two periods of reactivity. The first period, lasting up to 30 minutes after birth, reveals an alert, open-eyed, vigorously crying, fist-sucking infant whose vital signs and bowel sounds increase while body temperature decreases. This is followed by a decrease in responses and vital signs and a sleep period lasting 2 to 4 hours.

The second period of reactivity starts when the infant awakens (4 to 8 hours after birth). It is alert, with an increase in vital signs, secretions, and gagging. This period lasts 2 to 5 hours, concluding when secretions decrease and hunger, sucking, and a sleep and activity pattern become established.

This plan focuses on nursing care of the full-term infant. It includes interventions for possible abnormalities (related to immature systems) and interventions for maintaining normal physiologic function and meeting the infant's needs.

PHYSICAL FINDINGS
Maternal history
• prenatal care, age, and expected date of confinement
• genetic profile and familial tendencies
• abnormal conditions or disorders during pregnancy
• use of medications, over-the-counter drugs, street drugs, alcohol, tobacco or caffeine
• test results: amniotic fluid, blood type, Rh factor, Coombs', TORCH, sickle cell, tuberculosis, syphilis, and other screens
• description of delivery, especially if difficult

Infant status at birth
• gestational age 38 to 42 weeks
• Apgar score 7 to 10 at 1 minute and at 5 minutes after birth, indicating absence of abnormalities and normal adjustment to life

• weight: 5 lb, 8 oz to 8 lb, 13 oz (2,500 to 4,000 g)
• length: approximately 19″ to 21″ (48 to 53 cm)
• head circumference: 13″ to 14″ (33 to 35.6 cm), ¾″ to 1¼″ (2 to 3 cm) larger than chest

Cardiovascular
• heart rate ranging from 110 to 160 beats/minute at apical site with regular rhythm; decreases during sleep and increases during crying
• blood pressure ranging from 60 to 80 mm Hg systolic and 30 to 45 mm Hg diastolic
• apical pulse at third to fourth intercostal space at sternal edge
• S_2 of higher pitch and sharper than S_1
• possible murmur because of functional vibrations within the heart or major arteries
• pink nail beds with transient cyanosis

Gastrointestinal
• intact mouth, lips, and palate; normal sucking, swallowing, and gag reflexes as well as rooting reflex
• stomach capacity about 90 ml
• soft, cylindrically shaped abdomen
• liver palpable; spleen not palpable
• with clamp in place, cord at umbilicus has two arteries and one vein
• anus patent with meconium stool passing within 12 hours or history of meconium passage in utero

Integumentary
• red (not beefy red) and smooth skin, changing to pink, dry, and flaky
• edema and puffiness around eyes, face, arms and legs, and presenting parts
• acrocyanosis
• possible petechiae, nevi, spots, ecchymoses, rash, and milia
• fingernails and toenails; lanugo and vernix caseosa
• intact skin and mucous membranes

Musculoskeletal
• normal range of motion in arms and legs with good muscle tone
• flexion of head and arms and legs
• ear cartilage flexible
• equal muscle tone with symmetry; resists flexion
• creases on soles
• possible skeletal deformities resulting from fetal positioning
• soft skull and rib bones with fontanels and separations at suture lines present in head (fontanels soft, flat, and firm)
• more cartilage than ossified bone

Neurologic
• bilateral and equal Moro's, plantar, palmar grasp, and Babinski's reflexes; loud and lusty cry
• eyes usually closed, with vision the least developed and sensory function and touch the most developed; infant can taste, smell, and hear
• startle, blinking, pupillary, crawling, yawn, and cough reflexes apparent
• daily sleep and activity patterns: 1 to 4 hours of alertness, activity, and crying; 4 to 5 hours of regular sleep; 12 to 15 hours of irregular sleep
• skin temperature of 97° to 98.6° F (36° to 37° C); rectal temperature 1° F (0.6° C) degree higher

Pulmonary
• nasal patency and nasal breathing, thin white mucus, and sneezing
• respiratory rate ranging from 40 to 60 breaths/minute; chiefly abdominal breathing with slight sternal retractions during inspiration
• bronchial breath sounds bilaterally, with possible transient tachypnea and slight nasal flaring
• possible crackles for short period after birth
• possible irregular respirations or periodic breathing

Renal
• pale yellow urine, with voiding occurring within 24 hours after delivery
• volume of 200 to 300 ml voided every 24 hours, with bladder capacity of about 15 ml causing involuntary emptying
• kidneys palpable

Reproductive
• girl: larger labia minora than labia majora; edema of labia and clitoris
• boy: palpable testes in scrotal sac; scrotum edematous, large, and hanging with rugae present; urethral meatus at tip of penis

BEHAVIORAL FINDINGS
• alternates among behavioral sleep and awake states
• habituates to environmental stimuli
• responds to visual and auditory stimuli
• shows motor maturity within normal limits
• self-quiets effectively

DIAGNOSTIC STUDIES
Laboratory data
• tests related to findings of physical examination or observable changes in infant status
• blood tests—may include serum bilirubin levels, complete blood count, electrolyte analysis, blood type and Rh factor, and Coombs' test
• Chemstrip or Dextrostix testing—for glucose levels (followed by serum glucose study if glucose levels are low)
• Guthrie blood test—to identify possible phenylketonuria

Nursing diagnoses: *Ineffective breathing pattern related to irregular periodic breathing episodes and increased mucus secretion*

GOAL: Support respirations and maintain airway patency.

Interventions

1. Assess the infant's respiratory rate, regularity, depth, and ease every 15 minutes to 2 hours as appropriate. Auscultate breath sounds.

2. Assess for increased mucus production and for fluids, such as blood and amniotic fluid, swallowed during birth. Gently hand-suction oronasal areas as needed.

3. Position the infant on its abdomen or side with the head slightly lower or on its back supported by a small padded roll.

4. Assess the infant for tachypnea, nasal flaring, grunting, retraction, crackles or rhonchi, cyanosis, and tachycardia.

Rationales

1. An infant with an Apgar score between 7 and 10 at 1 and 5 minutes usually breathes at a rate ranging from 40 to 60 breaths/minute, with some irregularity, brief periods of transient crackles, and breathing rate changes followed by a period of sleep. Changes in breath sounds may indicate changes in respiratory status.

2. Hand-suctioning removes accumulated mucus and fluids and prevents aspiration. Parasympathetic nervous system stimulation increases saliva production, which is followed by gagging and vomiting. Increases in mucus and saliva occur by 6 hours after delivery.

3. This position facilitates chest expansion and mucus drainage.

4. These are signs and symptoms of respiratory distress; normal breathing is diaphragmatic and abdominal. The normal infant respiratory rate is 30 to 60 breaths/minute.

Interventions	**Rationales**
5. Keep infant's clothing, diaper, and blanket loose.	5. This action prevents constricted chest movement.
6. Have oxygen on hand to be administered if needed.	6. Oxygen should be available in case of respiratory distress.
7. Additional individualized interventions: _____	7. Rationales: _____

Nursing diagnosis: *High risk for altered body temperature related to fluctuations caused by the environment and increased activity*

GOAL: Establish and maintain stable infant temperature and thermoneutral environment.

Interventions	**Rationales**
1. Initially, assess the infant's core temperature and skin temperature by the appropriate method (per institutional policy) every 30 to 60 minutes and then every 2 to 4 hours for 8 to 12 hours.	1. Optimal skin temperature is about 97.7° to 98.6° F (36.5° to 37° C) for minimal oxygen consumption, with core (rectal) temperatures about 0.9° F (0.5° C) higher. After birth, the infant's body temperature falls; then it rises during periods of increased activity, muscle tone, and alertness because of sympathetic stimulation.
2. Monitor ambient nursery temperature and humidity.	2. Infants lose body heat to surrounding areas by convection. Ambient nursery temperature should be 75° to 78° F (24° to 25.6° C), and humidity should be 40% to 50%.
3. Maintain temperature stability by:	3. The objective is to minimize heat loss by conduction, evaporation, radiation, and convection after delivery by providing warmth when temperature decreases.
• drying the infant immediately after birth with a warm towel	• Drying the infant helps to prevent body heat loss from evaporation.
• wrapping the infant in a warmed blanket and placing the infant on a warm surface	• Warm blankets and surfaces conserve the infant's body heat and minimize heat loss from conduction.
• allowing the mother to cuddle the infant to provide warmth	• When the mother cuddles her infant, her body acts as a heat source. Cuddling also promotes bonding.
• placing the infant under a radiant warmer and avoiding drafts, cold surfaces, or other exposure to cold	• These actions help to prevent heat loss from evaporation and radiation.
• placing a cap on the infant's head	• The large surface area of the infant's head may promote heat loss if the head remains uncovered.
• postponing bathing and other procedures until the infant's body temperature stabilizes (about 4 hours after birth)	• These actions prevent heat loss.
• dressing the infant appropriately and covering it if the infant is placed in a bassinet.	• These actions provide warmth for the infant.
4. Provide a thermoneutral environment with a radiant warmer or an incubator. Use a Servo-Control device to monitor skin temperature if appropriate.	4. A thermoneutral environment maintains optimal core temperature with minimal oxygen consumption if the infant's temperature stability is a problem.
5. Assess for cold skin; a drop in temperature; pallor or cyanotic or red color; edema of the arms and legs; bradycardia; a feeble cry; lethargy; flaccid movements; slow, shallow, irregular breathing with expiratory grunt; poor feeding; vomiting; abdominal distention; and diminished activity or reflexes.	5. These are signs and symptoms of cold stress and require immediate physician notification.
6. Additional individualized interventions: _____	6. Rationales: _____

Nursing diagnosis: *Altered nutrition: less than body requirements related to high caloric requirement because of increased metabolic rate*

GOAL: Maintain and support nutritional requirements.

Interventions

1. Assess the infant's bowel sounds, clearing of mucus, and passage of meconium.

2. Weigh and measure the infant and calculate nutritional requirements, even though the infant takes what is needed with each feeding.

3. Perform a Chemstrip or Dextrostix test to establish the infant's glucose level on admission to the nursery. Follow the test with a serum glucose test if the glucose level is less than 45 mg/dl.

4. Assess for signs of readiness to feed:
• active bowel sounds
• absence of abdominal distention
• lusty cry that diminishes with rooting or sucking behaviors when a stimulus is placed near the lips.

5. Start feedings with 5% glucose in water in small amount (about 15 ml) if the infant's gag and swallowing reflexes are normal. Some infants start feedings with formula (physician preference); if tolerated, these formula feedings may be repeated.

6. If the infant tolerates glucose and water, start feeding with formula or breast milk. Breast-feeding may start soon after birth or when the infant can nurse.

7. Offer feedings every 3 to 4 hours, according to the infant's demand and needs.

8. Assess for regurgitation, choking, fatigue during feeding or refused feedings, abnormal stools, respiratory changes, and irritability.

9. Position the infant on the right side after feeding.

10. Additional individualized interventions: _____

Rationales

1. These processes usually occur between 2 and 6 hours after delivery and indicate possible readiness for feeding.

2. Daily caloric needs are based on the infant's weight and expected weight gain. Initially, infants lose weight because of physiologic changes required to adapt to extrauterine life and because they are poor feeders for the first day or two.

3. The infant's glucose stores are quickly depleted and must be replaced by feedings or by dextrose 10% in water ($D_{10}W$) given I.V., if necessary; early feedings increase the glucose level after the initial drop.

4. Readiness to feed enhances feeding and helps prevent complications.

5. Initial feeding with sterile water allows absorption of water by lung tissue if aspiration occurs. Feedings may be given at birth or 4 to 6 hours later as tolerated. Because the infant's stomach capacity averages 90 ml (about 2¾ oz), with an emptying time of 2½ to 3 hours, frequent small feedings are better tolerated.

6. Early feedings are advised, with breast-feeding preferred. (See Appendix 8: Fluid and Nutritional Needs in Infancy and Appendix 12: Parent Teaching Guides, for more information.) Breast-feeding soon after birth stimulates milk production, promotes maternal-infant attachment, and enhances success of breast-feeding.

7. Breast milk (or formula closely resembling breast milk in content) is given. Special formulas may be prescribed for special deficiencies.

8. Regurgitation caused by reverse peristalsis results in caloric loss. Feeding may also be affected by other conditions. Stool color normally changes from greenish meconium to greenish brown or yellowish brown and then to light yellow in bottle-fed infants and yellow-mustard and pasty in breast-fed infants.

9. This position promotes drainage and gastric emptying.

10. Rationales: _____

Nursing diagnosis: *High risk for fluid volume deficit related to sensible and insensible losses*

GOAL: Maintain fluid and electrolyte balance.

Interventions

1. Calculate fluid requirements based on the infant's weight, even though full-term infants tend to restrict their own fluids initially and regulate their own needs.

2. Monitor fluid intake and output accurately, and include all sources of intake and losses.

3. Assess the infant's first voiding and subsequent voiding pattern.

4. Assess for the absence of voiding, poor skin turgor, edema, and depressed fontanels.

5. Additional individualized interventions: _____

_____

Rationales

1. Fluid requirements depend on the infant's weight and condition (see Appendix 8: Fluid and Nutritional Needs in Infancy, for information on fluid needs).

2. Kidney function in the infant is immature, affecting concentration and reabsorption of water and electrolytes.

3. The first voiding occurs within 24 hours and is limited until fluid intake has been initiated. Bladder capacity averages 15 ml; voidings range from 2 to 3 ml/kg/hour or more with an approximate total of 170 ml daily. By age 3 days, the infant may void 10 to 20 times in 24 hours.

4. These are dehydration signs, which may be caused by warmers or phototherapy, vomiting, or poor feedings. These signs would be seen between age 3 and 7 days, not at birth or shortly thereafter.

5. Rationales: _____

_____

Nursing diagnosis: *High risk for impaired skin integrity related to rash, irritation, or use of skin-damaging substances*

GOAL: Maintain intact skin, free from injury or irritation.

Interventions

1. Assess all bony prominences for redness and pressure and buttocks and perineal area for erythema (redness) and rash.

2. Avoid using tape on skin.

3. Clean the infant's skin with water-soaked gauze initially after delivery and at each diaper change thereafter.

4. Bathe the infant during the 1st week with warm water. Perform following baths with soap and water (about once or twice weekly), using a low-alkaline, unscented soap, such as Neutrogena, Aveeno, or Oilatum.

5. Avoid using perfumed lotions, powders, and creams.

6. Use only warm water if the infant's skin is irritated or abraded.

7. Additional individualized interventions: _____

_____

Rationales

1. These areas are prone to injury because of the infant's inability to change position and because of irritation from urine and stool.

2. Removing tape from the infant's fragile skin may damage or actually remove the skin.

3. This promotes cleanliness and comfort without using irritating substances.

4. Bathing is limited for the first few days to retain the acid mantle (pH) of the skin for its bactericidal action. Alkaline soaps destroy this mantle by changing the pH for 1 hour after use (see Appendix 12: Parent Teaching Guides, for more information on infant bathing).

5. Most lotions, powders, and creams may be absorbed into the skin and may even cake on skin, creating irritation and a medium for microorganism growth.

6. Using any substance on irritated skin will increase the possibility of infection.

7. Rationales: _____

_____

Nursing diagnosis: *High risk for infection related to transmission of microorganisms to infant, umbilical cord stump, or circumcision*

GOAL: Prevent and minimize transmission of infectious agents.

Interventions

1. Assess the infant daily for skin breaks, rashes, and lesions.

2. Assess the umbilical cord and circumcision areas for redness, drainage, and foul odor. Observe also for edema and decreased urine output.
• Keep the umbilical area clean and dry; as ordered, apply alcohol or other preparation, such as triple dye or iodine-based solution (for instance, Betadine).
• Fold diapers below the umbilical area.

3. Exclude infants with infections from the nursery; isolate those with suspected infections.

4. Use gloves to care for infants with skin breaks or wounds. Discourage parents from kissing infant on the lips. Use proper handwashing methods as well as barriers when handling infants. Discourage others who may have or carry infections, such as family members, from handling the infant directly.

5. Follow handwashing and gown protocols before handling the infant.

6. Follow the protocol for care of equipment and supplies in the nursery. Maintain an individual unit and supplies for each infant.

7. Observe the infant for lethargy, poor feeding, apnea, tachypnea, hypothermia, weight loss, hypotension, jitteriness, hypertonia, hypotonia, jaundice, and vomiting.

8. Additional individualized interventions: _____

_____

Rationales

1. Breaks in the body's first line of defense, the skin, expose the infant to infection.

2. These are indications of infection.

• These agents promote drying. Betadine also provides a bactericidal effect.

• Wet or soiled diapers slow the drying process and increase the risk of infection.

3. Isolation prevents the exposure of infection-free infants to infectious agents.

4. An immature inflammatory response and phagocytic activity increase the infant's susceptibility to infection.

5. Handwashing removes transient flora and prevents cross-contamination. Proper gowning also prevents cross-contamination.

6. These measures prevent cross-contamination from infant to infant.

7. These are signs and symptoms of sepsis and other infectious processes.

8. Rationales: _____

_____

Collaborative problem: *High risk for complications (such as metabolic disorders, including hypoglycemia, hypocalcemia, and phenylketonuria [PKU], and other disorders, such as anemias, hypothyroidism, hyperbilirubinemia, and drug addiction) that may lead to brain damage*

GOAL: Prevent physiologic decreases in glucose, calcium, hemoglobin (Hb), and hematocrit (HCT) values and increases in bilirubin and phenylalanine values.

Interventions

1. Perform a heel-stick test or test capillary blood for bilirubin, glucose, and serum calcium levels; red blood cell count; and HCT and Hb values, based on presenting symptoms.

2. Perform blood tests for neonatal screening, PKU, and hypothyroidism.

Rationales

1. These tests identify abnormal levels of substances that may lead to shock, seizure activity, and subsequent brain cell damage (see plans for individual conditions for complete care of infant).

2. These are common neonatal screenings. In some states, they are required by law.

Interventions

3. Perform a drug screen to determine blood alcohol or drug content if the mother's history warrants the test or the infant manifests withdrawal signs.

4. Carry out interventions specific to the abnormal condition as presented in individual plans. Base your interventions on test results and the infant's signs.

5. Additional individualized interventions: _____

Rationales

3. A drug screen will identify the drug responsible for the infant's condition. This information is needed to determine treatment.

4. Care is specific to the particular cause of the disorder.

5. Rationales: _____

Nursing diagnosis: *Knowledge deficit related to infant care*

GOAL: Provide information and instruction in infant care.

Interventions

1. Inform the parents about their infant's condition, progress, and behaviors and about various changes that take place.

2. Give information appropriate to the parents' level of understanding and readiness to learn.

3. Instruct the parents about bathing, feeding, holding, and clothing the infant and trimming the nails.

4. Inform the parents about caring for the umbilical cord and circumcision site.

5. Inform the parents why an infant cries. Explain that holding and rocking calm the infant.

6. Explain the importance of calling the physician if necessary and of visiting the physician at prescribed times.

7. Additional individualized interventions: _____

Rationales

1. Knowledge decreases the parents' anxiety about caring for their infant.

2. Information given in simple language and in small amounts can be better accepted and understood.

3. Specific instructions about normal infant care relieves anxiety and promotes a feeling of adequacy and independence. See Appendix 12: Parent Teaching Guides for a complete set of guidelines to help parents care for an infant.

4. Parents may fear causing their infant pain if they touch these areas.

5. Giving information about crying and how to manage it will allay parental fears that the infant is ill.

6. Follow-up care is essential to ensure a well baby and to prevent complications.

7. Rationales: _____

ASSOCIATED PLANS AND APPENDICES

All plans have applications for caring for the full-term infant who may develop abnormal conditions or have congenital abnormalities listed in the Table of Contents. For specific information, refer to the appropriate plans.

ADDITIONAL NURSING DIAGNOSES

• Altered family processes related to infant feeding schedule
• Altered parenting related to the addition of new family member
• Family coping: potential for growth related to adjustment to new family member
• High risk for altered parenting related to lack of support from significant others, lack of knowledge, unrealistic expectations for self, infant
• Hypothermia related to cold stress
• Ineffective family coping: compromised related to temporary family disorganization and role changes and possibly to situational crisis of new baby

INFANT

Hip Dysplasia

DEFINITION
Hip dysplasia, a congenital malformation of the hip, occurs with various degrees of deformity. One aspect of hip dysplasia is the complete or partial displacement of the femoral head from the acetabulum (socket). These displacements are grouped into three types.
• *Preluxation,* the mildest form, does not involve actual dislocation but is a delay in acetabular development (oblique and shallow, with femoral head remaining in the socket but susceptible to dislocation by manipulation).
• *Subluxation,* the most common form, is an incomplete dislocation, with the femoral head in contact with the acetabulum, but a stretched capsule allowing the femoral head to become partially displaced.
• In *dislocation,* the most severe form, the femoral head is not in contact with the acetabulum but becomes displaced backward and upward over the rim.

The incidence of congenital hip dysplasia is about 10 in 1,000 live births. About 60% of cases involve the left hip, 20% involve the right hip, and 20% involve both hips. There is a familial tendency for the abnormality, with a higher incidence in girls, first-borns, and breech deliveries. The prognosis is good if the infant is treated in the first 6 months of life. The prognosis varies afterward, so early detection is vital to achieve a successful outcome.

This plan focuses on early identification and care of the neonate with hip dysplasia and on prevention of complications resulting from treatment.

ETIOLOGY AND PRECIPITATING FACTORS
• actual cause unknown
• possible genetic association because of familial tendency
• possible result of fetal position in utero or breech birth
• possible result of pelvic laxity caused by maternal hormones secreted late in pregnancy to prepare for labor

PHYSICAL FINDINGS
Maternal and family history
• other members of family with hip dysplasia

Infant status at birth
• infant's presentation at delivery (hip dysplasia more common in breech births)
• other congenital abnormalities, such as renal and other musculoskeletal anomalies
• hip joint laxity in one or both hips

Musculoskeletal
• failure to extend legs in breech presentation; possible joint abscess if pain is present
• positive Ortolani's sign with reduction of femur—a palpable, audible click can be felt and heard when affected limb is abducted; femoral head can be felt to slip forward into socket on pressure from behind, indicating dislocation
• Barlow's maneuver, indicating an unstable hip if the femoral head can be felt to slip over the lip of the acetabulum on pressure from the front and to slip back into the acetabulum on release of pressure
• Allis' sign—shortened limb on affected side
• restricted abduction of affected hip; asymmetry of thigh and gluteal folds may be apparent at birth

DIAGNOSTIC STUDIES
• X-ray (when examination discloses problem)—may reveal femur out of acetabulum, although femur may slip in or out with maneuvering
• ultrasonography of hips—to determine abnormalities

Nursing diagnosis: *High risk for injury related to delayed care or failure to provide appropriate care (2 goals)*

GOAL 1: Recognize hip dislocation.

Interventions

1. Assess for partial or complete dislocation, as follows.

• Inspect infant for laxity in one or both hips and for restricted hip abduction.
• Perform Barlow's maneuver by placing infant on back with hips flexed to a right angle and knees flexed; then

Rationales

1. Early diagnosis and treatment (before age 2 months) are important; otherwise, hip will develop abnormal configuration from failure of femoral head to remain in hip socket as growth and ossification occur.

• Laxity indicates possible dislocation.

• These maneuvers identify subluxation of hip if femoral head can be felt to slip into acetabulum on pressure

Interventions

place middle finger over greater trochanter and thumb over inner thigh; knees are midabducted and hip receives pressure forward and backward. Listen for audible click when femur is moved in or out of acetabulum, indicating Ortolani's sign.

• Inspect for Allis' sign by placing infant's feet flat on bed, with knees flexed, and noting whether one knee is lower than the other. Also inspect for asymmetry of thigh and gluteal folds.

• Inspect for broadened perineum if infant is a girl.

2. Additional individualized interventions: _____

Rationales

from behind (Ortolani's sign) or if femoral head slips back into place on pressure from front (Barlow's sign).

• Shortening of limb and asymmetry on affected side indicates hip displacement.

• This sign is found in bilateral dislocation.

2. Rationales: _____

GOAL 2: Maintain correct positioning of hip.

Interventions

1. Apply device for reduction of hip, as follows:

• Apply two or more diapers to achieve abduction, pinning snugly from front to back.
• Apply Frejka pillow splint over diapers and secure at shoulders in snug, not tight, position; cover with plastic; remove and reapply at each diaper change.
• Apply Pavlik harness (most commonly used type).

• Prepare for and assist with hip spica cast application, if indicated.

2. Care for the device or cast as follows.
• Apply plastic or waterproof substance around edges of cast if these are near perineal area.
• Remove and wash protective material each day.
• Report damage to cast, such as cracks or breaks.

3. Additional individualized interventions: _____

Rationales

1. Various methods of hip reduction are used, depending on severity of dislocation.
• Diapers help maintain femoral head in acetabulum and are used for borderline subluxation.
• Splint maintains thighs in flexion, abduction, and external rotation; plastic covering reduces soiling of splint appliance.
• Harness splints legs while maintaining thighs in position.
• A hip spica cast may be used to treat hip dysplasia when other methods of maintaining reduction are ineffective.

2. Plastic prevents soiling or damage to cast or device that may alter effectiveness; regular washing maintains cleanliness of cast or device; reporting damage ensures cast effectiveness by maintaining proper joint immobility.

3. Rationales: _____

Nursing diagnosis: *High risk for impaired skin integrity related to pressure and irritation from reduction device or cast*

GOAL: Prevent skin breakdown and irritation.

Interventions

1. Assess skin for the following:
• cleanliness, wetness, or soiling from elimination (urinary and fecal)
• redness, excoriation, abrasions, coolness, pallor, paresthesias, and pulselessness
• pressure against skin around cast edges (tightness)
• neurovascular changes in legs (nail beds and toes) every 2 to 4 hours.

2. If cast is used, petal its edges, if sharp, and protect them with plastic.

Rationales

1. Regular assessments allow for measures to prevent skin irritation and relieve pressure. Pressure may decrease circulation to tissues, leading to skin breakdown and possible infection.

2. This technique prevents cast from rubbing on skin; the plastic shields the cast from moisture and soil.

Interventions

3. Apply foam rubber around edges of cast.

4. Turn infant with cast or appliance every 2 hours (every 4 hours at night). Support with pillows.

5. Change diapers frequently.

6. Additional individualized interventions: _____

_____

Rationales

3. Foam rubber provides cushioning and prevents pressure or irritation from cast.

4. Turning and support prevent prolonged pressure on one area and promote proper positioning.

5. Frequent diaper changing minimizes the risk of skin irritation and breakdown.

6. Rationales: _____

_____

Nursing diagnosis: *Altered peripheral tissue perfusion related to constriction of cast or reduction device*

GOAL: Prevent circulatory impairment.

Interventions

1. Assess for signs and symptoms of circulatory impairment, including:
• tightness of cast or apparatus
• coolness and duskiness of toe skin with cast.

2. Perform neurovascular checks every 2 hours.

3. Additional individualized interventions: _____

_____

Rationales

1. Assessment data determine interventions to prevent complications. Changes in color and temperature of arms and legs indicate impaired circulation.

2. Neurovascular checks evaluate circulation to the arms and legs. Changes in assessment findings may indicate compromised status and allow prompt intervention.

3. Rationales: _____

_____

Nursing diagnosis: *Knowledge deficit (parental) related to deformity and care of infant*

GOAL: Provide appropriate information about infant's condition and care.

Interventions

1. Identify parental knowledge needs, interest in learning, and readiness and capability to learn.

2. Inform parents that treatment may be long and requires patience.

3. Encourage parents to fondle, hold, and cuddle infant regardless of cast or appliance.

4. Provide information regarding:
• infant's condition
• effect of early treatment
• how to apply appliance and how to remove for bathing and diaper changes
• care of cast, if used
• skin protection
• application of diapers if they are used as splint (snug but not tight)

Rationales

1. This provides a basis for teaching plan commensurate with parental needs and abilities.

2. Restrictive movement may make infant irritable; he needs help to adjust.

3. Contact with parents promotes infant's development and provides stimulation.

4. Providing information assures safe infant care and maintains correct hip positioning.

Interventions	Rationales
• feeding in supine position with infant's hips and legs supported on pillow at mother's side or held like a football with legs behind mother for breast-feeding • importance of follow-up care.	
5. Allow for questions, clarifications, and demonstration of care techniques.	5. These measures reinforce learning and decrease anxiety.
6. Refer parents to community and home health care.	6. Referrals to community and home health care provide continued support and instruction, promoting compliance with therapy and follow-up.
7. Additional individualized interventions: _____	7. Rationales: _____

ASSOCIATED PLANS AND APPENDICES
• Birth Trauma
• Skin Disorders
• Spinal Cord Defects and Hydrocephalus
• Talipes Deformity
• Parent Teaching Guides (Appendix 12)

ADDITIONAL NURSING DIAGNOSES
• Altered growth and development related to physical disability and stimulation deficiencies
• High risk for altered parenting related to lack of knowledge, lack of support from significant other, and unrealistic expectations for infant
• Impaired physical mobility related to cast
• Ineffective family coping (compromised) related to congenital defect
• Sleep pattern disturbance related to cast or reduction device

INFANT
Hyaline Membrane Disease – Respiratory Distress Syndrome (RDS I)

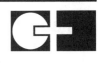

DEFINITION
Also known as idiopathic respiratory distress syndrome (RDS) Type I, hyaline membrane disease is an acute disorder found primarily in preterm infants at birth or shortly after birth, most often in infants under 32 weeks' gestation who weigh less than 3 lb, 4 oz (1,500 g). Roughly 60% of infants born before 29 weeks' gestation develop RDS.

Fetal lung development and surfactant production are necessary for normal respiratory function; lung development and surfactant production varies with each infant. The preterm infant is born before sufficient surfactant develops or with a lack of mature surfactant production. Surfactant, a lipoprotein that lines the alveoli, prevents alveolar collapse and decreases the work of respiration by decreasing surface tension. With a deficiency, surface tension increases, causing alveolar collapse and decreased lung compliance, which affects alveolar ventilation, leading to hypoxemia and hypercapnia with respiratory acidosis. The reduction in ventilation leads to a poor ventilation and perfusion ratio of the pulmonary circulation, resulting in hypoxemia. Tissue hypoxia and metabolic acidosis result with associated atelectasis and respiratory failure progression.

RDS, the leading cause of mortality and morbidity in preterm infants, usually lasts 3 to 5 days. The prognosis is poor if prolonged ventilatory support is needed; death is less likely after 3 days of treatment.

This plan focuses on care of the infant at risk for or with RDS and on all the associated respiratory support that may be needed.

ETIOLOGY AND PRECIPITATING FACTORS
• prematurity with immature lungs (ranges less than 32 to 35 weeks' gestation) and absence, alteration, or deficiency of pulmonary surfactants
• cesarean delivery of preterm infant
• decreased oxygen present in the fetus or at birth in term or preterm infants

PHYSICAL FINDINGS
Maternal history
• disorder such as diabetes mellitus
• condition such as placental bleeding
• type and length of delivery
• fetal or intrapartal stress

Infant status at birth
• prematurity, gestational age
• Apgar score noting asphyxia
• cesarean delivery of preterm infant

Cardiovascular
• bradycardia (less than 100 beats/minute) with severe hypoxemia

Integumentary
• pallor caused by peripheral vasoconstriction
• pitting edema in hands and feet within 24 hours
• mottling

Neurologic
• immobility, motionlessness; flaccidity
• decreased body temperature

Cardiovascular
• systolic murmur
• heart rate within normal limits

Pulmonary
• tachypnea (more than 60 breaths/minute; may be 80 to 100)
• expiratory grunting or whining
• nasal flaring
• intercostal, suprasternal, or substernal retractions
• cyanosis (circumoral followed by central) related to percentage of desaturated hemoglobin
• decreased breath sounds, crackles, apneic episodes

BEHAVIORAL FINDINGS
• lethargy

DIAGNOSTIC STUDIES
• serial chest X-rays—reveal clouded appearance with grainy look, areas of density or of atelectasis, and elevated diaphragm with overdistended alveolar ducts
• air bronchograms—reveal ventilation of the airway, not the alveoli

Laboratory data
• lung profiles—to determine lung maturity; done on amniotic fluid (for fetuses predisposed to RDS):
  □ lecithin/sphingomyelin (L/S) ratio of 2:1 or more indicates pulmonary maturity
  —1:1 before 35 weeks' gestation (L: 6 to 9 mg/dl, S: 4 to 6 mg/dl)
  —4:1 after 35 weeks' gestation (L: 15 to 21 mg/dl, S: 4 to 6 mg/dl)
  □ phosphatidylglycerol: elevated at 35 weeks' gestation
  □ phosphatidylinositol level
• arterial blood gas (ABG) levels—PaO_2 less than 50 mm Hg while on 100% oxygen, $PaCO_2$ less than 60 mm Hg, oxygen saturation 92% to 94%, pH 7.31 to 7.45
• potassium levels—increase as potassium is released from injured alveolar cells

Collaborative problem: *Respiratory insufficiency related to reduced lung volume and compliance, lung perfusion, and alveolar ventilation (2 goals)*

GOAL 1: Identify signs and symptoms of respiratory distress, deviations from desired functioning, and infant at risk for RDS.

Interventions

1. Assess for infant at risk for RDS, including:
• history of mother with diabetes or placental bleeding
• prematurity of infant
• fetal hypoxia
• cesarean birth.

2. Assess for changes in respiratory status, including:

• tachypnea (over 60—possibly 80 to 100—breaths/minute)

• expiratory grunting

• nasal flaring

• intercostal, suprasternal, or substernal retractions with use of accessory muscles
• cyanosis (circumoral followed by central) in room air

• apneic episodes, decreased breath sounds, and crepitant crackles.

3. Assess for associated signs of RDS, including:
• pallor and pitting edema in hands and feet within 24 hours
• flaccid muscles, motionlessness, or lying in frog-like position with head to the side
• heart rate of less than 100 beats/minute in late stage
• serial ABG values showing oxygen level less than 40 mm Hg, carbon dioxide level greater than 65 mm Hg, and pH less than 7.15
• grainy appearance and ground-glass appearance with air bronchograms.

4. Monitor transcutaneous PO_2 or pulse oximetry values continuously or every hour.

5. Additional individualized interventions: _____

Rationales

1. Assessment permits early interventions if infant displays signs of respiratory distress and, consequently, results in a better prognosis.

2. These changes indicate that RDS is present, calling for immediate treatment.
• Infant respiratory rate increases in attempt to increase oxygen level.
• This is the sound of the glottis closing to stop exhalation of air by forcing it against vocal cords.
• Flaring is an attempt to reduce resistance to respirations by narrow nostrils.
• Retractions indicate inadequate lung expansion during inspiration.
• Cyanosis becomes apparent as later sign, with PO_2 as low as 40 mm Hg.
• Apneic episodes and decreased breath sounds occur as respiratory distress becomes severer.

3. These signs occur with RDS.
• These signs result from peripheral vasoconstriction and altered vascular permeability.
• These signs result from exhaustion caused by energy expenditure during difficult breathing.
• Bradycardia results from severe hypoxemia.
• These signs indicate respiratory acidosis and metabolic acidosis if infant is hypoxic.

• This indicates RDS.

4. Transcutaneous PO_2 and noninvasive pulse oximetry devices measure oxygen percentage in inspired air. Monitoring these values ensures proper FIO_2 concentration and accuracy of readings.

5. Rationales: _____

GOAL 2: Maintain and maximize pulmonary function.

Interventions

1. Administer warm and humidified oxygen as follows:

• oxygen warmed to 89° to 93° F (31.7° to 33.9° C)
• humidity 40% to 60%

Rationales

1. Methods vary, depending on oxygen needs, infant acuity, and need for ventilatory assistance; these methods can also be used for other respiratory distress conditions.
• Warmed oxygen is provided to prevent hypothermia.
• Humidified oxygen prevents mucosal dryness.

Interventions

- small oxygen hood (Oxyhood) for infant of 2 lb, 8 oz (1,134 g) or less; medium hood for infant of 8 lb (1,135 to 3,629 g)
- Continuous positive airway pressure (CPAP), or continuous distending pressure, by endotracheal tube (using mechanical ventilation) to achieve intermittent buildup of positive pressure in the airway; nasal prongs, nasopharyngeal prongs, face mask, nasal mask, and head box are methods used for respiratory distress conditions other than RDS.
- positive end-expiratory pressure (PEEP), or continuous negative pressure, by same techniques to achieve intermittent negative pressure around the chest wall
- intermittent positive-pressure ventilation (IPPV) by endotracheal intubation (mechanical ventilation)

2. Prepare and administer pancuronium bromide (Pavulon).

3. Place infant in thermoneutral environment and monitor axillary temperature every hour.

4. Continually monitor vital signs electronically for changes in heart rate, respiratory rate, and blood pressure, and auscultate breath sounds every hour.

5. Observe for changes in skin color, movement, and activity.

6. Conserve infant's energy by spacing procedures and handling infant as little as possible.

7. Monitor serial ABG levels for PaO_2, $PaCO_2$, HCO_3, and pH levels at least hourly and every hour after any change; continuous monitoring of PaO_2 is ideal.

8. Obtain capillary blood for blood gas measurements from heelstick (warm heel for 5 to 10 minutes), if appropriate.

9. Start and maintain I.V. infusion of dextrose 10% in water ($D_{10}W$), depending on age and additional fluid requirements.

10. Additional individualized interventions: _____

Rationales

- Oxyhood, which delivers prescribed concentrations of oxygen, may be used if infant breathes spontaneously.

- CPAP is used for infant with recurrent apnea and RDS requiring more than 70% oxygen to maintain a PaO_2 of more than 60 mm Hg and to maintain breathing with positive pressure throughout respiratory cycle. Infants of 1,500 g are mechanically ventilated depending on other factors, such as gestational age.

- PEEP, like CPAP, prevents the collapse of alveoli by exerting positive pressure at end-expiratory phase, forcing the alveoli to retain air.
- IPPV is the best way of assuring effective ventilation; it is used when PaO_2 is not corrected by CPAP of 6 cm H_2O and 80% oxygen.

2. This drug may be ordered as a muscle relaxant to prevent infant from working against ventilation and causing injury.

3. A thermoneutral environment reduces oxygen requirements and carbon dioxide production by stabilizing temperature. As an initial step, this may prevent a life-threatening situation (see Hypothermia and Hyperthermia plan, page 229).

4. Changes can be observed without continually disturbing infant. Blood pressure is monitored to rule out hypovolemia respirations, to prevent long period of apnea.

5. Because changes in skin color, movement, and activity indicate increased metabolism of oxygen and glucose, additional information is necessary to meet changing fluid, caloric, and oxygen requirements.

6. Handling and performing procedures require the infant to use energy, increasing the need for oxygen, which may cause a drop in PaO_2 level.

7. PaO_2 level in the abdominal aorta of 60 to 80 mm Hg and pH above 7.25 are normal values; changes indicate potential for respiratory or metabolic acidosis.

8. Oxygen levels of 35 to 55 mm Hg in capillary blood are equal to oxygen levels of 40 to 65 mm Hg in arterial blood.

9. Infusion is given immediately to meet fluid and caloric requirements, based on calculations per kilogram of body weight, because poor gastric motility prevents oral feeding.

10. Rationales: _____

Collaborative problem: *High risk for complications related to medical therapy and treatments*

GOAL: Prevent complications of oxygen administration, assisted ventilation, mechanical ventilation, and high oxygen concentrations.

Interventions

1. Maintain safe use of Oxyhood and head box as follows:

• Do not plug holes or seal space between hood and neck.

• Ensure that hood does not touch infant and air does not blow directly into infant's face.

• Adjust oxygen to ordered flow rate, and measure amount that infant receives with oxygen analyzer, placing probe near infant's nose.

2. Maintain safe administration—by nasal or nasopharyngeal prongs—of Silastic device, as follows:

• Select prongs of appropriate size.

• Check for kinks in tube with nasopharyngeal prongs.

• Apply small amount of water-soluble lubricant to outside of prongs and insert into infant's nostrils.

• Secure prongs in infant's nostrils.

• Remove every 4 hours to check for redness and exudate, and clean and dry nostrils and prongs.

3. Maintain safe administration by face mask, as follows:

• Secure mask to face snugly.

• Check for skin trauma every 2 to 4 hours.

4. Maintain safe administration by endotracheal tube, as follows:

• Monitor pulse and respiratory rates during intubation and use Ambu bag for ventilation with 100% FIO_2.

• Based on infant's weight, select proper tube size:
  □ less than 1,000 g = 2.5 mm inner diameter
  □ 1,000 to 1,500 g = 3.0 mm inner diameter
  □ 1,500 to 2,200 g = 3.5 mm inner diameter
  □ greater than 2,200 g = 4.0 mm inner diameter.

• Have extra endotracheal tube, Ambu bag, and mask at hand.

• Place infant on flat surface with head tilted backward slightly and shoulders elevated slightly with a folded towel.

• After intubation by appropriate personnel, secure tube in proper position after placement is verified by X-ray or auscultation of air entering lungs.

• Connect tube to oxygen source or mechanical ventilator.

Rationales

1. Oxyhood has advantage of being noninvasive, but neck seal is difficult to achieve.

• Holes allow for escape of carbon dioxide.

• Danger exists of producing cold stress or of causing apnea by stimulating facial nerves.

• Proper adjustment ensures correct concentration of oxygen and prevents administration of higher amounts.

2. Prongs may injure turbinates and septum, causing excessive crying from discomfort. Sedation with chloral hydrate I.V. may be required; if so, change to assisted ventilation will be necessary.

• Appropriate size prevents irritation and leaks.

• Straight tubing ensures patency.

• Lubricant permits easier application and decreases mucosal excoriation. Infants with nasal prongs needing CPAP in addition to oxygen have problem maintaining constant pressure.

• Proper fit prevents air leak.

• Cleaning nostrils prevents breakdown of nasal mucosa from pressure; cleaning prongs ensures patency.

3. Face mask is a simple method of oxygen administration, but fixation is difficult.

• Proper fit prevents air leak.

• Pressure of mask on face may cause injury or skin breakdown.

4. Safety measures prevent complications.

• Monitoring ensures proper ventilation until tube and oxygen are in place.

• Proper fit is necessary to prevent injury to trachea. Tube size can also be determined by equating width of infant's little finger with diameter of trachea.

• Extra tube can be used in event of extubation or failure of ventilator.

• Hyperextension may close airway, so maintain appropriate position before intubation.

• Intubation procedure should be done by those trained in the technique. Verifying placement ensures that tube is not in the esophagus or positioned too far into the trachea. Securing tube prevents displacement, once it is verified.

• Connection to oxygen source permits oxygen flow.

Interventions

• Set alarms and maintain ON position; monitor and record all settings hourly, including changes made and who made them.

• Monitor both endotracheal and ventilator tubes to make sure they're patent, free of moisture, and not displaced.

5. Administer prescribed amount of CPAP or PEEP safely. One possible schedule is the following:

• Start with 3 to 4 cm H_2O.

• Monitor ABG measurements with each change of pressure or oxygen.

• Increase inspired oxygen in 5% to 10% increments if PaO_2 level remains below 50 mm Hg at pressures of 12 to 15 cm H_2O.

6. Maintain safe use of ventilator and document hourly as follows:

• Check that circuit to be used is leakproof.
• Check that heated nebulizer is working and that nebulization of inspired gas is correct.
• Check tubing to avoid condensation and accumulated moisture.

• Check tubes for kinking.
• Check ventilator settings for concentration and volume, and maintain as prescribed.

• Set alarms and maintain in ON position.
• Check manometer to maintain pressure and in-line thermometer for correct temperature.

7. Provide safe suctioning every 4 hours, using sterile technique for copious secretions, to prevent occluded endotracheal tube. Suctioning should be performed by one pass through tube with 5F or 6F suction catheter. Use no Ambu bag; reconnect to ventilator.

8. If hood or incubator is used or needed in other methods, place an oxygen analyzer with probe in area to be measured, such as near infant's nose.

9. If transcutaneous PO_2 or pulse oximeter is applied, monitor continuously or once every hour and record. Calibrate sensor each shift and rotate sensor position every 3 to 4 hours.

10. Additional individualized interventions: _____

Rationales

• Alarms provide warning that ventilator is not functioning or needs adjustment.

• This ensures patency for proper functioning and prevents suffocation from overhumidification or infection (moisture in tubing provides a growth medium for bacteria).

5. CPAP or PEEP prevents the collapse of alveoli by exerting positive pressure at end-expiratory phase. Procedures vary with hospitals and policy.

• Starting at lower pressure and increasing pressure, as appropriate, is a safety measure.
• This helps determine whether pressure needs to be adjusted; however, continuous monitoring is ideal.
• Oxygen increases must be made cautiously and according to protocol to prevent complications.

6. Ventilators used for infants are time-cycled or volume-cycled to assure adequate volume of gas to ventilate the lung and oxygenate and remove carbon dioxide from the blood. A respiratory therapist performs checks and documents chart.
• A leakproof circuit ensures safe functioning.
• This is necessary for safe ventilator function.

• This is another safety-related consideration; moisture in the tubing provides a good medium for bacterial growth.
• This ensures patency.
• This level varies according to type of ventilator and what is desirable for infant and ensures safe functioning.
• Alarm system ensures safety.
• These checks are necessary for safe ventilator function.

7. Suctioning may produce atelectasis or lesions by removing gas from small airways or may cause trauma from catheter tip. Infection may occur from introduction of contaminants. Hypoxia may also result.

8. Analyzer measures oxygen concentrations administered in a confined environment. Alarm sounds if oxygen is above or below desired concentrations.

9. Monitoring determines the fraction of oxygen in inspired air and ensures FIO_2 concentrations and accuracy of readings. Rotating sensor prevents skin burns. Electrode sites include chest, abdomen, and inner thigh. The oxygen diffusing through the skin from capillaries directly beneath the skin is measured. The oximeter is preferred because it doesn't produce heat.

10. Rationales: _____

Nursing diagnosis: *Altered nutrition: less than body requirements related to inability to ingest feedings, decreased gastric motility, and withholding of food and water*

GOAL: Maintain and support nutritional intake.

Interventions

1. Establish I.V. infusion of $D_{10}W$ at 65 to 80 ml/kg/day.

2. Insert nasogastric or orogastric tube (5F to 8F) to provide gavage feedings if indicated, to evaluate stomach contents, or to assist with placement of nasoduodenal or nasojejunal tube for feedings if prescribed.

3. Verify placement of tube as follows:
• Aspirate gastric contents.
• Inject minimal amount of air and auscultate for entry into stomach.
• Place tip in water; the tip will produce no bubbles if it is in the stomach.

4. Provide gavage feedings as follows:

• Elevate infant's head slightly.
• Allow breast milk or formula to flow into tube by low gravity from height of 6″ to 8″ above infant's head.
• Administer feedings at room temperature.

• Give 2 to 4 ml/minute as tolerated and then flush tube with sterile water.

• Place infant on side after feeding for 1 hour.

• Feeding schedules vary according to hospitals. A suggested schedule follows:
  □ Start with about 4 ml of formula every feeding for 1st day.
  □ Advance formula feeding 2 to 4 ml each day, depending on how well the infant tolerated the previous feeding.
  □ Advance feedings slowly with preterm infants. This helps prevent necrotizing enterocolitis. Reduce feeding at first indication of trouble.
  □ Check residuals before feedings and report to physician if more than 2 ml remain. Subtract residual amount from the amount to be given, provided it is a minimal amount. Residuals higher than 30% of previous feedings might mean that a next feeding will be omitted. If large residuals occur persistently, discontinue feedings.
  □ Add Pedi Mui to I.V. fluids if feedings cannot be achieved by 4 to 5 days and consider total parenteral nutrition (TPN) and intralipids.

5. Provide TPN when indicated.

6. Additional individualized interventions: _____

Rationales:

1. Rate is for initial caloric intake rather than for oral feedings.

2. A choice of routes for feedings is available when feedings are allowed, although feedings are withheld when umbilical arterial catheter is in place. The tube for gavage feedings must be placed cautiously; infant usually is too sick for feedings.

3. Verification prevents feedings from entering trachea.

4. Gavage feedings provide nutritional requirements with minimal energy expenditure.
• This position usually is used for feedings.
• Flow minimizes metabolic activity and reduces pressure on diaphragm by preventing distention.
• Feedings at room temperature are better tolerated and prevent body temperature changes.
• Small feeding amounts are supplied to accommodate infant's small stomach capacity; flushing maintains tube patency.
• Side position facilitates gastric emptying and prevents regurgitation.
• Feeding by gavage should include 20 kcal/30 ml, increasing to 120 to 144 ml/kg/day

5. TPN is an alternative method for maintaining nutrition if bowel sounds are not present and infant remains in acute stage (see Tracheoesophageal Fistula or Esophageal Atresia plan, page 297, for information on TPN).

6. Rationales: _____

Nursing diagnosis: *High risk for fluid volume deficit related to sensible and insensible fluid losses*

GOAL: Maintain fluid and electrolyte balance.

Interventions

1. Maintain I.V. infusion of $D_{10}W$ at 60 to 100 ml/kg/day.

2. Increase infusion by 10 ml/kg/day, depending on urine output, radiant heater use, and amount of enteral feedings.

3. Maintain I.V. at prescribed rate, using an infusion pump.

4. Monitor fluid intake and output by:
• weighing infant every 8 hours
• weighing diapers for urine output
• keeping track of number and amount of stools
• monitoring amount of fluid infused hourly.

5. Review electrolyte levels for sodium and potassium increases every 12 to 24 hours.

6. Additional individualized interventions: _____

Rationales

1. Initial fluid replacement prevents imbalance.

2. Maintain fluids based on patient's needs. Tachypnea and use of radiant warmer increase fluid loss.

3. Too rapid or too much fluid administration could cause circulatory overload, which may be fatal.

4. Fluid intake and output record indicates potential imbalance and serves as basis for fluid replacement.

5. Changes in electrolyte levels indicate dehydration and potential electrolyte imbalance.

6. Rationales: _____

Nursing diagnosis: *Ineffective family coping: compromised related to anxiety, guilt, and separation from infant as result of situational crisis*

GOAL: Minimize anxiety and guilt, and support bonding between parents and infant.

Interventions

1. Assess parents' verbal and nonverbal expression of anxiety and use of coping mechanisms.

2. Help parents verbalize feelings about sick infant, prolonged care in neonatal intensive care unit, and procedures and equipment used in infant care.

3. Provide consistent and accurate information concerning infant's condition and progress.

4. As appropriate, encourage parents to visit, stroke, and care for infant.

5. Refer parents to social services and community agencies.

6. Additional individualized interventions: _____

Rationales

1. This helps to identify and develop constructive coping strategies.

2. Encouraging parents to express feelings helps maintain a trusting, secure environment and shows acceptance of parents' concerns and fears.

3. Information reduces anxiety about course of disease and whether infant is improving.

4. Touching promotes bonding process.

5. Referrals offer additional support, information, and assistance to parents during the acute illness and after discharge.

6. Rationales: _____

ASSOCIATED PLANS AND APPENDICES
• Abruptio Placentae
• Air Leak Syndromes
• Bronchopulmonary Dysplasia
• Cesarean Section Birth
• Hypoglycemia
• Hypothermia and Hyperthermia
• Meconium Aspiration Syndrome
• Pregnancy Complicated by Diabetes Mellitus
• Preterm Infant, Less Than 37 Weeks
• Tracheoesophageal Fistula or Esophageal Atresia
• Aspects of Psychological Care—Maternal (Appendix 4)
• Assessing Vital Signs in the Infant (Appendix 9)
• Normal Lab Values for the Newborn Infant
(Appendix 10)

ADDITIONAL NURSING DIAGNOSES
• Altered cardiopulmonary tissue perfusion related to disease process
• Altered family processes related to critically ill infant
• Altered parenting related to interruption in bonding process and unrealistic expectations for self, infant
• Anticipatory grieving (parental) related to perceived potential loss of child
• Anxiety (parental) related to threat of infant's death
• Dysfunctional ventilatory weaning response related to lung immaturity and prolonged use of mechanical ventilation
• High risk for altered body temperature related to immaturity
• High risk for infection related to inadequate primary defenses, skin, mucous membranes, and invasive procedures
• Inability to sustain spontaneous ventilation related to respiratory distress
• Knowledge deficit (parental) related to lack of exposure to information regarding care of infant

Hyperbilirubinemia

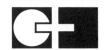

DEFINITION
Hyperbilirubinemia is greater-than-normal amounts of bilirubin in the blood, which, when the level is high enough (5 mg/dl in the full-term infant), produces jaundice, a visible yellowing of the skin, mucosa, sclerae, and urine.

Hyperbilirubinemia results from an alteration in the normal pathways of bilirubin metabolism and excretion. After bilirubin is produced, it is transported to the liver in its unconjugated form and bound to albumin in plasma (8.5 to 17 mg of bilirubin to 1 g of albumin) for action by the enzyme glucuronyl transferase, which converts it to conjugated bilirubin. It is then excreted through the biliary tree into the duodenum and also through the kidneys if serum levels become abnormally high. In the intestine, it is converted back to unconjugated bilirubin and absorbed by the intestinal wall into the enterohepatic circulation, which creates an additional load to be metabolized by the liver or excreted. Because the infant's capacity to excrete bilirubin is only 1% to 2% of the adult's during the first few days of life, all infants have elevated amounts of bilirubin with 25% to 50% of full-term infants and more than 50% of preterm infants experiencing jaundice.

Physiologic jaundice is the rise and fall in serum bilirubin (indirect) levels to 8 mg/dl (upper limit of 12 mg/dl) by the 4th day after birth, with gradual decreases to less than 1.5 mg/dl by the 10th day in normal infants (about 80% of infants). Jaundice occurs from 24 to 48 hours after birth, usually because of a breakdown of erythrocytes, which have a shorter life span in the infant than in the adult (specifically, one-half to one-third that of the adult's), resulting in an increased load to the liver. In the infant, bilirubin production is 6.5 mg/kg daily, or 35 mg per breakdown of each gram of hemoglobin (Hb). Bilirubin that is not formed from erythrocyte breakdown results from the destruction of early red blood cell (RBC) forms within the bone marrow or shortly after release from the bone marrow. Deficiency of glucuronyl transferase and reabsorption of unconjugated bilirubin from the intestine may contribute to elevated bilirubin levels in physiologic jaundice.

Breast-feeding jaundice, another type of hyperbilirubinemia, occurs in 1% to 5% of breast-fed, full-term infants. It is thought to be caused by inhibition of action of glucuronyl transferase by pregnanediol and a free fatty acid found in breast milk. This form of jaundice usually occurs by the 4th to 7th day after birth, with bilirubin levels rising as high as 15 mg/dl or more. Increased levels last 2 to 3 weeks before decreasing. The condition may require cessation of breast-feeding for 2 to 4 days; however, if the infant is healthy, bilirubin levels tend to decrease without treatment and are not associated with toxic complications.

Pathologic jaundice results from conditions that increase bilirubin production or reduce its excretion. It most often occurs within 24 to 36 hours after birth. Increased production results from hemolytic diseases, polycythemia, abnormal enterohepatic circulation, and extravascular bleeding. Decreased excretion results from decreased hepatic uptake of bilirubin, decreased bilirubin conjugation, impaired transport of conjugated bilirubin, and obstructed bile flow. Increased production and decreased excretion may result from prenatal infection or postnatal sepsis or prematurity with associated serious illnesses. Infants of diabetic mothers may also have this condition. Bilirubin levels that exceed 12 mg/dl (or a much lower level in preterm infants) and that increase by 5 mg/dl or more daily (determined by gestational age and weight) indicate a pathologic process.

Bilirubin encephalopathy, *(kernicterus)* results from deposits of unconjugated bilirubin in brain cells, which can result in mental retardation, behavioral disorders, delayed motor development, ataxia, and sensorineural hearing loss. Signs and symptoms appear between the 2nd and 10th days after birth, with bilirubin levels exceeding 20 mg/dl in full-term infants and 10 mg/dl in preterm infants (15 mg/dl in larger preterm infants). Variations depend on prematurity and vulnerability, illness, and other factors. Exact levels at which brain damage results in any one infant cannot be determined.

This plan focuses on care of the infant who displays signs and symptoms of hyperbilirubinemia with associated jaundice and on prevention of possible complications.

ETIOLOGY AND PRECIPITATING FACTORS
Physiologic jaundice
(believed to contribute to condition by presenting an increased load of bilirubin to the liver)
• shortened RBC survival
• destruction of early RBC forms
• deficiency or decreased activity of glucuronyl transferase
• enterohepatic reabsorption of indirect bilirubin from withholding of food and water or from late feedings, which cause intestinal stasis
• hyperalimentation or intralipid administration

Pathologic jaundice
• hemolytic diseases such as ABO and Rh incompatibility and severe erythroblastosis or use of certain drugs (such as vitamin K_3)
• genetic disorders, such as galactosemia, enzyme defects, hemoglobinopathies, and spherocytosis
• extravascular blood, such as blood swallowed during delivery, hematoma, petechiae, and cerebral hemorrhage
• polycythemia from fetal transfusions or fetal hypoxia
• severe enterohepatic circulation from bowel obstruction or reduced peristalsis

• decreased uptake of bilirubin by liver, such as with decreased protein levels, or drugs competing for sites to bind to albumin (maternal drug and alcohol abuse)
• decreased conjugation of bilirubin from such drugs as sulfonamides, salicylates, corticosteroids, and chloramphenicol, or congenital decrease in enzyme activity
• biliary obstruction from tumor, liver disease, or biliary atresia
• infection in infant, perinatal or prenatal infection, TORCH, syphilis, hepatitis
• preterm infant with or without serious illness
• infant of diabetic mother

PHYSICAL FINDINGS
Family and maternal history
• parent or sibling with neonatal jaundice or liver disease
• prenatal care
• maternal diabetes mellitus
• infections, such as toxoplasmosis, syphilis, hepatitis, rubella, cytomegalovirus, and herpes, which may be transmitted across the placenta during pregnancy
• maternal or paternal use of I.V. street drugs
• mother with Rh-negative blood and father with Rh-positive blood
• past transfusions of Rh-positive blood if mother is Rh-negative, causing production of anti-Rh antibodies by mother's immune system
• past abortions or deliveries of Rh-positive infant or fetus followed by treatment with immunoglobulin (RhoGAM) within 72 hours of delivery to destroy fetal RBCs passing into maternal circulation before they cause an immunogenic effect
• treatment during pregnancy with RhoGAM if mother is Rh negative and father is Rh positive
• medications, such as sulfonamides, nitrofurantoins, and antimalarials, taken during pregnancy
• oxytocin-induced labor
• vacuum extraction delivery
• possibility that mother had phenobarbital 1 to 2 weeks before delivery to stimulate protein synthesis, to provide increased binding sites, and to increase activity of glucuronyl transferase (no longer considered appropriate therapy because disadvantages outweigh advantages)

Infant status at birth
• prematurity or small for gestational age (SGA)
• Apgar score indicating asphyxia
• delayed cord clamping
• traumatic delivery with hematoma or injury
• neonatal sepsis, presence of foul-smelling fluid
• hepatosplenomegaly

Cardiovascular
• generalized edema or decreased blood volume, leading to cardiac failure in hydrops fetalis

Gastrointestinal
• poor oral feedings (refusal to take feeding or vomiting as bilirubin level rises)
• weight loss of up to 5% in 24 hours caused by low caloric intake from delayed bilirubin conjugation
• delay in passage of meconium or infrequent stools, causing increase in enterohepatic circulation
• hepatosplenomegaly in severely affected infant with anemia or infection

Integumentary
• jaundice (light to bright yellow hue) appearing within first 24 hours after birth (pathologic type), after first 24 hours (physiologic type), or after 1 week with breast-feeding; usually progresses from head to toe, with sclerae turning yellow before skin; in preterm infants, usually appears on trunk first
• pallor caused by anemia occurs only with severe hemolysis of RBCs

Neurologic
• hypotonia
• tremors, absent Moro and sucking reflexes, diminished deep tendon reflexes with encephalopathy
• downward gaze, irritability, elbows flexed with tight fists, rigid musculature, opisthotonic posture as central nervous system involvement progresses
• seizures

Pulmonary
• apnea, cyanosis, dyspnea later in kernicterus
• asphyxia, pulmonary effusion in hydrops fetalis

Renal
• dark-colored urine, which becomes more concentrated as bilirubin level rises

BEHAVIORAL FINDINGS
• lethargy (kernicterus)
• irritability (kernicterus)
• high-pitched cry (kernicterus)

DIAGNOSTIC STUDIES
Laboratory data
• blood typing and Rh factor—in mother and infant—to determine potential for incompatibility; father also tested if mother is Rh negative (test done prenatally)
• amniocentesis with amniotic fluid analysis—done if indirect Coombs' test on mother indicates increased anti-D antibody titer (1:32 or more in 4th or 5th month of pregnancy); bilirubin level in amniotic fluid increased to more than 0.28 mg/dl is considered abnormal (may indicate need for fetal transfusions)
• Coombs' test (direct) on cord blood after delivery— positive if antibodies (Rh-positive anti-A or anti-B) are attached to infant's RBCs
• Coombs' test (indirect) on cord blood—positive if antibodies (Rh-positive anti-A or anti-B) are present in mother's blood; may be done on mother at intervals during pregnancy to measure increases in anti-D antibody titer, which suggest incompatibilities

• serial total bilirubin levels—rise of more than 0.5 mg/hour to 20 mg/dl indicates risk for kernicterus and possible need for exchange transfusion, depending on infant's weight and gestational age; cord bilirubin level important, with increases of more than 4 mg/dl indicating need for exchange transfusion, depending on whether increase is 1 hour or 24 hours after delivery

• direct bilirubin level—increased (above 1 mg/dl) with infection or severe Rh hemolytic disease

• erythrocytes from peripheral smear—to determine numbers, immaturity, or abnormality revealing immaturity occurring with erythroblasts in Rh and spherocytes in ABO disorders

• reticulocyte count—increased with hemolysis; level of 12% with a hematocrit (HCT) of less than 40% indi-

cates need for exchange transfusion

• Hb and HCT—to measure concentration of Hb and percentage of RBCs in blood as Hb is released when RBCs are destroyed; HCT of less than 42% and Hb of less than 14 g/dl with hemolysis results in anemia; Hb in cord blood of less than 12 g/dl indicates need for exchange transfusion

• total proteins—to determine decrease in binding sites

• white blood cell count—decreases of less than 5,000/mm^3 or band forms increased to 2,000/mm^3 indicate infection

• urinalysis for specific gravity—to determine concentrating or reducing substance

• urinalysis—to detect glucose and acetone, pH and urobilinogen, and creatinine levels

---

Collaborative problem: *Increase in bilirubin level related to physiologic or pathologic conditions in newborn infant, placing infant at risk for long-term complications (2 goals)*

GOAL 1: Recognize signs and symptoms in infant at risk for hyperbilirubinemia.

Interventions

1. Assess for infant at risk for hyperbilirubinemia, including:

• mother and infant blood types and Rh factors; Coombs' test results; prematurity; infant size (SGA or large for gestational age); maternal illnesses or treatments that might affect infant; traumatic delivery; and severe infant illness, such as sepsis or asphyxia

• family and maternal history, infant's status at birth, and race

• color of amniotic fluid when membranes rupture

• cord bilirubin levels, reticulocyte count, HCT and Hb values.

2. Assess to determine physical signs and symptoms of hyperbilirubinemia, including:

• jaundice (yellowish skin, sclera, and mucosa).
Note: Use daylight or white fluorescent light for observation, blanching skin first over bony prominence to remove capillary coloration. Observe oral mucosa and conjunctival sac in dark-skinned infants.

• delayed stools

• dark-colored, concentrated urine

• poor feeding, lethargy, tremors, high-pitched cry, absent Moro reflex

• vomiting, irritability, rigid musculature, opisthotonos, elbows flexed with tight fists, seizures.

Rationales

1. The initial assessment performed for the infant at risk identifies abnormalities.

• Early identification of risk for hyperbilirubinemia allows preventive interventions and monitoring to ensure infant's safety.

• Infants of Native American and Asian descent have higher mean bilirubin levels.

• Yellow amniotic fluid indicates significant hemolytic disease.

• Increases in bilirubin level before 24 hours indicate pathologic hyperbilirubinemia; after 48 hours, physiologic hyperbilirubinemia. A serum bilirubin level increase of 5 mg/dl/day or more than 0.5 mg/hour or an increase in cord bilirubin level to 4 mg/dl indicates severe hemolysis or pathologic process. Increased reticulocytes and decreased HCT and Hb values are also significant and place infant at risk.

2. Recognizing physical signs of hyperbilirubinemia permits timely intervention and prevents complications.

• Almost all infants develop some degree of jaundice from increased hemolysis of RBCs.

• Bilirubin not excreted in stool is reabsorbed and sent back to liver in unconjugated form, creating an additional load to the liver.

• Dark, concentrated urine may be observable in full-term infants with more mature kidneys as bilirubin levels rise.

• These are first signs of bilirubin encephalopathy (kernicterus).

• These are later signs of encephalopathy, indicating potential for permanent damage.

Interventions

3. Evaluate physical signs, laboratory test results for bilirubin levels, and other changes as well as full-term or preterm status of infant.

4. Additional individualized interventions: _____

Rationales

3. These laboratory results and signs of infant maturity are significant in the context of time in determining treatment. A full-term infant with cord bilirubin level of 7 mg/dl at birth would be managed differently from a full-term infant with 7 mg/dl who is 24 hours old, for example.

4. Rationales: _____

GOAL 2: Minimize risk of hyperbilirubinemia and complications by decreasing bilirubin levels with phototherapy or exchange transfusion.

Interventions

1. Provide phototherapy based on bilirubin levels, infant age (under or over 24 hours), and hospital protocol. A possible guideline is to use phototherapy for an infant under 24 hours old if bilirubin level is 5 to 9 mg/dl and for infant over 24 hours old if bilirubin level is 10 to 14 mg/dl; check and update levels frequently.

• Note length of time determined by physician.

• Place infant nude, except for diaper, under special blue fluorescent lamps with Plexiglas shield to protect infant from ultraviolet rays.

• Cover infant's eyes when under light; remove cover when not under light. Use eye patches or Bilimask; do not apply mask too tightly.

• Monitor energy delivered; record as watts/cm² over 420 to 475 nm. For a single light, measure photointensity once per shift; for two lights, check each light separately and then both lights together once per shift.

• If a fluorescent light is applied, use 200 to 400 foot-candles, and record length of time the bulb is used and infant's exposure. Turn infant every 2 hours or as appropriate.

• Continue with feeding schedule.

• Remove infant from light when mother visits or feeds.

• Check bilirubin level every 4 to 8 hours. (Some institutions require bilirubin checks every 2 hours.) Turn light off when securing blood for test; otherwise, false low level may result.

2. Assess for adverse effects of phototherapy.

• Monitor temperature every 2 to 3 hours. If thermistor probe is used, shield it from light. Use Isolette for infant.

• Weigh infant every 8 hours for loss of 2% of body weight.

• Monitor urine output, specific gravity, and color every 1 to 4 hours.

Rationales

1. Phototherapy reduces bilirubin in the skin to a form that may be excreted in urine and feces by photo oxidation of bilirubin to biliverdin, then to yellow pigments, and then to colorless, nontoxic compounds. Each hospital has its own protocol and guidelines for phototherapy indications.

• After an initial rise, bilirubin levels usually start to decrease after 2 to 3 days of treatment and show a steady decline.

• Equipment emits most effective wavelengths (420 to 460 nm) while reducing exposure to other light that is ineffective in treating jaundice.

• High-density light may cause retinal injury and corneal burns. Irritation from patches may cause corneal abrasions and conjunctivitis.

• Relationship exists between energy and mean rate in fall of bilirubin level.

• Types of light used vary according to effectiveness. Documentation important for type and number of lamps, distance of lights from baby, time of exposure, and length of time each area is exposed. Lamps that have been used longer than 200 hours may be ineffective.

• Feeding is necessary to fulfill fluid and nutritional needs, and early feedings are thought to prevent delay in stool pattern.

• This encourages interaction and bonding between mother and infant.

• Assessing skin jaundice alone is not accurate enough to evaluate bilirubin level decreases during phototherapy.

2. Phototherapy can cause fluid losses, hyperthermia, eye damage, and rashes.

• Elevated temperature may result from heat and dehydration.

• Weight loss may be caused by fluid loss from evaporation or loose stools.

• Desirable urine output is 2 to 3 ml/kg/hour; green urine indicates photodegradation products that filter through glomeruli; specific gravity indicates degree of urine concentration.

Interventions

• Calculate fluid needs and replace fluids according to weight loss and fluid input and output. Offer dextrose 5% in water P.O. between formula or breast feedings.

• Monitor stools for looseness and green color.

• Observe skin for color or rash every 4 hours, turning off light to make assessment.

• Remove eye patches every 4 hours for observation.

• Shield gonads from light; keep diaper clean and dry.

• Monitor bilirubin levels as ordered after phototherapy.

• Monitor direct bilirubin level before each phototherapy treatment, noting any increases. Report adverse effects of therapy to physician.

3. Provide preparation and assistance for exchange transfusion based on bilirubin levels, infant age (under or over 24 hours), and hospital protocol. Check to make sure physician has obtained written informed consent. A possible guideline is to use exchange transfusion for an infant under 24 hours old if bilirubin level is 10 to 14 mg/dl and for an infant over 24 hours old if bilirubin level is 15 to 20 mg/dl.

• Assemble disposable exchange setup with appropriate-sized French catheter and cutdown set. Have extra unopened set and catheter available.

• Ensure sterility of all equipment and supplies, and maintain sterile technique during procedure.

• Carefully check (according to policy) type and Rh of donor blood for compatibility with infant's blood. For Rh incompatibility, may give infant's type or type O, Rh-negative blood; for ABO incompatibility, may give type O with infant's Rh factor.

• Ensure that blood is less than 48 hours old and has a pH of 7.1.

• Remove blood from refrigerator 1 hour before transfusion and allow to warm to room temperature. Use blood warmers to maintain blood at 98.6° F (37° C).

• Check type of anticoagulant used: heparin or acid citrate dextrose (ACD)- or citrate phosphate dextrose (CPD)-preserved blood.

• Have protamine sulfate ready to give at end of transfusion.

• Have calcium gluconate 10% ready to give (0.5 to 1.0 ml after each 100 ml of blood given) if ACD- or CPD-preserved blood used; give if irritability, tachycardia, or prolonged Q-T segment occurs.

• Have sodium bicarbonate available if needed.

• Restrain infant with Circumstraint.

• Prepare loading dose of 25% albumin.

• Observe as catheter is placed in umbilical vein, artery, or supraumbilical cutdown; placement is verified by X-ray.

Rationales

• Phototherapy lights may increase insensible fluid loss. Offer water P.O. or I.V. between feedings if infant is dehydrated.

• Products of photodegradation are excreted in bile.

• Macropapular rash may occur from light.

• Phototherapy may cause conjunctivitis.

• Shield protects genitals from injury and skin irritation.

• Infant may have rebound rise in bilirubin level after phototherapy.

• Increased direct bilirubin level may indicate possible liver disease, which may result in bronze baby syndrome if infant is exposed to lights. This syndrome results in bronze-tinted skin and urine; recovery occurs within several weeks in infant with normal liver function.

3. This process removes infant's blood in small amounts and replaces it with compatible blood. Whole blood is given to remove circulating antibodies, to replace sensitized erythrocytes, or to remove bilirubin. Each hospital provides guidelines for exchange transfusion indications.

• This ensures that all necessary supplies are available.

• Sterility prevents contamination and potential sepsis or infection at umbilical site.

• This prevents transfusion of mismatched blood and avoids hemolytic reaction.

• Older blood has high levels of potassium from hemolysis of old RBCs and may produce acidemia and cardiac arrest. Citrate content decreases pH of blood.

• Heat is not applied because it may traumatize and hemolyze RBCs close to surface of bag. Blood is maintained at 98.6° F (37° C) to prevent hypothermia or hyperthermia.

• Heparinized blood is preferred if acidosis or hypocalcemia is present; ACD- or CPD-preserved blood is preferred if they are not.

• Protamine sulfate is given if heparin anticoagulant is used to prevent hemorrhage from overheparinized blood.

• This prevents hypocalcemia during transfusion if symptoms appear.

• Sodium bicarbonate is given to correct acidosis if it should occur.

• Circumstraint immobilizes infant during procedure.

• Loading dose may be given 1 hour before transfusion to increase amount of bound bilirubin.

• Cutdown may be done if catheter cannot be inserted or if infection exists at umbilical area.

Interventions

• Infuse a small amount of saline solution after catheter is inserted.

• Assess bilirubin level, HCT and Hb values, and other test results on first 10 ml of blood drawn.

• Passes beginning with exchanges of 10 ml for the first 100 ml with increases to 15 to 20 ml if appropriate (computed by weight of infant).

• At completion, withdraw blood for bilirubin, HCT, Hb, electrolyte, and calcium measurement and for cross-matching.

4. Take measures to prevent complications of exchange transfusion.

• Provide radiant warmer and warm blankets (if needed) during procedure and monitor skin temperature.

• Remove stomach contents by nasogastric tube. Start I.V. infusion of fluids.

• Attach infant to monitors for blood pressure and heart rate, as indicated. Assess these signs every 10 minutes during procedure and then every 15 to 30 minutes after procedure.

• Maintain closed system for transfusion. Monitor stop-cock for proper position during procedure and before completion of infusion.

• Have resuscitation equipment at hand (oxygen, suction, breathing bag, endotracheal tubes, and laryngoscope).

• Assess infant for abdominal distention, bloody stools, pallor, hypotension, cyanosis, and vomiting, and report them as a critical condition.

• Monitor rate of infusion and amount infused. Adjust according to vital sign changes and slow rate of withdrawal and infusion if needed. If calcium is given, infuse slowly and assess for line patency.

• Assess transfusion site for bleeding, redness, swelling, and drainage every 2 to 4 hours as needed. To prevent catheter dislodgment, restrain infant if catheter is left in place.

• Monitor bilirubin, glucose, and platelet values.

• Measure bilirubin levels every 4 hours after procedure and HCT values every 4 hours for 24 hours after procedure, then every 8 hours.

• Resume feedings as soon as possible, or feed by nasogastric tube as prescribed.

• Assess for medications to be taken after transfusion.

5. Additional individualized interventions: _____

_____

Rationales

• Infusion clears catheter and measures venous pressure, which should be 4 to 19 cm H_2O during transfusion.

• Levels must be measured before transfusion.

• Total volume of blood used is twice volume of infant's blood; procedure lasts for 1 hour. Blood volume at birth averages 90 ml.

• Levels must be monitored after transfusion; bilirubin level should be half of what it was before procedure.

4. Complications may result from exchange transfusion and cause threat to life.

• Providing additional warmth to infant prevents hypothermia.

• Removing stomach contents prevents aspiration; I.V. fluids provide hydration when infant is not taking feedings.

• Monitoring reveals abnormalities such as cardiac dysrhythmias, signs and symptoms of hypocalcemia or hypervolemia as caused by rate of infusion.

• Closed system prevents air from entering catheter and possible air embolus.

• Equipment may be needed to treat cardiac arrest or another emergency.

• These are signs and symptoms of intestinal perforation and possibly peritonitis as result of catheter insertion.

• Too-rapid infusion or excessive replacement may result in heart failure from hypervolemia or dysrhythmias from forceful infusion. Extravasation of calcium infusion causes tissue necrosis.

• These may be signs of infection, especially if the catheter is left in place for repeat exchange; bleeding may occur with thrombocytopenia

• Bilirubin level after transfusion should be half the level before transfusion. Platelet count is likely to be decreased after the procedure. Glucose level will be decreased immediately after the procedure if heparinized blood was used and within 1 to 2 hours if ACD- or CPD-preserved blood was used.

• Rebound effect caused by binding of bilirubin to fresh albumin may necessitate repeat transfusion. Anemia may develop because remaining antibodies may continue to destroy cells.

• Feedings maintain infant's caloric needs.

• Some medications (phenobarbital, ampicillin, and gentamicin) should not be given after exchange, if they need to be cleared from the blood.

5. Rationales: _____

_____

Nursing diagnosis: *Altered parenting related to interruption in bonding between infant and parents because of separation or critical condition of infant*

GOAL: Promote optimal bonding between infant and parents.

Interventions

1. Assess parental perception of infant's condition and parental expectations.

2. Assist parents to identify and express feelings, needs, and fears.

3. Encourage parents to visit and care for infant as much as possible during treatment. Schedule parents' participation around the following infant needs:
• feeding
• holding and touching
• diapering and bathing.

4. Explain all procedures and treatments to parents.

5. Additional individualized interventions: _____

Rationales

1. This encourages parents to be realistic in their expectations of infant and themselves.

2. Discussing feelings offers emotional support to parents and an opportunity to change behaviors.

3. Parental involvement reinforces bonding through interaction and contact.

4. Information helps alleviate parents' fear and assists with parental involvement.

5. Rationales: _____

Nursing diagnosis: *Knowledge deficit (parental) related to lack of information about condition, treatments, and projected progress*

GOAL: Provide comprehensive information about infant's condition and needs.

Interventions

1. Assess parents' information needs and acceptance of infant's condition.

2. Using language appropriate to parents' level of understanding, provide information about infant's condition, its causes, aspects of care, and expected progress.
• Explain phototherapy treatment, precautions taken, and results expected.

• Use pamphlets and other written materials to improve understanding.
• Explain need for exchange transfusion if indicated and subsequent care using monitoring devices.
• Explain that blood to be transfused will be tested for human immunodeficiency virus.

• Keep parents informed of daily improvements in infant's condition.

3. Allow time for questions and clarifications, and reinforce information if needed.

4. Teach parents about signs and symptoms of hyperbilirubinemia.

Rationales

1. Parents may not know what information to ask for. Awareness of need for information allows for realistic teaching plan and increased comprehension.

2. This increases parents' knowledge and understanding as well as their cooperation in care.

• Phototherapy is expected to decrease jaundice. Safety measures are taken to protect infant and prevent complications.
• Visual aids enhance learning and reinforce verbal instruction.
• Some pathologic states causing elevated bilirubin levels require more invasive procedures.
• Parental concern about acquired immunodeficiency syndrome is common when blood transfusion is mentioned.
• This promotes parents' trust in caregiving staff and allays their anxiety.

3. Large amounts of information may be difficult to absorb at one sitting. An opportunity to review information improves understanding.

4. Knowledge of signs and symptoms improves parents' ability to identify problems and notify physician appropriately.

Interventions	**Rationales**
5. Instruct parents in use of home phototherapy equipment, such as bilirubin lights or fiberoptic light blanket.	5. Home phototherapy may be used to minimize the need for hospitalization. Understanding the procedure and knowing how to use equipment maximize compliance.
6. Refer parents to home health care agency for follow-up care of infant.	6. Referral to home health care agency allows additional support, follow-up, and instruction for parents.
7. Advise parents to notify physician if jaundice appears within 4 to 7 days if mother is breast-feeding infant. The condition resolves itself without complications.	7. Jaundice resulting from breast milk occurs later; mother may need to discontinue breast-feeding for 2 or 3 days.
8. Additional individualized interventions: _____	8. Rationales: _____

ASSOCIATED PLANS AND APPENDICES
• Abortion
• Anemia
• Birth Trauma
• Hypocalcemia
• Hypoglycemia
• Pregnancy Complicated by Diabetes Mellitus
• Preterm Infant, Less Than 37 Weeks
• Rh Isoimmunization
• Sepsis Neonatorum and Infectious Disorders
• Sexually Transmitted Diseases/TORCH
• Normal Lab Values for the Newborn Infant
(Appendix 10)
• Parent Teaching Guides (Appendix 12)

ADDITIONAL NURSING DIAGNOSES
• Anxiety (parental) related to jaundice of infant, possible interruption of breast-feeding, potential for complications
• Fear (parental) related to critical condition of infant at birth, possible death of infant from severe hemolysis and complications, acquired immunodeficiency syndrome exposure
• High risk for fluid volume deficit related to loss as result of phototherapy, reduced oral intake, vomiting, loose stools
• High risk for injury related to complications of encephalopathy leading to brain damage, adverse effects of phototherapy, complications of exchange transfusion
• Ineffective family coping: disabled related to fear, guilt over condition of infant

INFANT
Hypocalcemia

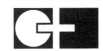

DEFINITION

Hypocalcemia is an abnormally low level of serum calcium (7 mg/dl or less or 3.5 mEq/liter or less), with symptoms occurring at less than 7 mg/dl. Measurements should be performed daily on all infants at risk for hypocalcemia; supportive treatment is considered when low levels are noted. Normally, calcium homeostasis begins soon after birth. Hypocalcemia usually is related to normal physiology and the infant's reaction to stress.

The most common reason for hypocalcemia is early neonatal low calcium levels that occur during the first 48 hours after birth. Infants at risk typically are preterm, those suffering trauma during delivery, those of low gestational age, those suffering neonatal illnesses, those suffering from neonatal asphyxia, and those with diabetic mothers. The result is a failure of homeostatic control of calcium partition between bone and serum.

A less common reason for hypocalcemia is associated with hyperphosphatemia, which occurs 5 to 7 days after birth (late onset). Infants at risk are those taking a formula with a high phosphorus content and low calcium-phosphorus ratio (for example, unmodified cow's milk) and those with immature renal function resulting in phosphorus retention, which produces a disturbance in calcium homeostasis known as tetany of the newborn. With breast-feeding and available commercial formulas, this condition is rare. A more likely cause of hypocalcemia occurring at this late date is parathyroid disease.

This plan focuses on care of the infant displaying signs and symptoms of hypocalcemia, supportive treatment for symptomatic and asymptomatic hypocalcemia, and prevention of complications after discharge.

ETIOLOGY AND PRECIPITATING FACTORS
Early-onset hypocalcemia
• preterm, small for gestational age (SGA), or low birth weight (infant has not accumulated calcium)
• trauma during delivery, such as use of forceps rotation, vacuum extraction, toxemia, abnormal presentation, breech delivery, maternal hemorrhage, treatment with magnesium sulfate, or birth by emergency cesarean section because of fetal distress
• asphyxia and associated I.V. sodium bicarbonate treatment for metabolic or respiratory acidosis because it decreases the ionized portion of serum calcium
• illnesses such as sepsis, hypoglycemia, cerebral injury, respiratory distress syndrome (witholding food and water because of illness prevents oral intake of calcium)
• diabetic mother exaggerating neonatal immaturity of parathyroid (mother has increased calcium levels that cross placenta and increase possibility of transient hypoparathyroid function in infant)
• maternal hyperparathyroidism causing hypocalcemia in infant

• exchange transfusion of infant with citrated blood because citrate combines with serum calcium, causing calcium to become nonionizable

Late-onset hypocalcemia
• with formula having high phosphorus content and low calcium-phosphorus ratio
• with formula having butterfat content may cause calcium malabsorption
• phototherapy
• maternal vitamin deficiency

PHYSICAL FINDINGS
Maternal history
• prenatal conditions, such as diabetes mellitus and hyperparathyroidism
• traumatic delivery
• severe calcium and vitamin D deficiencies

Infant status at birth
• preterm, SGA
• Apgar score indicates hypoxia and respiratory distress
• treatments received, such as administration of citrated blood as transfusion or sodium bicarbonate for acidosis
• severe illnesses with delay in feedings
• type of feedings: breast milk or formula

Cardiovascular
• cardiac dysrhythmias with prolonged Q-T interval seen on electrocardiogram at early onset

Gastrointestinal
• feeding intolerance or vomiting

Neurologic
• jitteriness, hypertonicity, localized twitching, seizures
• Chvostek's sign (spasm of facial muscle elicited by light taps on facial nerve) over either cheek

Pulmonary
• cyanosis, respiratory distress

BEHAVIORAL FINDINGS
• irritability, high-pitched cry

DIAGNOSTIC STUDIES
Laboratory data
• serum calcium level—7 mg/dl or less indicates hypocalcemia in infant
• ionized calcium level—decreased to below 4 mg/dl
• serum phosphorus level—increased in late onset to 8 mg/dl or more
• total protein (refractometer) with serum calcium levels—measured daily if infant is at risk for hypocalcemia

Collaborative problem: *High risk for decreasing calcium levels and associated complications in infants at risk for hypocalcemia (2 goals)*

GOAL 1: Recognize signs and symptoms of hypocalcemia.

Interventions

1. Assess infant for potential asymptomatic hypocalcemia; include the following:

• maternal history and infant's status at birth

• prematurity, neonatal illnesses, traumatic delivery, maternal diabetes or hyperparathyroidism, asphyxia, and transfusion

• daily review of serum calcium, ionized calcium, and total protein levels.

2. Assess for signs and symptoms of symptomatic hypocalcemia: irritability, vomiting, cyanosis or respiratory distress, seizure activity or twitching, incoordination of mouth and tongue movements, abnormal eye movements with blinking and staring, tonic posturing of a limb, and drooling. Review serum calcium and ionized calcium levels.

3. Additional individualized interventions: _____

Rationales

1. Infants at risk for hypocalcemia may receive supportive treatment as indicated by assessment.

• Serum calcium levels fall after birth for 24 to 48 hours; then levels stabilize without symptoms.

• High-risk infants must be monitored in anticipation of hypocalcemia so that supportive treatment can be initiated.

• A calcium level of 7 mg/dl or less or an ionized calcium level below 4 mg/dl with increases in total protein levels is an indication for treatment. Normal calcium level for full-term infant is 7 to 12 mg/dl (SI: 1.75 to 3.0 mmol/liter); for preterm infant, 6 to 10 mg/dl (SI: 1.5 to 2.5 mmol/liter). Normal ionized calcium level is 4.4 to 4.8 mg/dl. Normal total protein level for full-term infant is 4.6 to 7.4 g/dl; for preterm infant, 4.3 to 7.6 g/dl.

2. Symptomatic hypocalcemia requires immediate treatment. It is a life-threatening situation that often is accompanied by other problems in infant. Serum calcium levels below 7 mg/dl and ionized calcium levels below 2.8 mg/dl result in signs and symptoms of hypocalcemia.

3. Rationales: _____

GOAL 2: Maintain normal levels of calcium and minimize risk of life-threatening complications.

Interventions

1. Provide maximal rest and minimal activity. Avoid suddenly moving crib or handling or holding infant.

2. Prepare asymptomatic infant for oral calcium replacements; administer 10% calcium gluconate (drug of choice) orally at a rate of 75 mg elemental calcium/kg/day divided into six equal doses.

3. Prepare infant for infusion to treat symptomatic hypocalcemia with life-threatening potential; use infusion pump and avoid mixing with infusion of bicarbonate. Immediate treatment consists of 10% calcium gluconate at less than 1 mEq I.V., repeated every 1 to 3 days.

• Calculate accurate dose to be given as maintenance dose if needed.

• Monitor heart rate and pulse rate during I.V. infusion. Discontinue infusion and notify physician if heart rate falls below 100 beats/minute or if infant vomits.

• Monitor serum calcium level daily.

4. Administer dietary calcium for prolonged or late-onset hypocalcemia, tapering off in 2 to 4 weeks. Calcium supplement of 35 to 70 mg/dl enteral feeding in the form of calcium lactate (13% calcium), calcium gluconate (9% calcium), or calcium glubionate (23% calcium) to raise calcium-phosphorus ratio to 4:6.

Rationales

1. Unnecessary activity or stimuli may provoke tremors and seizures.

2. This is the treatment to replace calcium if serum calcium levels decrease to 7 mg/dl or ionized calcium levels fall below 4 mg/dl.

3. This is treatment for calcium replacement if levels decrease to 7 mg/dl or ionized serum calcium level falls below 2.8 mg/dl with associated symptoms.

• Treatment may continue with I.V. infusion of up to 50 mg/kg daily for 3 days.

• Bradycardia is an adverse effect of calcium administration and indicates hypercalcemia.

• This prevents hypercalcemia from calcium administration.

4. Administration of calcium supplement ensures appropriate serum calcium levels.

Interventions	**Rationales**
5. Additional individualized interventions: _____	5. Rationales: _____

Nursing diagnosis: *Impaired tissue integrity related to tissue necrosis as result of extravasation of chemical irritants by way of infusion*

GOAL: Prevent tissue damage from calcium administration.

Interventions	**Rationales**
1. Monitor administration of infusion, including:	1. Careful observation of infusion and discontinuation as necessary prevent sloughing of tissue.
• patency of infusion lines	• Patent line assures infusion of medication.
• prolonged use of same site	• Change site every 12 hours to prevent necrosis.
• precipitant in line	• Precipitant indicates incompatibility.
• movement of needle (secure with tape, if necessary).	• Movement may cause leakage during infusion.
2. Secure line with transparent occlusive dressing, and remove and replace carefully when changing I.V. line (use least amount of tape possible).	2. Dressing is a synthetic, transparent film that acts as a second skin, allowing view of site while protecting the skin.
3. Discontinue infusion by carefully removing needle and applying pressure to site for 1 minute.	3. This technique avoids extravasation of fluid into tissues during needle removal.
4. Additional individualized interventions: _____	4. Rationales: _____

Nursing diagnosis: *Knowledge deficit (parental) related to infant's condition and administration of calcium after discharge*

GOAL: Provide parents with appropriate information for safe infant care and safe medication administration.

Interventions	**Rationales**
1. Identify parents' knowledge needs, interest in learning, and readiness to learn.	1. This provides a basis for developing a teaching plan commensurate with parents' abilities and needs.
2. Provide information regarding: • infant's condition and progress • infant's need for rest (limit handling until calcium level is stable, then hold and feed) • any supplies that may be needed to maintain infant.	2. Information gives parents a more secure feeling in caring for infant. Stimuli may provoke tremors and seizures.
3. Instruct parents in oral administration of calcium, including:	3. Instructions ensure safe administration of medication and define when to report effects to physician.
• name of medication, how to measure it, how to add it to formula, and what formula to purchase	• Medications should not be given alone.
• amount and frequency of medications, including how to taper doses until discontinuation of medication	• Abrupt discontinuation of medications may cause rebound hypocalcemia.
• adverse reactions to report, such as vomiting and decreased heart rate, that may require discontinuation of medication	• Knowing what adverse effects to report may prevent complication of hypercalcemia.
• possibility of more frequent stools.	• Increased frequency of stools is common with calcium administration.

Interventions

4. Allow for questions, clarifications, and opportunities to prepare medication in formula and to feed infant.

5. Explain signs and symptoms of late-onset hypocalcemia, including:
• occurrence 6 to 10 days after discharge
• twitching, hypertonicity, irritability, eye and mouth movements
Note: This type of hypocalcemia seldom occurs when infants are breast-fed or receive formula that contains proper proportions of calcium.

6. Refer parents to home health care for follow-up.

7. Additional individualized interventions: _____

_____

Rationales

4. Discussion and practice help to reinforce instruction.

5. Providing information helps prevent complications after discharge.

6. Referral to home health care provides parents with additional physical and emotional support and added instruction to promote compliance.

7. Rationales: _____

_____

ASSOCIATED PLANS AND APPENDICES
• Birth Trauma
• Hypoglycemia
• Inappropriate Size or Weight for Gestational Age, Large
• Inappropriate Size or Weight for Gestational Age, Small
• Intracranial Hemorrhage
• Pregnancy Complicated by Diabetes Mellitus
• Preterm Infant, Less Than 37 Weeks
• Fluid and Nutritional Needs in Infancy (Appendix 8)
• Normal Lab Values for Newborn Infant (Appendix 10)
• Parent Teaching Guides (Appendix 12)

ADDITIONAL NURSING DIAGNOSES
• Altered growth and development related to environmental and stimulation deficiencies or separation from significant others
• High risk for altered parenting related to lack of information regarding infant care
• High risk for injury related to electrolyte imbalance
• Ineffective family coping: compromised related to infant's condition

Hypoglycemia

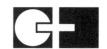

DEFINITION

Hypoglycemia is a condition of abnormally low levels of serum glucose (25 mg/dl or less in preterm infants and 35 mg/dl or less in full-term infants). Symptoms can occur at or near these levels, usually between 24 and 72 hours after birth or within 6 hours after birth in severely stressed infants. Actual practice dictates the need for immediate attention—either I.V. glucose administration or immediate feeding—in an infant with a serum glucose level under 45 mg/dl. Serum glucose levels are routinely measured within 1 to 2 hours after birth or more frequently if the infant is determined at risk for hypoglycemia. A glucose level of 45 mg/dl or more by 72 hours after birth is considered desirable despite infant weight, gestational age, and other factors.

Hypoglycemia may be symptomatic or asymptomatic. Little correlation exists between symptoms and blood glucose level. Each infant has his own "normal" level, so assessment and treatment must be highly individualized at this time, when a greater demand for glucose exists to maintain brain cells and to decrease risk of brain damage.

Transient hypoglycemia is common in intrauterine growth retarded (IUGR) infants, those small for gestational age (SGA), those with erythroblastosis fetalis, preterm infants suffering from low energy reserves or an immature liver, and those with increased demands because of diseases or ineffective gluconeogenesis. IUGR infants and infants with erythroblastosis fetalis have hyperinsulinemia. These infants are screened and monitored for hypoglycemia and receive supportive treatment immediately after birth (if indicated) to reduce potential for symptoms and complications. Hypoglycemia is also common in infants of diabetic mothers; they experience low glucose levels initially (1 to 2 hours after birth), followed by increases to acceptable levels by 4 to 6 hours after birth because of hyperinsulinism and increased number and activity of pancreatic beta cells. Less than 20% of these infants have symptoms.

The prognosis for hypoglycemia, if treated, is good; if hypoglycemia remains untreated or if the infant experiences seizures, hypoglycemia can cause significant sequelae, including cerebral damage and mental retardation. The prognosis of infants with asymptomatic hypoglycemia remains controversial. Hypoglycemic infants with diabetic mothers do well and usually recover without complications.

Hyperglycemia is a condition of increased glucose levels of more than 150 mg/dl, usually occurring in preterm infants receiving glucose infusions of 10% or greater at 100 ml/kg/day. The result may be glucose levels as high as 450 mg/dl, causing osmotic diuresis or dehydration with intraventricular hemorrhage from brain volume changes (fluid shifts) and sepsis. Treatment and prevention consist of adjusting and carefully monitoring glucose infusion rates (not to exceed 5 to 8 mg/kg/minute, as tolerated). Sick preterm infants may be given 2.5% instead of 10% glucose; they have a poor insulin response to increased glucose levels in the blood.

This plan focuses on the infant at risk for hypoglycemia after birth, supportive treatment, and prevention of complications.

ETIOLOGY AND PRECIPITATING FACTORS
• low economic status, no prenatal care
• preterm, SGA, IUGR, low birth weight (infant has not had benefit of storing glycogen)
• illness, such as sepsis, respiratory distress, asphyxia, hemolytic disease, hypothermia, galactosemia
• diabetic mother
• delayed feedings in which glucose is not replaced
• pancreatic disorders, such as adenoma or nesidioblastosis, causing overproduction of insulin
• administration of blood preserved with acid citrate dextrose (ACD)
• adrenal insufficiency, causing inadequate carbohydrate-regulating hormone
• cesarean delivery

PHYSICAL FINDINGS
Maternal history
• little or no prenatal care
• prenatal or gestational diabetes mellitus or toxemia during pregnancy
• depressed nutritional status during pregnancy
• medications or drugs taken or abused during pregnancy, such as tolbutamide, chlorpropamide, alcohol, or street drugs

Infant status at birth
• preterm, SGA, IUGR
• Apgar score indicating asphyxia
• such conditions as cold stress, congenital cardiac defects, sepsis, or central nervous system (CNS) injury
• hypocalcemia

Gastrointestinal
• poor feeding, delayed feeding, refusal to suck

Neurologic
• hypotonia, limpness
• jittery movements, muscle twitching, tremors
• hypothermia, diaphoresis
• seizures

Pulmonary
• cyanosis, respiratory distress, apnea, irregular respirations

BEHAVIORAL FINDINGS
• lethargy
• high-pitched cry
• irritability

DIAGNOSTIC STUDIES
Laboratory data
• Dextrostix (performed on admission) — color change

indicating glucose level less than 45 mg/dl or Chemstrip testing for a more accurate glucose reading, followed by serum glucose test
• Serum glucose test — to confirm concentrations by laboratory analysis of two specimens

---

Collaborative problem: *High risk for decreasing glucose levels and associated complications in infants at risk for hypoglycemia (2 goals)*

GOAL 1: Recognize signs and symptoms of hypoglycemia.

Interventions

1. Assess infant for potential or actual hypoglycemia.

• Identify infant at risk by assessing maternal history; infant's status at birth; parental economic status; history of little or no prenatal care; maternal diabetes, toxemia, alcohol or drug abuse.

• Assess physiologic factors related to hypoglycemia, including prematurity, SGA, IUGR, perinatal sepsis; neonatal illnesses; asphyxia, cold stress; exchange transfusion with ACD-preserved blood; and multiple congenital anomalies.

• Warm heel to dilate vessels and secure capillary blood sample. *Note:* Test immediately with Dextrostix or Chemstrip and appropriate glucose monitoring device.

• Test 1 hour after birth (this is when serum glucose level falls) and secure blood for laboratory; test twice if levels are below safe margin. If infant is at risk, test immediately.

• Repeat glucose level test as indicated every 30 minutes for three times, then every 2 hours for two times, and then before meals for the first 24 hours.

2. Assess for symptoms of hypoglycemia, including:
• irritability, tremors
• jittery movements, twitching
• lethargy or hypotonia
• irregular respirations, apnea, cyanosis
• refusal to suck, high-pitched or weak cry
• hypothermia, diaphoresis
• seizure activity with uncoordinated movements of mouth and tongue (chewing, sucking), abnormal eye movements with blinking of eyelids, staring, tonic posturing of limbs, drooling.

3. Additional individualized interventions: _____

Rationales

1. Infants at risk for hypoglycemia may be given supportive treatment before symptoms appear or as indicated by assessment.

• These are factors identified with infants at risk for developing hypoglycemia. In full-term infants, serum glucose levels usually fall 1 to 2 hours after birth to between 35 and 40 mg/dl and then rise between 45 and 60 mg/dl within 6 hours after birth; hepatic glucose production is 5 to 8 mg/kg/minute (25 to 45 calories/kg/hour).

• In preterm, SGA, malnourished, or sick infants, energy stores are inadequate at birth. Existing energy stores are compromised or rapidly depleted by abnormal conditions in infant. Preterm infants usually are the first to be treated for hypoglycemia.

• Securing sample from unwarmed heel may cause underestimation of glucose level because of stasis; levels may fall to 18 mg/dl/hour at room temperature.

• On infants with levels below 45 mg/dl, repeat test by laboratory analysis for more accurate determinations. Overreliance on Dextrostix alone can lead to difficulties.

• Repeat tests are necessary to confirm rise in glucose levels in normal infant or failure of levels to rise in preterm infant, especially if food and water are withheld. Normal ranges for serum glucose levels are 30 to 125 mg/dl for full-term infants and 20 to 100 mg/dl for preterm infants; 45 mg/dl is the lowest level considered safe.

2. The brain's requirement for glucose is continuous; decreases cause CNS symptoms and, if untreated, lead to cerebral damage or retardation.

3. Rationales: _____

GOAL 2: Maintain normal glucose levels, and minimize risk of life-threatening or long-term complications.

Interventions

1. Provide early feedings. Allow infant to breast-feed as soon as possible and supplement breast milk with formula or I.V. solution of dextrose 10% in water ($D_{10}W$). Offer bottle-fed infant glucose 5% in water at birth or within 2 hours if infant is preterm or suspected of being hypoglycemic.

2. Prepare infant at risk for hypoglycemia for glucose infusion when indicated, using infusion pump to regulate rate.

3. Prepare infant with acute hypoglycemia (serum glucose level of less than 30 mg/dl in full-term infant), using infusion pump to regulate rate for constancy of glucose infusion. Administer push dose of $D_{10}W$ I.V. at rate of 1 to 2 ml/kg (less if infant has diabetic mother), followed by I.V. of 100 to 200 ml/kg/day (glucose, 7 to 8 mg/kg/minute), with rate increased according to glucose levels and infant response.

4. Using Chemstrip, Dextrostix, or serum glucose level, monitor glucose levels hourly or more frequently during therapy until condition is stabilized; verify levels every 4 to 8 hours with serum glucose measurement.

5. Maintain rest, reduce activity, and provide optimal thermal environment with Isolette or over-bed warmer.

6. Prepare for administration of steroids as an additional or alternative treatment; give glucagon as an emergency treatment, especially in infants of diabetic mothers; and supply insulin I.V. as another alternative treatment.

7. Additional individualized interventions: _____

_____

Rationales

1. Early feedings and supplementation provide nutrition, serving as a preventive measure against hypoglycemia. If infant is hypoglycemic, colostrum alone is inadequate for feeding.

2. Asymptomatic treatment is given to prevent hypoglycemia. Constancy of amount of glucose delivered affects response, so using a pump to regulate I.V. infusion is advisable.

3. Symptomatic treatment is given for acute hypoglycemia.

4. Monitoring glucose levels prevents possibility of hyperglycemia while correcting hypoglycemia.

5. Rest and relaxation reduce infant's energy requirements and need for increased glucose.

6. Steroids may be administered to stimulate gluconeogenesis in the liver; glucagon stimulates insulin release (usually a last-ditch effort); this is dangerous because glucose levels rise and then drop precipitously to lower than they were originally. Administration of insulin would be preferred treatment if more insulin were needed.

7. Rationales: _____

_____

Nursing diagnosis: *High risk for injury related to hyperglycemic response*

GOAL: Prevent hyperglycemia and associated complications.

Interventions

1. Assess for factors suggesting infant at risk, including:
• immaturity (less than 30 weeks' gestation with weight of 1.1 kg or less)
• age 3 days or less
• infusion therapy with rate over 7 mg/kg/minute
• increased serum glucose level
• glycosuria (more than a trace).

2. Monitor infusion carefully by:
• using infusion pump to regulate rate
• adjusting rate according to individual infant, usually 5 to 8 mg/kg/minute, as tolerated
• ensuring patency of line and keeping site free of extravasation.

Rationales

1. Condition is common in infants with illnesses and in immature infants receiving I.V. therapy because of slower insulin response and failure of decrease in liver glucose release and in infants with illness at birth. Serum glucose level of 130 mg/dl or more is considered hyperglycemic; level of 450 mg/dl results in osmotic changes that lead to brain damage, intraventricular hemorrhage, or glycosuria.

2. These actions prevent hyperglycemia and tissue necrosis.

Interventions	**Rationales**
3. Monitor blood and urine glucose levels for changes.	3. This is essential to determine safe glucose levels and response to glucose therapy.
4. Additional individualized interventions: _____	4. Rationales: _____

Nursing diagnosis: *High risk for altered parenting related to interruption in bonding between infant and parents caused by separation and concern over infant condition and treatment*

GOAL: Promote optimal bonding between infant and parents.

Interventions	**Rationales**
1. Assess parents' perception of infant's condition and what to expect.	1. Assessment clarifies what parents need to know about infant.
2. Help parents identify feelings, needs, and fears, and provide an opportunity to express them.	2. Parents may feel guilty, especially if infant has other problems or abnormalities.
3. Offer information about infant's condition, progress, and behavior.	3. Providing timely information is important to allay parent's anxiety because infant may not behave (for example, in feeding or response to parents) as they expect.
4. Allow maximal contact between infant and parents.	4. Touching and physical contact reinforce bonding.
5. Refer parents to social service and community resources.	5. Referrals provide emotional and physical support.
6. Additional individualized interventions: _____	6. Rationales: _____

ASSOCIATED PLANS AND APPENDICES
• Congenital Heart Disease
• Hypocalcemia
• Hypothermia and Hyperthermia
• Inappropriate Size or Weight for Gestational Age, Large
• Inappropriate Size or Weight for Gestational Age, Small
• Intracranial Hemorrhage
• Pregnancy Complicated by Diabetes Mellitus
• Preterm Infant, Less Than 37 Weeks
• Sepsis Neonatorum and Infectious Disorders
• Fluid and Nutritional Needs in Infancy (Appendix 8)
• Normal Lab Values for the Newborn Infant (Appendix 10)
• Parent Teaching Guides (Appendix 12)

ADDITIONAL NURSING DIAGNOSES
• Altered nutrition: less than body requirements related to difficulty feeding
• Anxiety (parental) related to potential for complications
• Fear (parental) related to condition of infant at birth, potential loss of infant
• Ineffective family coping: disabled related to fear, guilt over condition of infant
• Knowledge deficit (parental) related to disease process

INFANT

Hypothermia and Hyperthermia

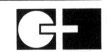

DEFINITION

Hypothermia is an abnormally low body temperature (below 97° F [36.1° C]); hyperthermia is an abnormally high body temperature (above 98° F [36.7° C]). Both conditions depend on the neonate's age, weight, and general condition. Maintaining a normal body temperature is essential to extrauterine adaptation. However, limited subcutaneous fat and a large body surface relative to mass predispose the neonate to an abnormal body temperature. Other factors also may alter body temperature, including an excessively warm or cold environment, brown fat, inability to shiver, reduced metabolism per unit area, and peripheral vessels that are dilated and close to the body surface. Most of the infant's body heat is produced through nonshivering thermogenesis as a result of lipolysis of brown fat (2% to 6% of total body weight), which is located at the nape of the neck and around the adrenal glands. This fat has a greater concentration of energy-producing mitochondria in its cells, which enhances heat production. Full-term infants generate heat by motor activity. Sick or preterm infants have little muscle activity; they cannot sustain contractions, have smaller muscle mass, and lack subcutaneous fat for heat production.

The infant's environment is affected by airflow, proximity to heat or cold, air temperature, and humidity. Heat may be lost from within the body to the body surface (internal gradient) and from the body surface to the environment (external gradient). The internal gradient may be altered by such physiologic control mechanisms as vasomotor changes, which function to deliver heat to the epidermis via blood flow from the core to subcutaneous tissues. The external gradient consists of heat loss through convection, radiation, evaporation, or conduction. Excessive environmental temperature results in dilatation of peripheral vessels, causing more heat to be delivered to the skin and lost through the body surface. The infant also attempts to remove more heat by evaporation, which is accomplished through insensible water loss and visible perspiration. In warm environments, heat gain is increased when physiologic limits of heat loss have been reached.

A complication of hypothermia is cold stress. Occurring most commonly in the preterm infant, cold stress leads to hypoxia, hypoglycemia, and metabolic acidosis. These conditions are caused by the release of norepinephrine in response to chilling. Norepinephrine release stimulates metabolism and uses oxygen and glucose to raise body temperature. After these resources are used up, glycogen is converted without oxygen, causing metabolic acidosis and pulmonary vasoconstriction, leading to impaired pulmonary function from decreased blood flow and gas exchange. These conditions may be irreversible, even with rewarming. Untreated hyperthermia may lead to brain damage or death.

After birth, the infant's core temperature may drop as much as 0.2° F (0.1° C) a minute. A neutral thermal environment is provided, depending on the infant's needs. This environment includes a room temperature that usually is higher than normal and adjusted so that the infant has to use the least amount of oxygen and the fewest calories to maintain normal core temperature.

This plan focuses on caring for the full-term and preterm infant at risk for altered thermoregulation and maintaining a neutral thermal environment.

ETIOLOGY AND PRECIPITATING FACTORS
• hypothermia
  □ prematurity
  □ asphyxia, with resuscitation procedures performed
  □ sepsis
  □ neurologic conditions, such as meningitis and cerebral hemorrhage
  □ inadequate drying and warming of infant after birth (wet infant in cold environment)
  □ exposure to cold environmental conditions
• hyperthermia
  □ excessive environmental temperature
  □ dehydration
  □ infections
  □ phototherapy
  □ central nervous system (CNS) damage from trauma or drugs

PHYSICAL FINDINGS
Maternal history
• difficult delivery with trauma to infant
• drug use
• type of anesthesia or analgesia used by mother

Infant status at birth
• prematurity
• low Apgar score
• asphyxia with resuscitation
• CNS anomalies or damage
• skin temperature below 97° F (36.5° C) or core temperature below 96° F (35.5° C) (hypothermia)
• skin temperature above 98.6° F (37° C) or core temperature above 99.5° F (37.5° C) (hyperthermia)
• maternal fever precipitating neonatal sepsis

Cardiovascular
• bradycardia
• tachycardia in hyperthermia

Gastrointestinal
• poor feeding
• vomiting or abdominal distention
• weight loss

Integumentary
- central cyanosis or pallor (hypothermia)
- bright (beefy) red color (hyperthermia)
- edema of face, arms, and legs
- cold to touch on trunk and extreme cold at arms and legs (hypothermia)
- perspiration (hyperthermia)

Neurologic
- feeble cry
- decreased reflexes and activity
- temperature fluctuations above or below normal range for age and weight

Pulmonary
- nasal flaring or decreased, irregular, and shallow respirations
- retractions
- expiratory grunt
- apneic episodes or tachypnea (hyperthermia)

Renal
- oliguria

BEHAVIORAL FINDINGS
- irritability
- lethargy
- restlessness

DIAGNOSTIC STUDIES
Laboratory data
- serum glucose levels—to identify decrease because reserves are used in response to chilling
- arterial blood gas studies—to determine increased carbon dioxide and decreased oxygen levels, indicating potential for acidosis
- blood urea nitrogen levels—to note increase, indicating impaired renal function and potential oliguria
- electrolyte studies—to identify potassium increases associated with impaired renal function
- cultures of body fluids—to identify infection

Collaborative problem: *Abnormal temperature related to extremes in gestational age and weight, abnormal disorders at birth, and exposure to cool or warm environments (4 goals)*

GOAL 1: Identify infant at risk for potential or actual temperature instability.

Interventions

1. Assess factors related to infant's risk of temperature fluctuations; include the following:
- prematurity
- sepsis and infections
- asphyxia and hypoxia
- CNS trauma
- fluid and electrolyte imbalance
- high or low environmental temperature
- trauma during delivery
- maternal drug use.

2. Assess for potential or actual hypothermia or hyperthermia:

- Monitor core temperature according to institutional protocol. Take axillary temperature and apply a thermostatic skin probe. Monitor both (axillary and skin) methods every 30 to 60 minutes or as needed during rewarming and then every 2 to 3 hours for 8 to 12 hours. Correlate the axillary and skin temperatures to ensure accurate temperature readings.

- Monitor environmental temperature hourly and record according to hospital policy, correlating the infant's temperature and the environment's.

- Be alert for environmental factors that can cause infant heat loss, for example:

Rationales

1. Assessment offers an opportunity to prevent cold stress. Infants are prone to temperature changes, and heat loss and production depend on increased metabolic activity. This ability may be compromised in the premature or sick infant with poor metabolic reserves, smaller ratio of body mass to surface area, lack of subcutaneous fat, and poor ability to shiver. Both full-term and preterm infants are at risk for hypothermia, which increases their metabolism and need for oxygen.

2. These assessment data indicate whether hypothermia or hyperthermia may develop.

- Optimal skin temperature is 97.7° to 98.6° F (36.5° to 37° C) for minimal oxygen consumption, with core temperature about 0.9° F (0.4° C) higher. Axillary temperatures may be falsely high because of friction between skin and thermometer. Skin probe placed on abdomen over the liver is best indicator of cold stress because the probe responds to peripheral vasoconstriction.

- Nursery temperature should be regulated at about 77° F (25° C). Heat may be lost by conduction, radiation, convection, or evaporation in response to environment temperatures.

- Infant body heat may be lost by conduction, radiation, convection, or evaporation in response to environmental temperatures. Nursery temperature should be stable.

Interventions

- □ use of cold sheets, scale, or table
- □ wet linens or wet infant
- □ placement near cold incubator sides or a window
- □ exposure to drafts, cold environment, oxygen, or improper humidification.
- Check respiratory rate (tachnypea), depth, and ease.

- Observe skin for pallor, mottling, coolness, or warmth.

- Monitor for irritability, tremors, and seizure activity.

- Monitor for flushing, respiratory distress, apneic episode, skin moisture, seizure activity, fluid loss, elevated temperature, and hypotension.

3. Additional individualized interventions: _____

Rationales

- □ causes heat loss through conduction
- □ causes heat loss through evaporation
- □ causes heat loss through radiation
- □ causes heat loss through convection

- Increased respiratory rate occurs with increased need for oxygen.
- Peripheral vasoconstriction causing these signs results from hypothermia.
- These signs of hypoglycemia result from increased use of glucose reserves.
- These signs of hyperthermia may indicate infection or overheating. Infants with temperatures (axillary) higher than 99.5° F (37.5° C) have hyperthermia.

3. Rationales: _____

GOAL 2: Prevent conditions that precipitate temperature fluctuation.

Interventions

1. Carry out the following procedures at birth:
- Dry infant immediately.
- Wrap infant in warmed blanket.
- Allow mother to cuddle infant to provide warmth.
- Place infant under radiant warmer without allowing infant to touch any metal or other surface until temperature stabilizes.
- Avoid placing infant in drafts.
- Transport infant to nursery in warmed blankets or use incubator if needed.
- Place infant under the radiant warmer in the nursery.
- Place the preterm infant and the full-term infant with unstable temperatures in an incubator. The infant should be naked with a warm cap on head and a plastic (Saran) wrap blanket around body to reduce heat loss. A Saran wrap prevents insensible water loss.

2. To prevent heat loss while caring for infant:
- Remove infant from radiant warmer and then dress, place in bassinet, and cover with blankets in 1 to 2 hours.
- Warm linens before use.
- Maintain hood temperature for oxygen equal to Isolette temperature.
- Dress infant in cap, diaper, booties, and shirt if observation is needed.
- Refrain from bathing infant if heat source is needed or for at least 3 hours if not needed.
- Use portholes for access to infant in Isolette.
- Use over-bed warmer with probe when infant is cared for in external environment.
- If infant is admitted to open bassinet in nursery, dress and cover infant with two or more blankets.

3. Additional individualized interventions: _____

Rationales

1. These procedures prevent heat loss, provide warmth, and prevent infant temperature fluctuations, especially if nursery is a distance from delivery room. Core and skin temperatures decrease as much as 0.2° F (0.1° C) and 0.5° F (0.3° C) a minute, respectively, from evaporation as the infant's moist body is exposed to the cold air in the delivery room after birth.

2. These measures maintain infant's temperature and prevent cold or heat stress.

3. Rationales: _____

GOAL 3: Provide neutral thermal environment.

Interventions

1. Place infant under radiant warmer and set temperature dial to desired temperature. Cover infant with plastic blanket when intubated, attaching Servo-Control device to infant's abdomen.

2. Place naked infant in incubator with Servo-Control device attached.
• Warm incubator before using, adjusting temperature dial according to infant's weight and age.
• Check alarm function on Servo-Control and attach device to abdomen.
• Keep portholes closed as much as possible.

3. Attach Servo-Control device, if used, to infant's abdomen (right upper quadrant) over liver but never over bone, as follows:
• Attach with heat-reflective adhesive.
• Set desired temperature.
• Keep skin probe uncovered.
• If infant lies prone, place probe on infant's back.
• Make sure to raise incubator's side panels.

4. Alleviate hyperthermia by:
• reducing environmental temperature
• reducing clothing and bundling
• sponging infant gently with tepid water
• decreasing temperature on warming device.

5. Provide appropriate environment to prevent or alleviate hypothermia as follows:
• Move infant from radiant warmer to incubator.
• Move infant from incubator to bassinet or to radiant warmer when performing procedures.
• Assess for optimal temperature hourly or as needed.
• Use low-reading thermometer for axillary temperature in low-birth-weight infants.

6. Additional individualized interventions: _____

Rationales

1. A neutral thermal environment permits optimal core temperature with minimal oxygen use. External heat needed depends on infant's weight, age, maturity, and physical condition. Radiant warmers may be used for temporary warming and for procedures.

2. Incubator provides heat by convection and control of temperature manually or automatically. The Servo-Control device monitors infant's temperature continuously.

3. This device is used in radiant warmers and incubators to control temperature and maintain a neutral thermal environment. Heat will be increased if skin temperature goes down.

4. These measures provide cooling for the hyperthermic infant.

5. Environmental support ensures a neutral thermal status.

6. Rationales: _____

GOAL 4: Prevent complication of cold stress.

Interventions

1. Assess infant for signs of cold stress, including:
• drop in core temperature, as low as 90° F (32.2° C)
• early restlessness and irritability
• poor feeding and lethargy
• pallor, central cyanosis, or mottling
• skin cold to touch
• beefy red color
• bradycardia
• slow, shallow, irregular breathing with expiratory grunt
• diminished activity and reflexes
• flaccid movements and feeble cry
• vomiting and abdominal distention
• edema of face, arms, and legs.

2. Perform treatments for actual or potential cold injury as follows:

Rationales

1. These are signs of cold stress complication of extreme hypothermia. Although most signs of cold stress emphasize the infant's decreasing activity, early cold stress manifests itself in increased activity as the infant attempts to compensate with movement to increase heat production.

2. Cold stress increases oxygen and caloric metabolism.

Interventions

• Warm infant slowly and record skin temperature every 15 minutes.

• Set ambient temperature about 3° F (1.1° C) warmer than skin temperature.

• Prepare and administer plasma protein fraction (Plasmanate) over 30 minutes.

• Administer warmed and humidified oxygen.

• Monitor serum glucose levels to identify decreases.

• Prepare and administer sodium bicarbonate for metabolic acidosis.

• Withhold food and water; administer I.V. dextrose 10% in water, or supply gavage feedings until infant's temperature reaches 95° F (35° C).

3. Additional individualized interventions: _____

Rationales

• If infant warms rapidly, apnea may result from increased oxygen consumption.

• This optimal ambient temperature prevents cold stress.

• Plasmanate is used when a volume expander is needed.

• This supplies oxygen if cold stress increases oxygen use.

• Detecting decreased glucose levels helps to identify hypoglycemia, which results in anaerobic metabolism; this condition, in turn, causes metabolic acidosis.

• Sodium helps to correct metabolic acidosis and improve circulation if infant is not responding to treatments to provide warmth.

• If infant's temperature drops below 95° F (35° C), nothing-by-mouth status is maintained to minimize oxygen expenditure. Then alternative feeding methods provide nutrition and fluids.

3. Rationales: _____

Nursing diagnosis: *Knowledge deficit (parental) related to infant's condition and maintenance of appropriate body temperature*

GOAL: Provide parents with appropriate information about infant's condition and care given to maintain infant's temperature.

Interventions

1. Inform parents about:
• temperature fluctuation causes
• infant's condition
• temperature stabilization treatments
• length of time infant may be out of temperature-regulated environment
• appropriate covering and protection for infant when holding and visiting—emphasize need to keep infant away from drafts and to ensure that infant wears a cap to prevent heat loss through the head's large surface area.

2. Teach parents how to take axillary temperature and have them demonstrate the procedure.

3. Inform parents that when infant's weight and condition allow, the infant will be weaned from the incubator before going home.

4. Encourage parents' questions, requests for clarifications, and demonstrations.

5. Additional individualized interventions: _____

Rationales

1. Informing the parents helps relieve their anxiety and concern about their infant's condition. Teaching them about heat conservation procedures ensures that infant will be appropriately protected when they are caring for the infant.

2. This allows parents to obtain an accurate temperature reading and thus monitor increases or decreases in temperature.

3. Weaning the infant from the incubator allows infant's temperature to be reduced safely to that of the nursery.

4. Honest and open discussion promotes better understanding.

5. Rationales: _____

ASSOCIATED PLANS
• Anemia
• Birth Trauma
• Hypoglycemia
• Inappropriate Size or Weight for Gestational Age, Small
• Intracranial Hemorrhage
• Preterm Infant, Less Than 37 Weeks
• Sepsis Neonatorum and Infectious Disorders

ADDITIONAL NURSING DIAGNOSES
• Altered peripheral tissue perfusion related to cold stress
• High risk for fluid volume deficit related to loss from radiant warmer
• Hyperthermia related to exposure to hot environment
• Hypothermia related to exposure to cool environment, illness or trauma, inability to shiver
• Ineffective thermoregulation related to immaturity, fluctuating environmental temperature

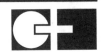

Inappropriate Size or Weight for Gestational Age, Large

DEFINITION

Infants who are large for gestational age (LGA) include those with birth weights above the 90th percentile on the intrauterine growth chart at any gestational week, regardless of whether they are preterm, full-term, or postterm. A weight of 8 lb, 13 oz (4,000 g) or more is considered LGA for full-term or preterm infants. The mortality is higher for LGA infants if delivery is difficult and cesarean birth is necessary, which may lead to trauma and other complications during birth. Postterm infants are those born after 42 weeks' gestation, regardless of birth weight. They appear long, thin, and wasted and look more like infants 1 to 3 weeks old. Cesarean birth or labor induction usually is performed to avoid the risk of an overdue birth, with its potential for hypoxia and meconium aspiration associated with placental insufficiency.

This plan focuses on the identification and care of the LGA infant and the prevention of complications associated with this condition.

ETIOLOGY AND PRECIPITATING FACTORS

• mother with diabetes mellitus
• maternal size, overnutrition, weight gain during pregnancy
• genetic predisposition to large size
• erythroblastosis fetalis, transposition of great vessels, Beckwith's syndrome (genetic condition associated with neonatal hypoglycemia and hyperinsulinism)

PHYSICAL FINDINGS
Maternal history

• such conditions as diabetes mellitus, toxemia, vascular or renal disease
• nutritional status, including overweight, excessive weight gain during pregnancy
• multiparity or past delivery of LGA infants
• possible miscalculation of expected date of confinement (EDC)

Infant status at birth

• weight and length at birth
• cesarean birth or oxytocin-induced labor
• low Apgar score
• asphyxia or use of resuscitation
• birth trauma from use of midforceps and difficulty in delivery, causing shoulder dystocia, fractured clavicle, depressed skull fracture, facial paralysis, brachial plexus palsy
• congenital heart defect, including transposition of great vessels
• congenital anomalies

Gastrointestinal

• poor feeding and bloated, prominent abdomen
• weight greater than 8 lb, 13 oz (4,000 g)

Integumentary

• reddish complexion or possible jaundiced appearance
• obese, plump-looking, with generous fat deposits; plethoric fat deposits in infant of diabetic mother
• loose, baggy look in postterm infant (from use of fat for energy)
• dry, peeling, parchment-looking skin, with long nails in postterm infant
• hematoma resulting from traumatic birth

Pulmonary

• sighing respirations

BEHAVIORAL FINDINGS

• listlessness

DIAGNOSTIC STUDIES
Laboratory data

• Dextrostix or Chemstrip by heelstick—to identify glucose levels less than 45 mg/dl within 1 to 2 hours after birth; test repeated frequently for 2 days after birth
• serum glucose measurement—to identify and confirm decreases if Dextrostix or Chemstrip results are below normal
• serum bilirubin levels—to check for increase resulting from additional load to liver caused by breakdown of blood from hematoma, hemorrhage caused by birth trauma, or polycythemia associated with hypoxia
• serum calcium levels—to check for decrease 1 to 3 days after birth

Collaborative problem: *High risk for complications from physiologic changes associated with LGA status, with or without diabetic mother (2 goals)*

GOAL 1: Recognize infant at risk for complications common with LGA.

Interventions

1. Assess infant for risk factors, including:

• maternal diabetes mellitus, EDC, size, maternal weight gain during pregnancy

• low Apgar score, asphyxia, respiratory distress syndrome, bone fractures, soft tissue paralysis, congenital anomalies

• bilirubin level, increased red blood cell count

• capillary blood sample from lateral aspect of heel; after warming heel for 15 minutes, test immediately for glucose level with Dextrostix or Chemstrip and meter, using fresh reagent strip and accurate glucometer

• continued Dextrostix or Chemstrip testing for 2 to 3 days after birth with serum glucose analysis if levels fall below 45 mg/dl

• signs of hypoglycemia, such as twitching, lethargy, irritability, apnea, hypothermia, and seizures

• serum calcium level for decreases.

2. Additional individualized interventions: _____

Rationales

1. Because of their size, LGA infants often are not considered at risk for complications. However, they need careful assessment and close attention because their mortality is higher than that of averaged-sized infants.

• LGA infants have a higher mortality rate and higher risk for complications and, for those of diabetic mothers, a higher risk of abnormalities unless delivered before EDC.

• LGA infants are prone to these problems because of intrauterine stress caused by decreased placental efficiency and delivery difficulty because of their large size or premature status if delivered early (an elective procedure, as for the infant of a diabetic mother).

• Increases because of polycythemia in infants of diabetic mothers are thought to be associated with hypoxia, which causes blood hyperviscosity. This increases the risk for cardiopulmonary and circulatory congestion and emboli.

• Securing the sample from an unwarmed heel may lead to an underestimation of the glucose level. Because of stasis, the level may fall as much as 18 mg/dl/hour at room temperature.

• When Dextrostix or Chemstrip testing reveals glucose levels below 45 mg/dl, glucose measurement should be repeated by laboratory analysis to confirm an accurate reading. This double testing should not delay treatment.

• In infants of diabetic mothers, a state of hypoglycemia exists 2 to 4 hours after delivery. When the glucose supply from the mother is removed at birth, insulin production continues and depletes the existing glucose level; these sudden drops may cause neurologic symptoms and central nervous system damage.

• Decreased calcium levels occur after delivery and may be accentuated in infants of diabetic mothers with asphyxia. A measurement of less than 7 mg/dl indicates hypocalcemia.

2. Rationales: _____

GOAL 2: Maintain infant's physiologic stability and minimize effects of LGA status.

Interventions

1. Maintain respiratory function by:

• noting abnormalities in rate, depth, or ease; distress or cyanosis

• suctioning nasopharynx area as appropriate

• providing vibration, percussion, and postural drainage if indicated

Rationales

1. Maintaining adequate respiratory function prevents hypoxia.

• Infants who are asphyxic at birth, who have decreased surfactant levels, or whose mothers have diabetes are more likely to have respiratory distress. The infant delivered by cesarean birth is at risk for wet lung.

• Suctioning ensures airway patency by removing potential obstruction.

• These interventions mobilize secretions for removal.

Interventions

• providing warm, humidified oxygen

• monitoring arterial blood gas (ABG) results.

2. Maintain nutritional status by:

• initiating feedings, as tolerated, as soon as possible after birth

• weighing infant daily and evaluating weight in light of caloric intake and fluid intake and output

• providing treatment for hypoglycemia or hypocalcemia, as indicated, based on glucose and serum calcium levels.

3. Maintain a neutral thermal environment for infant.

4. Maintain freedom from effects of trauma during birth by:

• noting birth injuries, such as hematoma, paralysis, and fractures

• monitoring serum bilirubin levels for increases.

5. Additional individualized interventions: _____

Rationales

• This action promotes adequate oxygenation; humidified oxygen helps prevent drying of the mucous membranes; warm oxygen minimizes heat losss.

• Monitoring ABG levels identifies potential for hypoxemia and hypercapnia, which lead to acidosis.

2. Physiologic stability requires adequate nutrition.

• Feedings prevent hypoglycemia and provide for nutritional needs.

• Monitoring weight and fluid intake and output ensures caloric and fluid needs and helps prevent fluid imbalance.

• This prevents continuing decreases in glucose and calcium levels, which may lead to brain damage (see Hypoglycemia and Hypocalcemia plans on pages 225 and 221, respectively, for administration of medications and treatment).

3. A neutral thermal environment assures metabolic stability and prevents hypothermia and hyperthermia, both of which increase the infant's energy needs.

4. Birth trauma can potentially cause physiologic complications.

• Most injuries caused by traumatic birth resolve within 2 to 3 days. Severe injuries that involve nerves or the spinal cord require more complex medical and nursing care.

• Hyperbilirubinemia is possible in infants with hematoma because the breakdown of blood from bleeding adds to the liver's bilirubin load.

5. Rationales: _____

Nursing diagnosis: *Knowledge deficit (parental) related to infant's condition and care*

GOAL: Provide appropriate information about the infant's condition and growth patterns.

Interventions

1. Inform the parents about the following:

• infant's condition and progress toward stability

• infant's feeding and nutritional needs

• effects of trauma during delivery, which usually are temporary.

2. Answer questions and clarify any information as needed.

3. Encourage parents to have physical contact with infant, allowing them to participate in the infant's care.

4. Additional individualized interventions: _____

Rationales

1. Information allays parental anxiety and enhances infant care.

• This information about the infant's condition and progress reduces parental anxiety and concerns.

• This information ensures the infant's intake of proper nutrients to replace deficiencies.

• Obvious bruising, paralysis, or fractures increase parental fear about the loss of the "perfect child."

2. This promotes better understanding.

3. Contact with infant reinforces bonding and increases their comfort in caring for the infant.

4. Rationales: _____

ASSOCIATED PLANS
• Birth Trauma
• Cesarean Section Birth
• Congenital Heart Disease
• Drug Addiction and Withdrawal
• Hyperbilirubinemia
• Hypocalcemia
• Hypoglycemia
• Hypothermia and Hyperthermia
• Meconium Aspiration Syndrome
• Pregnancy Complicated by Diabetes Mellitus

ADDITIONAL NURSING DIAGNOSES
• High risk for impaired skin integrity related to trauma
during difficult delivery
• High risk for injury related to difficult delivery of LGA
infant
• Ineffective family coping: compromised related to fear,
guilt

Inappropriate Size or Weight for Gestational Age, Small

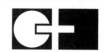

DEFINITION

A neonate is considered small for gestational age (SGA) if its birth weight is below the 10th percentile on the intrauterine growth chart at any week of gestation, whether preterm, full-term, or postterm. A more definitive description of an SGA or intrauterine growth-retarded (IUGR) infant is based on more than two standard deviations below the mean gestational age, circumference, and length greater than two standard deviations from mean, or as follows:
• mild IUGR—weight more than two standard deviations below mean, with a reduced weight-length ratio
• moderate IUGR—weight-length ratio greater than two standard deviations below mean
• severe IUGR—weight, length, and head circumference all greater than two standard deviations below mean. A full-term infant with a weight of 5 lb, 8 oz (2,500 g) or less fits into the IUGR category.

Early in fetal development, all growth is the result of increases in cell number (hyperplasia). Cells are fewer in number but are normal in size, causing below-normal growth. Later in fetal development, cells increase in size (hypertrophy), with cell numbers normal. Outcome and appearance of the infant at birth depend on the period (early or late development) of intrauterine insult on the fetus.

Maternal, placental, and fetal factors may all contribute to SGA, low birth weight (LBW), and IUGR problems in newborn infants. Whether the infant is labeled SGA, LBW, or IUGR is determined during the assessment for gestational age done on all neonates, using the Dubowitz or a similar system and plotting the information on the Denver intrauterine growth curve.

The prognosis depends on the cause, severity, and duration of the intrauterine insult to the fetus and on the care the infant receives after birth. The mortality rate decreases as gestational weeks increase and increases as birth weight decreases, except for postterm infants, whose mortality and morbidity increase greatly past 42 weeks.

This plan focuses on identifying and caring for the SGA infant and preventing complications associated with this condition. It also applies to infants who are small for date or who have LBW or IUGR.

ETIOLOGY AND PRECIPITATING FACTORS

• genetic factors (small or short parents, chromosomal abnormalities, multiple anomalies, anencephaly)
• twin fetuses
• maternal malnutrition
• maternal use of alcohol, cigarettes, or narcotics or mother living in high altitude
• maternal infection, such as TORCH
• placental insufficiency caused by diabetes, renal disease, toxemia, hypertension
• congenital anomalies
• medications, such as antimetabolites and anticonvulsants, taken by the mother
• congenital fetal infections and inborn errors of metabolism

PHYSICAL FINDINGS
Maternal history
• small stature or past SGA infants in family
• mother's age (adolescent or advanced)
• amount of prenatal care, socioeconomic status, nutritional status
• conditions, such as diabetes, heart disease, renal hypertension, toxemia, TORCH
• such disorders as placenta previa and abruptio placentae
• past use of alcohol, cigarettes, narcotics or other drugs or medications taken during pregnancy

Infant status at birth
• one of multiple births
• low Apgar score, asphyxia, use of resuscitation, acidosis
• possible wasted appearance, with smaller body parts and symmetry
• weight, length, and head circumference disproportionate
• congenital or chromosomal anomalies

Gastrointestinal
• sunken abdomen
• possible hungry appearance, with sucking of hands or clothing

Integumentary
• pale, dry skin
• sparse hair
• loose, baggy skin and widened skull sutures

Musculoskeletal
• lack of adipose tissue and poor muscle growth on trunk, arms, and legs, with long, thin appearance

Neurologic
• possible flaccidity
• possible activity
• hypothermia

Pulmonary
• tachypnea, gasping respirations, crackles, or cyanosis if meconium aspiration is present

BEHAVIORAL FINDINGS
• lethargy
• vigorous cry
• alertness

DIAGNOSTIC STUDIES
• chest X-ray—to determine pulmonary complication changes associated with asphyxia, such as pneumonia and pneumothorax, caused by aspiration

Laboratory data
• maternal serial estriol levels—to reveal decreases if placenta is dying, resulting in poor intrauterine environment
• Heelstick glucose measurement—to indicate levels of 45 mg/dl within 1 to 2 hours after birth and frequently for 2 to 3 days after birth; or Chemstrip testing with meter for more accurate glucose levels
• serum glucose measurement (after heelstick testing)—to be done on two specimens for verification
• hematocrit (HCT) and hemoglobin (Hb) values—to indicate HCT increased to 70% in polycythemia (increased viscosity) and Hb increased to 20 g/dl
• bacterial and viral cultures and TORCH screen—to rule out infections
• bilirubin levels—to reveal increase in polycythemia associated with hypoxemia
• immunoglobulin (IgM) levels—to reveal increases suggesting infection; possible increased or decreased white blood cell count; decreased platelet count; possible abnormal prothrombin time or partial thromboplastin time
• arterial blood gas (ABG) studies—to determine oxygen and carbon dioxide levels in asphyxia
• serum electrolyte levels—to detect decreases in sodium and calcium levels

---

Collaborative problem: *High risk for complications caused by physiologic changes associated with SGA infant (2 goals)*

GOAL 1: Recognize the infant at risk for complications common with SGA.

Interventions	Rationales
1. Assess the infant at risk, including:	1. Anticipating and recognizing complications of LBW, SGA, and IUGR allows for preventive measures to ensure infant's stability.
• review of maternal history and delivery events	• Maternal conditions predispose infant to complications.
• low Apgar score, asphyxia, meconium-stained skin or nails, or fluid (monitor respirations every 4 hours for tachypnea, gasping, and cyanosis indicating respiratory distress)	• Asphyxia may be caused by hypoxia in utero or during labor, causing the fetus to pass meconium and producing meconium aspiration or other respiratory disorders. Preterm infants are not meconium-stained but still may have significant asphyxia.
• signs of hypoglycemia (twitching, lethargy, irritability, apnea, hypothermia, seizure activity, low glucose level) by warming heel for 15 minutes to dilate vessels and securing blood sample from lateral aspect (test immediately for glucose level and then every 3 to 4 hours)	• Lack of glycogen stores at birth may cause hypoglycemia within 48 to 72 hours. Glucose levels should be maintained between 45 and 120 mg/dl; if levels are low, two serum glucose tests should be done in laboratory for accurate assessment. Drops in glucose levels may cause neurologic symptoms and central nervous system (CNS) damage.
• signs of hypothermia (cold skin, lethargy, poor feeding) by measuring axillary temperature every 2 to 3 hours	• Hypothermia may be caused by reduced glycogen and fat stores, resulting in infant's decreased ability to maintain normal heat and reduced energy level.
• polycythemia by measuring red blood cell (RBC) count and HCT value at birth and as needed and by checking skin for pallor, petechiae, bruising, and bleeding at I.V. sites	• This potential complication is caused by a prolonged lack of oxygen in utero, sometimes creating a need for partial exchange or plasmapheresis transfusion using plasma in exchange for infant's blood to reduce viscosity and maintain HCT value below 65% on central venous blood sample (not arterial).
• vital signs, peripheral pulses, capillary refill.	• Changes in vital signs and vascular status may signal complications.
2. Additional individualized interventions: _____	2. Rationales: _____

GOAL 2: Maintain the infant's physiologic stability and minimize the effects of SGA status.

Interventions

1. Maintain respiratory function by:

• preparing for immediate resuscitation at birth

• suctioning nasopharynx, as needed

• providing warm, humidified oxygen via hood, mask, or mechanical ventilation, as appropriate

• monitoring ABG values and pH

• providing chest physiotherapy and postural drainage.

2. Maintain nutritional status by:
• initiating feedings as soon as possible, within 4 hours after birth, if asphyxia is not present or if food and water have been withheld for 24 hours and infant is receiving I.V. feeding

• weighing the infant at the same time on the same scale daily and comparing weight with caloric intake

• monitoring fluid intake and output every 4 hours or more frequently

• preparing to give 10% to 12.5% glucose I.V. to infant with asphyxia who cannot be fed orally.

3. Maintain neutral thermal environment by:
• placing infant in Isolette and checking and adjusting temperature every 2 to 3 hours
• avoiding drafts and placing infant on cold surfaces or in drafty areas
• using additional blankets, if needed
• warming the infant gradually and monitoring for hyperthermia.

4. Maintain circulatory status by:
• preparing and assisting with exchange transfusion
• monitoring bilirubin level every 8 hours
• initiating phototherapy, if indicated (see Hyperbilirubinemia plan, page 213).

5. Additional individualized interventions: _____

Rationales

1. Adequate respiratory function supports physiologic stability.
• Neonatal asphyxia is common in SGA infants, so anticipate respiratory distress in infants at risk.
• Suctioning ensures airway patency by removing potential obstruction.
• This action prevents gas exchange imbalances leading to respiratory acid-base problems.
• Monitoring identifies potential for hypoxia, hypercapnia, and acidosis.
• Respiratory physiotherapy enhances mobilization and removal of secretions.

2. Adequate nutrition is essential to physiologic stability.
• Early feedings prevent continued weight decreases, with potential for hypoglycemia and hypocalcemia. The infant with asphyxia needs to rest the gut before feeding is started because he may have suffered an anoxic episode to the gut.
• Daily weighing measures whether caloric and fluid needs are being met.
• An accurate comparison is important to maintaining fluid balance with increased fluids.
• If the infant cannot tolerate oral intake, an I.V. prevents hypoglycemia by maintaining glucose level.

3. These precautions prevent hypothermia by maintaining a temperature of 97° to 98° F (36.1° to 36.7° C). SGA infants do not have adequate fat stores and adipose tissue for insulation, so they are prone to hypothermia, which produces feeding intolerance. Proper monitoring of temperature and equipment prevents hyperthermia. Thermoregulation is difficult because SGA infants are unable to conserve body heat.

4. Polycythemia may result from stimulation of RBC production by hypoxic condition. The increased production of RBCs increases bilirubin load to liver and causes jaundice with possible CNS involvement.

5. Rationales: _____

Nursing diagnosis: *Knowledge deficit (parental) related to infant's condition and care*

GOAL: Provide appropriate information regarding the infant's condition and growth patterns.

Interventions

1. Keep the parents informed, as follows:

• Review the infant's condition and progress toward stability, and reinforce the cause and effect of the underlying problem that the physician presented.

Rationales

1. Information about the infant reduces parental anxiety.

• Information about the SGA infant's condition, progress, and diagnosis helps reduce parental concern about the infant's welfare.

Interventions

• Review the infant's feeding, nutritional needs, and potential for normal weight pattern.

• Give rationales for the treatments needed and for follow-up care.

2. Listen to parental questions and clarify information, as needed.

3. Encourage parents to have physical contact with the infant, allowing them to participate in the infant's care.

4. Refer parents to community services for follow-up.

5. Additional individualized interventions: _____

Rationales

• Some SGA infants have a large initial weight deficit to make up in the first 6 months, unless a complicating condition exists.
• Some treatments may have to be continued to maintain the infant's status.

2. Information enhances parental understanding.

3. Participating in the infant's care reinforces bonding and increases the parents' confidence in their ability to care for their infant.

4. Referrals provide the parents and family with additional support before and after infant's discharge.

5. Rationales: _____

ASSOCIATED PLANS
• Congenital Heart Disease
• Hyperbilirubinemia
• Hypoglycemia
• Hypothermia and Hyperthermia
• Inappropriate Size or Weight for Gestational Age, Large
• Meconium Aspiration Syndrome
• Multiple Gestation
• Preterm Infant, Less Than 37 Weeks
• TORCH and Sexually Transmitted Diseases

ADDITIONAL NURSING DIAGNOSES
• Altered nutrition: less than body requirements related to LBW, malnutrition, nothing-by-mouth status, I.V. fluid support, low glycogen and fat stores at birth
• High risk for altered parenting related to infant's need for specialized care
• High risk for injury related to future growth patterns, immune factors leading to infection, abnormal blood profile leading to circulatory deficiencies, hyperbilirubinemia, altered clotting factors
• Hypothermia related to malnutrition
• Impaired gas exchange related to altered oxygen supply (hypoxia)
• Ineffective family coping (compromised) related to fear, guilt

Intracranial Hemorrhage

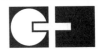

DEFINITION

Intracranial hemorrhage is bleeding within the cranium that affects the brain. Arising during the perinatal period, it typically occurs in preterm infants.

Periventricular/intraventricular (P/IVH) hemorrhage is hemorrhage of capillaries in tissue adjacent to the ventricular wall (germinal matrix) that remains in place or bursts into the cerebrospinal fluid (CSF) and circulates into the ventricular system. These fragile capillaries can be ruptured by hypoxia or ischemia in the brain. If CSF flow becomes obstructed, the ventricles dilate from the accumulation of fluid and pressure. If the obstruction is not relieved, hydrocephalus may result. The most common type of intracranial hemorrhage arising during the neonatal period, P/IVH is a major cause of morbidity and mortality in infants. It is the most serious and most common neurologic disorder in preterm infants, seen almost exclusively in those who were born at less than 32 weeks' gestation or who weigh less than 3 lb, 5 oz (1,500 g).

Primary subarachnoid hemorrhage—bleeding into the subarachnoid space without involving other areas—occurs predominantly in preterm infants. The condition may be mild, with complete recovery expected within 1 week of life, or severe and associated with neural damage. The prognosis depends on the extent of the injury.

Subdural hemorrhage, occurring most frequently in the full-term infant 1 week or later after birth, is bleeding in the subdural space caused by tearing of the dural sinuses or small superficial cerebral veins. Signs and symptoms may be mild or severe and are caused by the localized, space-occupying accumulation of subdural fluid. The prognosis depends on the severity and extent of tearing.

This plan focuses on caring for the infant with mild or severe intracranial hemorrhage and preventing neurologic damage.

ETIOLOGY AND PRECIPITATING FACTORS

• P/IVH
  □ prematurity
  □ hypoxia and ischemia to brain from maternal toxemia, maternal drug addiction or therapy, placental insufficiency, or birth trauma
  □ respiratory distress syndromes, pneumothorax, sepsis, or positive pressure ventilation causing increased venous pressure
  □ increased cerebral blood flow from excess fluid or volume expanders, vasopressors, and hyperosmolar drugs, such as sodium bicarbonate, that cause fluid shift and pressure on cerebral capillaries when given in improper dilution
  □ coagulopathies

• subarachnoid hemorrhage
  □ birth trauma
  □ asphyxia
  □ prolonged or difficult labor
  □ fetal distress
• subdural hemorrhage
  □ mechanical trauma from difficult delivery of the head, causing tearing of the dural sinuses, superficial cerebral veins, or tentorium
  □ bleeding from coagulation problems or thrombocytopenia
  □ shaken baby syndrome

PHYSICAL FINDINGS
Maternal history
• such conditions as diabetes and toxemia
• drug use, history of addiction

Infant status at birth
• prematurity and postmaturity
• low Apgar score showing asphyxia
• head trauma from birth

Cardiovascular
• decreased blood pressure in P/IVH
• sudden decrease in hematocrit (HCT) values

Integumentary
• abrasions or hematoma on the head in subdural or subarachnoid hemorrhage

Neurologic
• mild P/IVH
  □ possibly asymptomatic
  □ hypotonia or intermittent opisthotonos
  □ focal seizures that pass rapidly
  □ head enlargement with increase in circumference, tightness of anterior fontanel, or separation of sutures in 1 to 2 weeks
• severe P/IVH
  □ temperature difficult to maintain
  □ cyanosis and severe hypotonia
  □ increased intracranial pressure (ICP)
  □ seizures after hemorrhage onset or within a few hours; the time of seizure onset tells if bleeding occurred before, during, or after birth
• mild subarachnoid hemorrhage
  □ possibly asymptomatic
  □ hypotonia
• severe subarachnoid hemorrhage
  □ hypotonia, hyporeactivity
  □ seizures for several days
• subdural hemorrhage
  □ usually asymptomatic in neonatal period

Pulmonary

• apnea or cyanosis in severe IVH and, if infant is preterm, in subarachnoid hemorrhage
• irregular breathing

BEHAVIORAL FINDINGS

• lethargy
• irritability
• high-pitched cry

DIAGNOSTIC STUDIES

• computed tomography (CT) scan—to reveal type of intracranial hemorrhage

□ In P/IVH, CT scan shows high-density cast. Lesions are graded from I to IV (least to most severe). Procedure requires moving infant to X-ray department; if infant is on a ventilator, this is inadvisable.

□ In subarachnoid hemorrhage, lumbar puncture reveals blood in CSF. CT scan reveals increased ventricular size.

□ In subdural hemorrhage, CT scan reveals fluid accumulation.

• transillumination—to reveal abnormalities
• cranial ultrasonography (when P/IVH is suspected)—to detect bleeding; test must be performed within 2 weeks of bleeding to detect it; otherwise, bleeding resolves, leaving no abnormality or increased ventricular size

Laboratory data

• CSF studies—to identify bleeding; CSF may be red-brown, indicating old blood from past P/IVH
• HCT values—to identify falls from 20% to 60%, indicating P/IVH
• arterial blood gas (ABG) studies—to detect hypercapnia and hypoxemia even with ventilatory support in P/IVH

Collaborative problem: *High risk for neurologic impairment related to intracranial hemorrhage caused by trauma, asphyxia, hypoxia, or ischemia (3 goals)*

GOAL 1: Identify intracranial hemorrhage and altered neurologic status.

Interventions

1. Assess infant for changes in neurologic function; include the following:
• apnea or irregular respirations
• decreased activity or hypotonia
• decreased spontaneous and elicited movements
• opisthotonos and other abnormal positions
• lethargy
• tremors, shrill cry, or jittery movements
• cyanosis
• fixed and dilated pupils or pupil inequality or sluggishness
• unstable temperature
• variable heart rates or bradycardia
• increased ICP with tight, bulging anterior fontanel, separation of sutures, or head enlargement
• seizure activity with tonic manifestations, including horizontal deviation of eyes, blinking, limb posturing, staring, drooling, chin movements, chewing, or sucking.

2. Review CT scan, skull X-ray, CSF analysis, and other study results.

3. Assess for other conditions that cause neurologic changes, such as seizures, including:
• hypoglycemia, hypocalcemia, or hypomagnesemia
• sepsis, meningitis, and encephalitis
• hyponatremia or hypernatremia
• hypoxia
• drug withdrawal
• brain tumor or malformation
• hyperbilirubinemia.

4. Review serum glucose, calcium, bilirubin, and magnesium levels, drug panel, culture results, CSF analysis, ABG measurements, and electrolyte levels.

Rationales

1. Intracranial hemorrhages can occur without signs or symptoms or they may appear and disappear intermittently (with P/IVH) until stopping or occur with more frequency than had been suspected. Recovery and survival are common.

2. Results may confirm hemorrhage and fluid retention.

3. Assessment rules out other common conditions that may cause seizures.

4. Test results may indicate abnormal conditions causing signs.

Interventions

5. Additional individualized interventions: _____

Rationales

5. Rationales: _____

GOAL 2: Prevent or minimize neurologic impairment.

Interventions

1. Prepare and assist with serial lumbar puncture and intraventricular taps.

2. Prepare and administer I.V. anticonvulsants, as ordered:
• for mild and infrequent seizures: phenobarbital I.V. initially, with a repeat dose after 8 to 12 hours, followed by maintenance dose I.V. in two to three doses
• in refractory cases: phenytoin with phenobarbital I.V. initially, followed by a maintenance dose I.V., or orally in two separate doses.

3. Prepare and administer diazepam I.V., a muscle relaxant, as ordered.

4. Prepare and administer I.V. steroids, such as dexamethasone, as ordered, to reduce cerebral edema.

5. Review blood studies (phenobarbital and phenytoin levels) for possible drug toxicity, and observe for adverse reactions to anticonvulsants, including decreased activity, diarrhea, and increased motor seizures.

6. Additional individualized interventions: _____

Rationales

1. These procedures reduce pressure in ventricles.

2. Phenobarbital is given for its sedative effect. Maintaining therapeutic range of 20 to 30 mg/liter for phenobarbital and 20 mg/liter for phenytoin is essential for desired effect.

3. Diazepam is given when additional relaxation is needed, although it is not administered in jaundiced infants.

4. Although dexamethasone use is controversial, it may be ordered to reduce CSF levels.

5. Adverse reactions and inappropriate blood levels of drug require that the medication be discontinued and the reaction reported to the physician for possible medication or dosage changes. Decreased activity, diarrhea, and increased motor activity are adverse reactions to phenobarbital.

6. Rationales: _____

GOAL 3: Control and maintain ICP.

Interventions

1. Elevate the head of the bed slightly; place the infant in a prone or side-lying position, with the head midline or to the side. Do not flex the infant's neck.

2. Avoid a tight, encircling phototherapy mask, if ordered.

3. Administer I.V. volume expanders, as ordered, at the prescribed rate; use an infusion-control device to prevent overly rapid infusion.

4. Continuously monitor the infant's vital signs, especially blood pressure.

5. Suction only as needed.

6. Avoid measures that may make the infant cry; minimize excessive handling and manipulation.

7. Monitor ABG values.

Rationales

1. Such positioning helps minimize ICP; placing the infant's head midline or to the side prevents cerebral blood flow obstruction.

2. Pressure on the occiput can increase ICP by impeding venous drainage.

3. Rapid increases in intravascular volume may cause rupture of cerebral capillaries and increase ICP.

4. Changes in vital signs may indicate changes in ICP; early detection of such changes allows prompt treatment.

5. Suctioning increases cerebral blood flow and raises ICP.

6. Crying can impede venous return and increase cerebral blood volume and ICP.

7. Acid-base imbalances can further impair the infant's compromised ability to regulate cerebral blood flow and ICP.

Interventions	Rationales
8. Additional individualized interventions: _____	8. Rationales: _____

Nursing diagnosis: *Anxiety (parental) related to infant's condition, prognosis, and risk for permanent brain dysfunction*

GOAL: Minimize parental anxiety with support and information during crisis.

Interventions	Rationales
1. Assist parents to appraise the crisis in terms of their needs and the infant's needs.	1. This identifies necessary changes and possible coping strategies needed to deal with crisis.
2. Maintain calm and accepting environment.	2. This environment allows parents to feel comfortable expressing their feelings and asking questions.
3. Encourage questions, give honest and accurate answers, and provide information regarding: • condition's cause; its severity or mildness • infant's condition • procedures and rationales • possible prognosis and ongoing report of problem resolution • rarity of permanent brain damage if condition is monitored and treated effectively while the infant is hospitalized (unless condition is extremely severe).	3. Informative interaction promotes trust and lessens parental anxiety and fear, especially of the unknown. Parents often blame themselves for a sick infant or one with abnormal conditions or defects.
4. Allow parents to visit and participate in infant's care.	4. Parental participation promotes contact and bonding.
5. Assist parents to verbalize their fears and concerns about their infant's welfare. Assure them that their response is normal.	5. Verbalization decreases anxiety by externalizing feelings.
6. Inform the parents that caregiver will be present whenever needed for support and information.	6. Expressing the availability of caregiver validates caring, acceptance, and support.
7. Refer parents to community resources for assistance.	7. Referrals provide the parents with continued support, guidance, and follow-up.
8. Additional individualized interventions: _____	8. Rationales: _____

ASSOCIATED PLANS
• Birth Trauma
• Drug Addiction and Withdrawal
• Hyperbilirubinemia
• Hypocalcemia
• Hypoglycemia
• Postoperative Care
• Pregnancy-Induced Hypertension
• Preoperative Care

ADDITIONAL NURSING DIAGNOSES
• Anticipatory grieving (parental) related to potential loss of infant experiencing severe hemorrhage or potential loss of normal infant functioning

• High risk for caregiver role strain related to infant's condition
• High risk for infection related to lumbar puncture that may introduce microorganisms
• High risk for injury related to neurologic dysfunction
• Ineffective breathing pattern related to apnea or irregular breathing
• Ineffective family coping: compromised related to situational crisis of sick infant
• Knowledge deficit (parental) related to limited exposure to information regarding infant care

INFANT
Meconium Aspiration Syndrome

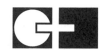

DEFINITION
Meconium aspiration syndrome is a condition in which meconium that has entered the amniotic fluid is aspirated before, during, or after delivery. This syndrome usually occurs in full-term infants. Meconium is found in the amniotic fluid of 10% of all neonates, indicating some degree of in utero asphyxia. The asphyxia causes an increase in intestinal peristalsis because the diminished oxygenated blood flow relaxes the anal sphincter, allowing the meconium to be released. The sickest, most severely distressed fetuses, while making gasping attempts to save themselves in utero, suck meconium so deeply into their airways that it cannot be retrieved by normal suctioning after delivery. Aspiration of the meconium causes partial or complete airway obstruction and pulmonary vasospasm. Bile salts in the meconium act as detergents, producing chemical burns of lung tissue. As the condition progresses, atelectasis, pneumothorax, persistent pulmonary hypertension, and bacterial pneumonia may develop.

With intervention, this disorder usually subsides in a few days, but death occurs in at least 28% of those affected. The prognosis depends on the amount of meconium aspirated, the degree of lung infiltration, and immediate and effective suctioning. Suctioning should include aspiration of the nasopharynx as the infant's head appears during birth and also direct suctioning of the trachea through an endotracheal tube immediately after birth if meconium is present.

This plan focuses on the care of the infant who has aspirated meconium and is at risk for pulmonary complications.

ETIOLOGY AND PRECIPITATING FACTORS
• fetal asphyxia
• prolonged labor

PHYSICAL FINDINGS
Maternal antenatal history
• intrauterine stress

Infant status at birth
• full-term, preterm, or small for gestational age
• Apgar score lower than 5
• meconium in amniotic fluid
• suctioning, resuscitative measures, or oxygen administration

Pulmonary
• respiratory distress with gasping, tachypnea (more than 60 breaths/minute), grunting, retractions, and nasal flaring
• possible increased breath sounds with crackles, depending on meconium spread to lungs
• cyanosis, if severe
• barrel chest with increased anteroposterior (AP) diameter
• rhonchi

BEHAVIORAL FINDINGS
• diminished activity

DIAGNOSTIC STUDIES
• chest X-ray—to reveal patches of density representing atelectasis, increased AP diameter, hyperinflation, flattened diaphragm, and possible pneumothorax

Laboratory data
• arterial blood gas (ABG) test results—to identify respiratory or metabolic acidosis with decreased PO_2 and increased PCO_2 levels

---

Collaborative problem: High risk for respiratory insufficiency related to meconium aspiration (2 goals)

GOAL 1: Prevent and remove meconium aspirated at birth and later.

Interventions

1. Observe for immediate need to suction nasopharynx when the infant's head appears during birth (performed by physician).

2. Suction the infant's trachea through an endotracheal tube immediately after birth.

3. Continue to suction the infant's mouth to remove larger meconium particles.

Rationales

1. Meconium in the amniotic fluid is an indication for suctioning before the infant takes a breath.

2. Procedure should be performed before stimulating infant, if meconium is noted, to prevent further aspiration.

3. The infant who aspirates meconium needs resuscitation, especially if the infant is in respiratory distress.

Interventions

4. Continue mouth suctioning as endotracheal tube is withdrawn.

5. Provide rest and quiet for the infant.

6. Additional individualized interventions: _____

Rationales

4. Continued suctioning retrieves meconium that clings to the tube's tip.

5. Crying or agitation may increase intrathoracic pressure, causing pneumothorax.

6. Rationales: _____

GOAL 2: Identify and minimize respiratory compromise after birth.

Interventions

1. Assess respiratory status; include the following:

• rate, depth, and ease of breathing with tachypnea (rate more than 60 breaths/minute)

• grunting

• nasal flaring

• retractions with accessory muscle use

• cyanosis

• ABG levels showing increased PCO_2 and decreased PO_2

• serial lung X-ray results.

2. Administer oxygen therapy and mechanical ventilation with positive pressure.

3. Set mechanical ventilator to provide higher distending pressures with short inspiratory rates (60 to 70 breaths/minute).

4. Maintain hyperoxygenation and pH and ABG values at 7.45 to 7.55, with PCO_2 of 22 to 30 mm Hg, respectively.

5. Provide physiotherapy with percussion and vibration every 1 to 2 hours. Use percussor or fine vibrator if infant can tolerate treatments.

6. Prevent infection complication (pneumonitis) by administering I.V. antibiotics, if ordered, such as ampicillin.

7. Slowly administer I.V. aminoglycosides, if ordered, such as kanamycin. Monitor serum peak and trough levels.

Rationales

1. All are indications that meconium was aspirated and that immediate treatment must begin.
• Respiratory rate increases to enhance oxygen level.

• The grunting sound results from the glottis closing to stop the exhalation of air by forcing the air against the vocal cords.
• Narrowing of the nostrils produces resistance to respirations; flaring is an attempt to reduce this.
• Retractions indicate inadequate distention of lungs during inspiration.
• Cyanosis results as oxygen levels decrease.
• These values indicate impending acidosis.

• X-rays may indicate atelectasis, hyperinflation, or pneumothorax.

2. Mechanical ventilation may or may not be needed. Positive pressure is administered after bronchoscopy or laryngotracheal therapy to prevent pushing meconium down into smaller airways (see Hyaline Membrane Disease—Respiratory Distress Syndrome [RDS I], page 205, for oxygen therapy and mechanical ventilation procedures).

3. These settings are needed to ventilate distal alveoli in infants with severe meconium aspiration.

4. Hyperoxygenation prevents persistent fetal circulation. A state of respiratory alkalosis helps to reduce pulmonary vasoconstriction in infants with meconium aspiration.

5. Procedure helps remove secretions, but procedure and equipment use depends on the infant's condition.

6. Antibiotics destroy bacteria by binding to the bacterial cell wall, resulting in cell death.

7. Aminoglycosides destroy bacteria by prohibiting protein synthesis, resulting in cell death. Slow administration prevents renal toxicity or ototoxicity. Monitoring peak and trough levels maximizes effectiveness of drug therapy.

Interventions

8. If ordered, administer steroids to reduce inflammatory response to meconium.

9. Prepare infant for transfer to an agency for surgery and for attachment to extracorporeal membrane oxygenation (ECMO) pump if the infant has severe aspiration and lung involvement. If ECMO is used:

• Assess the infant's fluid intake and output.

• Monitor transcutaneous blood oxygen tension (PO_2) or pulse oximetry values.

• Assess the infant's neurologic status.

• Suction the endotracheal tube, as ordered.

10. Additional individualized interventions: _____

Rationales

8. Although hydrocortisone is the drug of use is controversial.

9. CCMD maintains gas exchange and p lected hospitals provide this technology is performed to implant two thick tubes in the neck. These tubes are attached to an ECMO machine that pumps blood through an artificial lung. This procedure keeps the infant alive until the lungs can be supported with mechanical ventilation.

• Maintaining fluid balance is essential to preventing fluid overload.

• These readings evaluate tissue oxygenation and alert caregivers to changes in the infant's status.

• Neurologic signs and symptoms may reflect changes in the infant's oxygenation status.

• Suctioning maintains airway patency, aiding treatment. (For details on ECMO, see *Extracorporeal membrane oxygenation*.)

10. Rationales: _____

EXTRACORPOREAL MEMBRANE OXYGENATION

In major neonatal care facilities, extracorporeal membrane oxygenation (ECMO) may be used to maintain gas exchange and perfusion during preoperative management of diaphragmatic hernia or for selected neonates with refractory respiratory failure or meconium aspiration syndrome. ECMO maintains ventilation and oxygenation by oxygenating the neonate's blood outside the body through an arterial shunt. This permits cardiopulmonary recovery at low fractions of inspired oxygen (FIO_2) and reduced mechanical ventilator settings.

In the neonate, ECMO usually involves venoarterial bypass. A cannula is inserted into the right atrium via the right internal jugular vein; the aortic arch is cannulated via the right common carotid artery. After circulating through the tubing via a pumping device, blood circulates through a membrane oxygenator. The oxygenated blood then flows through a heating device and into the carotid cannula. The neonate remains on mechanical ventilation during ECMO, with ventilator settings reduced to the lowest level required.

Nursing diagnosis: *Ineffective family coping: compromised related to anxiety, guilt, and possible long-term care*

GOAL: Minimize parental anxiety and guilt, and support coping during situational crisis.

Interventions

1. Assess parents' verbal and nonverbal expressions, feelings, and use of coping mechanisms.

2. Assist parents to verbalize their concerns about their sick infant, the prolonged care, and the procedures and equipment used in that care.

3. Provide consistent and accurate information concerning their infant's condition and progress, future care, and potential for pulmonary problems.

4. Encourage parents to visit, to give care if appropriate, and to telephone for information.

5. Inform parents of care needed after discharge and instruct in procedures if they are candidates for carrying out procedures.

Rationales

1. Assessment data enable caregiver and the parents to identify and develop constructive coping strategies.

2. Verbalization helps to maintain a trusting, secure environment and acceptance of parents' concerns and fears.

3. Information reduces anxiety about disease course and rate at which infant is improving.

4. Visitation, communication, and participation in the infant's care promote the bonding process.

5. Some infants need ventilatory assistance after discharge to home.

Interventions

6. Refer parents to community agencies and inform them of available home care resources.

7. Additional individualized interventions: _____

_____

Rationales

6. Referrals provide the family wtih additional support and follow-up. Equipment and supplies needed for home care are available to buy or rent.

7. Rationales: _____

_____

ASSOCIATED PLANS
• Bronchopulmonary Dysplasia
• Hyaline Membrane Disease—Respiratory Distress Syndrome (RDS I)

ADDITIONAL NURSING DIAGNOSES
• Altered nutrition: less than body requirements related to increased caloric needs
• Fear (parental) related to possible death of infant, responsibility of long-term care, and providing ventilatory assistance at home
• High risk for fluid volume deficit related to insensible water losses from increased respirations
• High risk for infection related to pneumonia as result of meconium in lungs
• High risk for injury related to complications of pneumothorax, atelectasis
• Impaired gas exchange related to chemical pneumonitis and respiratory compromise resulting from meconium aspiration
• Ineffective airway clearance related to meconium aspiration
• Ineffective infant feeding pattern related to respiratory compromise
• Knowledge deficit (parental) related to infant's long-term care needs after discharge

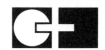

Necrotizing Enterocolitis

DEFINITION

Necrotizing enterocolitis (NEC), also called inflammatory bowel disease, primarily affects preterm and low-birth-weight (LBW) infants. Its development seems to be linked to ischemia and bacterial invasion, along with certain conditions created by infant feeding.

NEC is characterized by ischemia of the gut, mucosal damage, edema, ulceration, and perforation. Hypoxemic, hypothermic, or shock states cause blood to be shunted to vital organs, decreasing mesenteric circulation, which damages the mucus-producing cells that protect the bowel wall. This allows bacteria to invade areas in the intestinal wall and proliferate in the poorly functioning bowel. If the infant has been fed, the milk also sits in the gut and provides the perfect medium for bacterial growth. Free gas accumulates in the intestine, causing pneumatosis intestinalis and necrosis. Disease onset usually is within 72 hours after the first feeding.

NEC is associated with such disorders as respiratory distress syndrome (RDS), asphyxia, patent ductus arteriosus, sepsis, and polycythemia or with such procedures as catheterization of the umbilical artery or vein and exchange transfusions. If medical management does not contain the infection or if severe acidosis persists and perforation occurs, the perforated area is surgically resected and ileostomy or colostomy is performed. The survival rate has dramatically increased with improved medical and surgical care and use of total parenteral nutrition. Overall mortality is 33%, but this varies with treatment. The long-term prognosis is good; the survival rate depends on how much of the bowel is resected. If the small intestine or a significant portion of it (including the ileocecal valve) is lost, severe feeding problems develop.

This plan focuses on care of the infant with NEC or at risk for NEC, with emphasis on preventing progression or complications of the disease.

ETIOLOGY AND PRECIPITATING FACTORS

• uncertain, may be caused by ischemic insult to the bowel and the effect of microorganisms on this vascular insult
• possibly caused by reestablishment of circulation
• type of feeding (hyperosmolar formula), volume of feeding, and effect of microorganisms on formula
• bacterial infection caused by *Escherichia coli*, *Klebsiella*, *Clostridium*, *Salmonella*, and others
• viral infection

PHYSICAL FINDINGS
Maternal history
• such conditions as placenta previa, abruptio placentae, sepsis, pregnancy-induced hypertension, drug abuse, and diabetes mellitus
• prolonged rupture of membranes

Infant status at birth
• prematurity and LBW
• low Apgar score, asphyxia, and respiratory distress
• breech or cesarean birth

Cardiovascular
• murmur
• delayed capillary filling time
• heart failure

Gastrointestinal
• bile-colored (bilious) vomitus
• possible retention of feedings from poor absorption
• abdominal distention
• blood in stools
• decreased or absent bowel sounds (ileus)

Integumentary
• possible jaundice

Neurologic
• temperature instability

Pulmonary
• apnea with bradycardic episodes

BEHAVIORAL FINDINGS
• lethargy
• irritability

DIAGNOSTIC STUDIES
• X-ray (left lateral decubitus, upright) studies—to reveal bubbles or gas in wall of bowel, portal venous gas, or pneumatosis intestinalis (free air in peritoneum may mean perforation of bowel)

Laboratory data
• Clinitests—to detect glucose (reducing substances)
• Hematest or guaiac test—to identify occult blood in emesis, nasogastric (NG) tube aspirate, or stool
• platelet count—to indicate severe infection and deterioration if decreased to 100,000/mm³ or below
• complete blood count (CBC)—to detect white blood cell (WBC) count less than 5,000/mm³ or greater than 25,000/mm³; absolute neutrophil count less than 5,000; ratio of immature to mature neutrophil count greater than 13
• clotting profile of prothrombin time (PT), partial thromboplastin time (PTT), and fibrinogen—to indicate coagulation complication
• typing and crossmatching of blood—to prepare for exchange transfusion if needed
• electrolytes—to determine levels for correction (with vomiting and gastric decompression)
• culture of blood, urine, stool, cerebrospinal fluid, and peritoneal fluid—to determine causative organism

Collaborative problem: *High risk for extension of bowel injury related to continued or further bowel infection and to necrosis (2 goals)*

GOAL 1: Identify presence and progression of bowel involvement.

Interventions

1. Assess the infant at risk, and monitor for early symptoms of NEC, as follows:
• Review maternal history.
• Be alert to onset of signs and symptoms in an infant with asphyxia, RDS, sepsis, or other illnesses or in infant undergoing exchange transfusions.
• Note onset of vomiting, lethargy, change in feeding pattern, jaundice, apnea, or temperature instability within 72 hours after first formula feeding.
• Review stool Hematest and Clinitest results.

2. Assess for later signs, including:
• abdominal distention
• bile-colored vomitus
• decreased or absent bowel sounds and bowel movements.

3. Review X-rays, cultures of body fluids and stools, platelet count, WBC, segmented cell count, and electrolyte levels.

4. Additional individualized interventions: _____

Rationales

1. Early recognition of the disease increases the survival rate, and nursing observations of subtle changes are essential for early intervention or preventive therapy. Early, nonspecific signs and symptoms are similar to those of other conditions.

2. Later signs usually appear 12 to 24 hours after retained gastric contents are noted because of poor absorption.

3. These studies identify infection and infectious agents. Platelet count decreases in infection; WBC count increases or decreases; and neutrophil count decreases.

4. Rationales: _____

GOAL 2: Reduce or minimize the infectious process.

Interventions

1. Discontinue oral feedings for 7 to 14 days.

2. Insert an NG tube and attach it to low intermittent suction, or aspirate by hand at frequent intervals. Measure abdominal girth every 4 to 8 hours.

3. Start I.V. infusion of dextrose 10% in water ($D_{10}W$) at 150 ml/kg/24 hours.

4. Prepare and administer I.V. antibiotic therapy, such as ampicillin or aminoglycosides, as prescribed.

5. Additional individualized interventions: _____

Rationales

1. This provides rest to the injured bowel.

2. These actions maintain gastric decompression to eliminate vomiting and distention. Abdominal girth measurements provide information about changes in distention.

3. An infant 3 to 4 days old needs volume expansion to reperfuse. An I.V. of $D_{10}W$ at 60 ml/kg/24 hours may be given initially for first 24 hours. An electrolyte replacement of minerals and sodium may also be considered.

4. These broad-spectrum antibiotics inhibit protein biosynthesis of bacterial cell wall.

5. Rationales: _____

Collaborative problem: *Nutritional deficiency related to infant's inability to ingest and absorb nutrients because of bowel infection*

GOAL: Restore and maintain adequate nutritional intake to meet infant's needs.

Interventions

1. Maintain I.V. parenteral nutritional support for 2 weeks as follows:

Rationales

1. Parenteral nutrition supplies nutritional needs while allowing the bowel to rest. Poor absorption of feedings

Interventions

• Start with $D_{10}W$, using an infusion control device.
• Add amino acid mixture to $D_{10}W$ infusion.
• Add a supplement of fat administered via another setup and device.

2. Administer total parenteral nutrition (TPN) after sepsis is controlled.

3. Resume feedings slowly and in small amounts by gastric gavage.

4. Aspirate gastric contents before each feeding.

5. Measure abdominal girth before feedings and note increases. Note presence or absence of bowel sounds, tone of stomach, and abdominal musculature.

6. Weigh the infant every 8 hours. Record and report losses.

7. Calculate the infant's caloric needs to be given intermittently or continuously by NG tube.

8. Additional individualized interventions: _____

Rationales

and the need to rest injured bowel make withholding of food and water necessary. Formula feedings also contribute to production of hydrogen gas, which increases gas-forming bacteria.

2. Parenteral nutrition is continued to maintain nutritional intake until the infant can take oral feedings (see Tracheoesophageal Fistula or Esophageal Atresia plan, page 297, for the correct TPN procedure).

3. This prevents exacerbation of GI symptoms caused by retained gastric contents.

4. Increasing gastric residual contents may indicate poor absorption and cause distention and vomiting if feeding is given.

5. Girth measurement helps determine increasing distention. Presence of normal bowel sounds indicates an adequately functioning bowel.

6. Weight measurements help determine adequate growth and fluid status.

7. Identifying caloric needs ensures appropriate nutrient administration. Formula or breast milk (preferred) is given in amounts needed for growth and in progressive amounts as tolerated.

8. Rationales: _____

Nursing diagnosis: *High risk for fluid volume deficit related to fluid loss through gastric decompression and to withholding of food and water*

GOAL: Prevent fluid and electrolyte imbalance.

Interventions

1. Monitor fluid intake for comparison with output:
• I.V. infusion
• feedings via NG tube or other route
• TPN.

2. Monitor fluid output, including:
• weight of diapers (1 g = 1 ml) and oliguria
• weight loss
• gastric aspirate and emesis
• insensible water loss.

3. Review electrolyte levels, osmolality, and urine specific gravity and osmolality.

4. Assess for dehydration, including:
• hot, dry skin and poor skin turgor
• depressed fontanels
• elevated temperature
• increased urine specific gravity
• dry mucous membranes.

Rationales

1. Comparison of fluid intake and output prevents imbalance, dehydration, and overhydration.

2. Urine output should be at least 1 ml/kg/hour, with a low specific gravity of 1.005 to 1.010. Weight is the best indication of fluid loss in the infant.

3. Assessment reveals imbalance in sodium, potassium, and urine concentration, indicating dehydration. Specific gravity and sodium and potassium levels increase with dehydration.

4. Signs and symptoms of dehydration are related to third-space fluid shifting associated with NEC.

Interventions	Rationales
5. Additional individualized interventions: _____	5. Rationales: _____
_____	_____

Collaborative problem: *Physiologic injury and infection related to failure of disease to resolve (2 goals)*

GOAL 1: Identify actual or potential complications of NEC.

Interventions

1. Assess for signs and symptoms of disseminated intravascular coagulation (DIC), including:
• bleeding or oozing from any site (such as incision and I.V. puncture) or in stools, urine, and vomitus
• pallor or presence of petechiae, ecchymoses, or poor capillary filling time
• frank bleeding from intestine.

2. Review serial laboratory results for decreased hemoglobin (Hb) and fibrinogen levels and platelet count; CBC, WBC, and differential; serial laboratory results for increased PT, activated partial thromboplastin time (APTT), and thrombin time.

3. Assess for signs of septic shock, including:
• decreased blood pressure with wide pulse pressure
• tachycardia
• warm arms and legs.

4. Assess for signs of peritonitis, including:
• listlessness and "rag-doll" limpness
• apnea
• bradycardia
• hypothermia
• abdominal rigidity and distention; shiny red abdomen.

5. Additional individualized interventions: _____

Rationales

1. DIC is a possible complication of NEC. DIC develops in infants with NEC because infections are the most common stimuli that activate the clotting process; thromboplastin is released by the damaged bowel.

2. A decreased Hb indicates blood loss from bleeding. A decreased platelet count (100,000/mm³ or less) increases the risk of DIC. A reduced fibrinogen level slows the clotting process. Increases in PT, APTT, and thrombin time indicate a clotting abnormality and potential bleeding.

3. The infectious process may eventually extend to severe systemic involvement.

4. Continued inflammation and damage to the intestinal mucosa may cause perforation and peritonitis.

5. Rationales: _____

GOAL 2: Reduce or minimize the effects of complications.

Interventions

1. Treat DIC as follows:

• Record the amounts of blood taken for frequent testing.
• Avoid I.M. injections; monitor heelsticks and I.V. sites.
• Administer phytonadione (vitamin K) I.V.

• Apply pressure to bleeding sites.
• Prepare and assist with transfusion of volume expanders, such as plasma protein fraction (Plasmanate).
• Prepare and assist with transfusion of packed red blood cells (RBCs).
• Prepare and assist with transfusion of platelets and crystalloids.

Rationales

1. Therapy for coagulopathy may prevent life-threatening hemorrhage.
• Frequent testing may result in significant additional blood loss.
• Puncture wounds may predispose infant to blood loss.
• Vitamin K is given in an emergency to aid liver synthesis of clotting factors.
• Pressure helps control bleeding.
• A volume expander is given if clotting factors are the problem.
• Packed RBCs are given if bleeding is a problem and hematocrit value is decreased.
• Platelets and crystalloids are given if PTT and WBC count are low in sick infants.

Interventions

2. Treat for septic shock as follows:

• Prepare and administer hydrocortisone sodium succinate (Solu-Cortef) (not always used because it may mask infection).

• Monitor the infant's blood pressure and heart rate electronically and continuously.

• Prepare and assist with administration of transfusion.

3. Treat perforation and peritonitis as follows:

• Remove the umbilical artery catheter (UAC) if present and if possible.

• Limit palpation of abdomen.

• Handle infant minimally.

• Measure abdominal girth for increases every 2 hours.

• Assist with paracentesis, and collect a specimen for culture.

• If the culture is positive for gram-negative or -positive rods, give additional I.V. antibiotic. The usual drugs of choice are ampicillin and gentamicin, oxacillin, and methicillin.

• Prepare infant for surgery.

4. Additional individualized interventions: _____

Rationales

2. Septic shock may complicate NEC.

• A corticosteroid is given to increase cardiac output and peripheral perfusion.

• Increased heart rate and decreased blood pressure indicate shock.

• Whole blood transfusion, plasma, or crystalloid infusion may be given to maintain blood pressure and urine output.

3. Perforation may complicate uncontrolled NEC.

• Removal of UAC prevents additional injury, but it is not possible if the infant is critically ill and the UAC is needed for monitoring.

• Palpation may cause additional trauma to abdomen.

• Unnecessary handling may cause injury.

• Increases in girth indicate distention.

• Paracentesis relieves distention by removing fluid; culture identifies infection in peritoneal cavity.

• An antibiotic specific for these organisms is given to inhibit protein biosynthesis of bacterial cell wall.

• Perforation and peritonitis may require surgical intervention (see Preoperative Care plan, page 263).

4. Rationales: _____

Nursing diagnosis: *Anxiety (parental) related to the uncertain outcome of surgical intervention*

GOAL: Minimize parental anxiety and support the parents through the crisis.

Interventions

1. Maintain calm and accepting environment.

2. Encourage the parents to ask questions, and give honest and accurate answers or obtain needed information regarding:
• surgery involving resection of affected parts and reconnection of bowel
• possibility of ileostomy or colostomy (usually temporary) and accompanying short-bowel syndrome
• care being given before and after surgery and its rationale. (See Postoperative Care, page 257, and Preoperative Care, page 263, for details on knowledge deficit.)

3. Spend as much time as possible with the parents, keeping them informed of the infant's care and progress.

4. Assist the parents to appraise the crisis in terms of their needs and the needs of their infant.

5. Refer parents to community agencies for follow-up.

Rationales

1. This allows the parents to feel comfortable in expressing their feelings.

2. An open discussion with honest information promotes trust and decreases anxiety.

3. This involvement shows caring and support.

4. This appraisal identifies needed changes caused by the crisis.

5. Referral provides the family with continual support and guidance.

Interventions	Rationales
6. Additional individualized interventions: _____	6. Rationales: _____
_____	_____

ASSOCIATED PLANS
- Abruptio Placentae
- Cesarean Section Birth
- Hyperbilirubinemia
- Hypothermia and Hyperthermia
- Placenta Previa
- Postoperative Care
- Pregnancy-Induced Hypertension
- Premature Rupture of Membranes
- Preoperative Care
- Preterm Infant, Less Than 37 Weeks
- Sepsis Neonatorum and Infectious Disorders
- Tracheoesophageal Fistula or Esophageal Atresia

ADDITIONAL NURSING DIAGNOSES
- Altered nutrition: less than body requirements related to short-bowel syndrome
- Altered parenting related to compromised bonding process, misunderstanding, or lack of information
- Altered body temperature related to infection affecting regulation
- Impaired skin integrity related to injury, irritation of NG tube
- Impaired tissue integrity related to surgery
- Ineffective family coping related to guilt, anxiety about sick infant
- Ineffective infant feeding pattern related to bowel infection
- Knowledge deficit (parental) related to care of infant after surgery

Postoperative Care

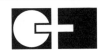

DEFINITION

Postoperative care in this plan consists of the care given to infants after surgical interventions for palliative or corrective procedures. The potential for altering each infant's physiologic status depends on the type of surgical procedure, the organ involved, and the system most severely affected by the surgery.

This plan presents general information on infant care after surgery and focuses on preventing complications related to surgery. Postoperative care for specific surgical procedures is also included, but each infant has individual needs based on the infant's status and the disorder's severity. Specific nursing diagnoses and interventions may need to be modified to fit a specific infant.

ETIOLOGY AND PRECIPITATING FACTORS

• congenital defect that produces a life-threatening situation in the infant and requires immediate correction (some surgeries require more extensive follow-up procedures when the infant is older and in better condition to undergo permanent correction)
• conditions such as gastroschesis, myelomeningocele, and patent ductus arteriosus (PDA) ligation that require immediate surgery but no further surgical procedures

• conditions that develop later and require surgical procedures, such as gastrostomy tube insertion, shunting when intraventricular hemorrhage results in hydrocephalus, and retinopathy

PHYSICAL FINDINGS
Infant status at birth
• congenital anomalies that threaten any system functions
• conditions that develop soon after birth because of abnormalities

Body systems
• signs and symptoms included in the assessment of each system noted in the plan

BEHAVIORAL FINDINGS
• depend on condition necessitating surgery (see specific plan for more information)

DIAGNOSTIC STUDIES
• See Preoperative Care plan, page 263, for appropriate tests; postoperative tests are included in this plan as they relate to the system affected by surgery.

Collaborative problem: *Respiratory compromise related to inadequate spontaneous respirations, with decreased lung expansion and increased tracheobronchial secretions from trauma or surgical anesthesia*

GOAL: Maintain and support respiratory effort and oxygenation after surgery.

Interventions

1. Assess infant's respiratory status hourly;
• rate, depth, and ease of respirations greater than 60 breaths/minute
• return of respiratory effort
• vital signs, including hourly blood pressure
• apneic episodes
• chest retractions and movements
• decreased or absent breath sounds with auscultated crackles or rhonchi
• skin color for central and peripheral cyanosis
• abdominal distention.

2. Have ventilatory support ready for the infant's return from surgery.

3. Monitor FIO_2 hourly.

4. Provide suction, if needed.

Rationales

1. Infants going to surgery usually receive pancuronium bromide (Pavulon), a skeletal muscle relaxant; this drug, combined with an anesthetic, affects respiratory status. Continual assessment can identify problems before they become serious. Infants usually are intubated preoperatively and not extubated until respiratory status is controlled.

2. Having ventilation support on hand minimizes delays in beginning treatment, if a problem should arise. Information from surgery ensures proper ventilation.

3. This identifies oxygen levels, ensuring proper oxygenation and preventing hypoxia.

4. Suction removes excess secretions that interfere with breathing ease by obstructing airways.

Interventions

5. Avoid restraining the infant, and minimize handling.

6. Maintain a neutral thermal environment by incubator or radiant warmer, which should be warm and ready for use when the infant returns from surgery.

7. Monitor arterial blood gas (ABG) values after establishing patent airway and ventilation.

8. Review complete blood count (CBC) results, electrolyte analyses, chest X-ray, and Chemstrip test for glucose level.

9. Check if the chest tube was inserted in OR.

10. Perform chest physiotherapy, unless the infant had chest surgery or is still intubated.

11. Allow the parents to see the infant as soon as possible after surgery.

12. Additional individualized interventions: _____

_____

Rationales

5. Minimizing movement helps the infant to stabilize.

6. A neutral thermal environment reduces metabolic expenditure of energy and oxygen demands. Hypothermic infants may develop disseminated intravascular coagulation if they get cold in the operating room (OR).

7. Monitoring ABG levels helps identify the adjustments needed in oxygen administration and helps prevent acid-base imbalances.

8. Test results establish a baseline for comparison with future test results. Deviations may indicate improvement or abnormalities.

9. Specific interventions ensure tube patency if surgery was performed in chest area.

10. Chest physiotherapy helps loosen secretions. This procedure may be considered 2 to 3 days postoperatively; small percussors with cup may be used.

11. Seeing the infant alive reassures the parents and helps relieve their anxiety.

12. Rationales: _____

_____

Collaborative problem: *Decreased cardiac output related to anesthesia, an inadequate shunt, or PDA ligation*

GOAL: Maintain optimal cardiac output after surgery.

Interventions

1. Monitor cardiovascular status every 1 to 2 hours, assessing for:
• irregular apical pulse
• blood pressure changes and narrowing pulse pressure
• capillary refill time greater than 5 seconds
• diminishing peripheral pulses and cool arms and legs
• distant heart sounds
• skin mottling
• oliguria.

2. Monitor ABG and hematocrit (HCT) values, X-ray results, and serum calcium and potassium levels.

3. Provide calcium or other electrolyte replacement as indicated.

4. Prepare and administer digoxin or other medications, as ordered.

5. Prepare and administer prostaglandin E and titrate at lowest dose.

Rationales

1. These measures ensure optimal cardiac function to permit oxygen and nutrient delivery to body tissues, thereby enhancing recovery.

2. Monitoring laboratory results helps to promptly identify changes. Abnormal results may indicate complications.

3. Reduced electrolyte levels may cause cardiac dysrhythmias.

4. Digoxin improves cardiac output and is given to treat congestive heart failure that results from cardiac dysfunction.

5. This drug is given if the shunt is functioning improperly.

Interventions	Rationales
6. Attach a cardiopulmonary monitor, turn on the alarm, and observe the infant's status as appropriate.	6. Continuous monitoring allows prompt assessment and intervention if changes should occur. An alarm warns of inappropriate oxygenation and cardiac changes.
7. Additional individualized interventions: _____	7. Rationales: _____

Nursing diagnosis: *High risk for infection related to surgical incision*

GOAL: Ensure intact surgical wound and healing without infection.

Interventions	Rationales
1. Assess the incisional site for infection, including: • skin for redness, breaks, irritation, or edema • drainage from wound for color, type, amount, and odor • chest tubes, if present, for inflammation at insertion site.	1. An infant is more susceptible to infection because of deficient phagocytic action and immune systems, which decrease the inflammatory response. Postoperatively, the infant is further compromised by decreased resistance.
2. Perform proper handwashing before approaching infant, using an antiseptic cleansing agent.	2. Handwashing removes transient bacteria and prevents the transmission of contaminants.
3. Change gown before caring for the infant. Follow hospital protocol for reverse isolation if indicated.	3. These measures protect infant from infection and cross-contamination.
4. Take the infant's axillary temperature hourly or monitor temperature electronically until infant's temperature stabilizes. Be alert for increases over 96.8° F (36° C) and poor temperature control.	4. Temperature increases indicate possible infectious process.
5. Review results of cultures from wound exudate and results of white blood cell count and differential.	5. When infection is suspected, cultures identify the infecting organism and blood tests confirm infection process.
6. Maintain absolute sterile technique when caring for the wound or performing dressing changes, irrigations, and other procedures.	6. Sterile technique helps prevent contamination that predisposes the infant to infection.
7. Additional individualized interventions: _____	7. Rationales: _____

Collaborative problem: *Nutritional deficiency related to withholding food and fluid and to inadequate nutritional intake from parenteral infusion*

GOAL: Maintain optimal nutrition after surgery.

Interventions	Rationales
1. Assess for changes in nutritional status: • Weigh the infant daily to determine loss or gain. • Note vomiting. • Determine how long the infant has gone without food or water. • Note lethargy and irritability. • Monitor glucose levels with Chemstrip and Dextrostix; monitor serum calcium levels. • Begin an I.V. infusion, gavage feedings, or total parenteral nutrition (TPN), as ordered.	1. An infant has the potential for developing hypoglycemia and hypocalcemia because of limited glucose and calcium reserves. Because of limited stores and rapid use by the compromised infant, caregivers must be alert for signs of developing disorders and intervene promptly to restore balance.

Interventions

2. Maintain nutritional requirements as follows:
• Calculate the infant's caloric needs and document the infant's fluid intake and output hourly.
• Weigh the infant daily unless condition prohibits it.
• Administer and monitor I.V. glucose, gavage feedings, or TPN as ordered.

3. Additional individualized interventions: _____

Rationales

2. Proper nutrition may be achieved by the most appropriate route, based on the infant's condition and the type of surgery. Initially, an I.V. infusion is provided followed by other methods as tolerated by the infant (see Tracheoesophageal Fistula or Esophageal Atresia plan, page 297, for procedures).

3. Rationales: _____

Collaborative problem: *Fluid imbalance related to withholding food and fluid or to blood or fluid loss*

GOAL: Maintain hydration and prevent fluid and electrolyte imbalance.

Interventions

1. Document infant's fluid intake every 1 to 2 hours, recording the following:
• parenteral fluids
• fluids received in OR
• volume expanders or blood products given
• medications given I.V. or P.O.
• oral feedings, including breast, bottle, or gavage.

2. Document infant's fluid output every 1 to 2 hours, recording the following:
• urine output, including that in OR
• liquid or loose stools
• nasogastric or thoracic drainage or drainage from other routes
• blood loss in surgery, from blood tests, or from other bleeding sites.

3. Compare fluid intake and output for positive or negative fluid balance.

4. Monitor ABG, HCT, CBC, and blood urea nitrogen values; creatinine and electrolyte levels; and urine specific gravity.

5. Monitor heart rate, blood pressure, and central venous pressure every 1 to 2 hours.

6. Ensure hydration:
• Administer I.V. fluids as ordered.
• Provide electrolyte replacement as needed and ordered.
• Administer blood or volume expanders as ordered.
• Monitor urine output of at least 2 to 3 ml/kg/hour, indicating adequate output.
• Monitor urine specific gravity of 1.005 to 1.015, indicating normal urine concentration.

7. Additional individualized interventions: _____

Rationales

1. These records help predict the infant's potential for imbalances before they occur, allowing for appropriate replacement therapy.

2. These records help predict potential for excess losses.

3. Fluid intake-output ratio identifies or predicts fluid imbalances.

4. These tests indicate changes in cardiac output, renal function, and fluid and electrolyte losses to be reported for appropriate interventions.

5. These parameters indicate changes in cardiac and renal functions.

6. Proper fluid replacement is essential to preventing or minimizing fluid losses. See Appendix 8: Fluid and Nutritional Needs in Infancy for fluid requirements.

7. Rationales: _____

Nursing diagnosis: *Altered parenting related to separation from infant because of surgery*

GOAL: Establish and support parent and infant relationship and bonding.

Interventions

1. Frequently and accurately inform parents of the infant's condition and progress after surgery. Permit parental visits as soon as possible.

2. Allow for expressions of parental feelings and fears, and show acceptance of them.

3. Allow the parents to visit frequently, to participate in infant care, and to telephone around the clock.

4. Reassure the parents that they can care for the infant after discharge by teaching them how to provide appropriate care.

5. If appropriate, inform the parents that the surgical outcome may be temporary and future hospitalization for additional procedures may be needed, if the physician's information needs reinforcement.

6. Additional individualized interventions: _____

Rationales

1. Informing the parents helps decrease their anxiety and increase their comfort level with the infant.

2. This establishes a trusting nurse and parent relationship.

3. Visitation, participation, and communication promote bonding.

4. Proper infant care instructions and assurance that support is available if needed enhance parental comfort in providing care.

5. Adequate information enhances compliance and alleviates further stress. Some procedures are temporary measures until the infant is old enough for permanent corrective surgery.

6. Rationales: _____

Nursing diagnosis: *Knowledge deficit (parental) related to postoperative care of infant at home*

GOAL: Provide information about the disease, surgery, and follow-up care.

Interventions

1. Teach parents (and reinforce information) about:
• infant's disease and surgery
• treatments and procedures
• signs and symptoms of complications
• follow-up care and therapy.

2. Teach parents about ordered treatments and infant care, which may include:
• home oxygen therapy and chest physiotherapy
• drug, nutritional, and fluid therapy
• incisional care and dressing changes
• skin care.

3. Encourage the family to participate in the infant's care.

4. Teach parents and family about signs and symptoms of infection, such as:
• fever
• redness, warmth, and inflammation at surgical site
• foul-smelling, purulent drainage from incision.

5. Have parents return demonstrations of all required procedures.

Rationales

1. Providing information alleviates parents' anxiety and helps them prepare adequately for the infant's discharge.

2. Proper instruction promotes compliance and helps dispel parents' fears about equipment and procedures.

3. Participation in care helps relieve feelings of inadequacy and prepares the family to care for the infant at home.

4. Early identification of signs and symptoms of infection allows prompt intervention.

5. Return demonstrations foster parental feelings of adequacy and independence in caring for the infant and may alert the nurse to the need for more instruction.

Interventions	**Rationales**
6. Teach parents and family how to balance activities with rest and how to evaluate the infant's tolerance for activities.	6. Stimulation of activity is crucial for normal infant growth and development, which may be delayed from prolonged hospitalization. Activity tolerance varies from one infant to the next.
7. Arrange for home health care follow-up.	7. Home health care referral provides the parents and family continued support outside the hospital.
8. Additional individualized interventions: _____	8. Rationales: _____

ASSOCIATED PLANS
• Bowel Obstruction, Small or Large
• Cleft Lip and Cleft Palate
• Congenital Heart Disease
• Intracranial Hemorrhage
• Necrotizing Enterocolitis
• Preoperative Care
• Spinal Cord Defects and Hydrocephalus
• Tracheoesophageal Fistula or Esophageal Atresia

ADDITIONAL NURSING DIAGNOSES
• Anticipatory grieving (parental) related to possible loss of infant during or as a result of surgery or loss of the anticipated perfect child
• Fear (parental) related to separation from infant
• High risk for altered body temperature related to extremes in age and weight
• High risk for aspiration related to anesthesia
• High risk for fluid deficit related to withholding of fluids postoperatively
• Impaired adjustment (parental) related to infant requiring surgery
• Impaired gas exchange related to anesthesia
• Impaired skin integrity related to drainage from colostomy, ileostomy
• Ineffective breathing pattern related to anesthesia
• Ineffective family coping: disabled related to guilt, anxiety
• Knowledge deficit (parental) related to lack of exposure to information or care of infant after surgery
• Pain related to surgical tissue trauma

Preoperative Care

DEFINITION

Preoperative care is given to an infant before surgical intervention for palliative or corrective procedures. Preparatory procedures depend on the infant's chronologic and gestational age and the defect or abnormal condition to be corrected. In most cases, the decision to intervene surgically is based on the infant's condition, the disorder's acuity (or life-threatening potential), the surgeon's and neonatologist's diagnoses and evaluations of the infant, and parental desires.

This plan focuses on the preoperative needs of most infants undergoing surgery for congenital defects, obstructions, relief of intracranial pressure, and other abnormalities. Because each infant's needs vary according to health status and severity of the disorder to be corrected, the following plan is general rather than specific to any disease or condition.

ETIOLOGY AND PRECIPITATING FACTORS

• cardiac defects, such as tetralogy of Fallot, truncus arteriosus, coarctation of the aorta, hypoplastic heart syndrome, and any of the ductal-dependent lesions
• GI defects, such as gastroschesis, omphalocele, imperforate anus, strangulated inguinal hernia, volvulus, intestinal atresia or stenosis, necrotizing enterocolitis, tracheoesophageal fistula or esophageal atresia, and cleft lip or cleft palate
• musculoskeletal defects, such as talipes deformity
• neurologic defects, such as meningocele and hydrocephalus (shunt placement)
• pulmonary defects, such as choanal atresia and diaphragmatic hernia

PHYSICAL FINDINGS
Infant status at birth
• immaturity, low birth weight and height, or, possibly, full-term infant with cardiac defects not identified at birth

• visible congenital anomalies, such as umbilical cord with only two vessels, cleft lip or cleft palate
• low Apgar score, asphyxia

BEHAVIORAL FINDINGS
• depend on condition necessitating surgery (see specific plan for more information)

DIAGNOSTIC STUDIES
• X-ray — to determine presence and extent of abnormality and area dependent on assessment
• computed tomography scan or magnetic resonance imaging — to detect abnormalities
• cardiac catheterization — to determine nature and extent of cardiac defects

Laboratory data
• serum glucose levels — to identify hypoglycemia
• electrolyte studies — to identify hypocalcemia and hypernatremia
• prothrombin time, partial thromboplastin time, and blood typing and crossmatching — to prepare for blood replacement if needed
• complete blood count — to identify changes indicating blood loss or infection
• TORCH screen — to identify possible viral infections
• arterial blood gas studies — to identify changes indicating altered gas exchange
• chromosomal studies — to identify genetic abnormalities

Nursing diagnosis: *Anxiety (parental) related to uncertain outcome of surgery*

GOAL: Minimize parental anxiety and support the parents through the crisis.

Interventions

1. Maintain a calm and accepting environment.

2. Encourage parents to ask questions; give honest and accurate answers and obtain necessary information, as needed.

Rationales

1. A calm environment allows the parents to feel comfortable expressing feelings and asking questions.

2. This interaction promotes trust by decreasing parental anxiety and fear of the unknown.

Interventions

3. Use pamphlets and drawings to reinforce the physician's information about the infant's surgical procedure, prognosis, and postsurgical care.

4. Stay with the parents or spend as much time as possible with them.

5. Inform the parents if the infant must be moved to another hospital, and explain the methods of safe transfer. The father or other family members may be allowed to accompany the infant and visit if the mother is still hospitalized.

6. Keep the parents informed of the infant's care and progress. Allow them unlimited time for contact with the infant as condition permits.

7. Additional individualized interventions: _____

Rationales

3. This information may need to be repeated or reinforced because parents may be too anxious to integrate previous information. This also ensures more fully informed consent before surgery.

4. The caregiver's presence shows support and caring.

5. Some hospitals do not have intensive care nursery (ICN) facilities. Although transferring the infant to a hospital with an ICN will benefit the infant, the move may cause additional parental anxiety because of separation. (See Appendix 11: Transporting an Infant to Another Hospital.)

6. Providing reports about the infant's condition and care alleviates parental anxiety. Facilitating their contact with the infant promotes bonding.

7. Rationales: _____

Nursing diagnosis: *High risk for fluid volume deficit related to withholding of food and water or to gastric decompression*

GOAL: Maintain hydration and prevent a fluid and electrolyte imbalance.

Interventions

1. Assess hydration status as follows:
• Weigh infant daily as condition permits.
• Compare urine output with fluid intake. Note urine output less than normal 2 to 3 ml/kg/hour.
• Note urine specific gravity greater than 1.013.
• Take axillary temperature, watching for increases over 100.2° F (37.9° C).
• Observe for changes in skin turgor; for dry, hot skin and mucous membranes; and for depressed anterior fontanel.
• Review electrolyte values for sodium and potassium increases or decreases.
• Note diarrhea.

2. Maintain hydration as follows:
• Calculate fluid needs based on infant's age and defect.
• Prepare, administer, and monitor I.V. infusion of fluids and electrolytes as ordered.
• Compare fluid intake and output amounts hourly. Include gastric drainage, insensible and urinary loss, and all parenteral intake for accurate calculation of infant's fluid needs.

3. Additional individualized interventions: _____

Rationales

1. Fluid loss resulting from withholding of food and water or a nasogastric or orogastric tube attached to suction may cause an imbalance and dehydration (hyponatremia and hypokalemia). Electrolyte levels may decrease with gastric decompression.

2. Combined with weight loss or gain, fluid intake and output are sensitive indicators of fluid imbalance. For an infant scheduled for surgery, accurate fluid intake and output records are essential to correcting fluid imbalance preoperatively. Fluid replacement may be essential for fluid balance and must be calculated individually in milliters per kilogram per 24 hours; a rule of thumb is cc/cc (ml/ml) over 4 to 8 hours.

3. Rationales: _____

Nursing diagnosis: *Altered nutrition: less than body requirements related to withholding of food and water and parenteral infusion of nutrients (I.V. and total parenteral nutrition [TPN])*

GOAL: Maintain optimal nutrition preoperatively.

Interventions

1. Assess changes in infant's nutritional status as follows:
• Weigh every 8 hours to determine loss, if any.
• Record vomiting and diarrhea.
• Note irritability and restlessness.
• Note length of time infant goes without food and water.
• Monitor I.V. glucose and TPN infusion.
• Monitor infusion and caloric content.
• Review heelstick blood glucose levels, such as Chemstrip and Dextrostix, in relation to maintaining normal glucose level.

2. Maintain nutritional requirements as follows:
• Calculate caloric needs.
• Monitor and document caloric intake and weight every 4 to 8 hours, or as needed.
• Monitor I.V. administration of fluid and glucose.
• Monitor TPN administration, if given.

3. Additional individualized interventions: _____

Rationales

1. The infant has limited stores of glucose. Other factors may also contribute to a nutrient deficiency.

2. Maintaining nutritional requirements helps the infant withstand the added stress of surgery and provides for continued growth and development. Caloric needs are supplied in calories per kilogram per 24 hours. They usually are administered with fluids parenterally.

3. Rationales: _____

Nursing diagnosis: *High risk for infection related to a break in skin integrity from surgery or from a defect in which a sac protrudes from the skin surface*

GOAL: Reduce risk of infection.

Interventions

1. Before approaching the infant, wash hands properly with an antiseptic cleansing agent.

2. Take axillary temperature every 2 to 4 hours. Note temperature over 96.8° F (36° C) or poor temperature control.

3. Monitor skin cultures.

4. Note changes such as lethargy, irritability, dyspnea, and cyanosis.

5. Maintain absolute sterile technique when caring for infants with such defects as gastroschesis or myelomeningocele. Clean the equipment and supplies used on infant daily or as hospital policy dictates. Cover the sac with a moist sterile saline dressing.

6. Additional individualized interventions: _____

Rationales

1. Handwashing removes transient bacteria and prevents transmission of contaminants.

2. Temperature increases indicate possible infection.

3. Culture results identify infectious organisms.

4. Early identification of these signs may reveal that the infant has an infection and allows prompt treatment.

5. These actions prevent contamination, which predisposes the infant to infection.

6. Rationales: _____

Nursing diagnosis: *Knowledge deficit (parental) related to lack of familiarity with hospital procedures and perioperative routines*

GOAL: Prepare the infant and family for surgery.

Interventions

1. Determine parents' readiness to learn.

2. Assess effect of the infant's medical problem on parents and on family's lifestyle.

3. Determine each parent's stage of adaptation to infant's condition (such as shock and disbelief, developing awareness, or resolution and reorganization). Base teaching approach on that stage.

4. Assess parents' knowledge of infant's disorder, its implications, and potential complications.

5. Determine parents' learning needs.

6. Determine realistic goals and work with family to ensure that goals are mutually acceptable.

7. Set priorities and divide teaching content into information to teach now and information to teach later.

8. Determine the best time for teaching sessions.

9. Use various teaching strategies and tools, including:
• discussions
• demonstrations
• booklets
• films and videotapes
• models or dolls.

10. Teach family about infant's perioperative care, such as:
• food and fluid restrictions
• time of surgery
• type of anesthesia
• insertion of I.V. or intra-arterial lines
• operating room and postanesthesia care unit personnel and environments
• equipment and procedures, such as monitors, tubes, drains, dressing changes, and respiratory therapy.

11. Evaluate parents' response to teaching.

12. Additional individualized interventions: _____

Rationales

1. This assessment helps guide choice of teaching method and type and amount of material to be presented.

2. This assessment helps determine extent of teaching required. Teaching should be structured according to the areas most affected.

3. Focus and issues differ with the stage of adaptation, necessitating a different teaching approach.

4. Adults learn best when teaching is based on knowledge or previous experience.

5. Learning needs determine appropriate teaching content. Responding to these needs conveys sensitivity to family's concerns.

6. Goals affect teaching content. Family participation in goal setting improves the chance of success.

7. Setting priorities and dividing teaching content into these categories ensure coverage of important information without overwhelming the family.

8. Choosing appropriate times for teaching sessions enhances parents' attention and receptivity, aiding their retention of information.

9. Parents are more likely to retain information when learning engages multiple senses.

10. Such teaching reduces parents' fears and anxieties by informing them of what to expect. Also, parents are more likely to remember and comply with perioperative care if they understand the rationales for equipment and procedures.

11. This evaluation determines whether goals have been met and may reveal the need for further teaching.

12. Rationales: _____

ASSOCIATED PLANS
• Bowel Obstruction, Small or Large
• Cleft Lip and Cleft Palate
• Congenital Heart Disease
• Hypothermia and Hyperthermia
• Intracranial Hemorrhage
• Necrotizing Enterocolitis
• Spinal Cord Defects and Hydrocephalus
• Tracheoesophageal Fistula or Esophageal Atresia

ADDITIONAL NURSING DIAGNOSES
• Altered growth and development related to environmental and stimulation deficiencies
• Fear (parental) related to possible separation from infant or death of infant as result of surgery
• High risk for altered body temperature related to extremes in age and weight
• Ineffective family coping related to guilt and anxiety
• Ineffective infant feeding pattern related to withholding of food and fluids

Preterm Infant, Less Than 37 Weeks

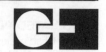

DEFINITION

An infant whose gestational age is 37 weeks or less at birth is called preterm. Although small, the preterm infant may be appropriately sized for its gestational age, but poor intrauterine growth may complicate the postnatal period of the already compromised infant.

An infant whose birth weight is about 5 lb, 8 oz (2,500 g) or less and whose gestational age is more than 37 weeks is considered small for gestational age (SGA) rather than preterm, although about 75% of neonates who weigh less than 2,500 g are born prematurely. Preterm births constitute 8% to 10% all live births in the United States.

Clinical problems occur more often in the preterm infant than in the full-term infant. Prematurity results in immaturely developed and functioning systems, limiting the infant's ability to cope with problems and illnesses.

Common problems include respiratory distress syndrome (RDS), necrotizing enterocolitis, hyperbilirubinemia, hypoglycemia, thermoregulation, patent ductus arteriosus (PDA), pulmonary edema, and intraventricular hemorrhage. Additional stressors for infant and parents include separation and prolonged hospitalization for the high-risk or critically ill infant. Parental responses and coping mechanisms may create deficits in their relationship; special allowances and planning may be needed to support the bonding process.

The preterm infant's survival depends on weight, gestational age, and illnesses or abnormalities. Preterm delivery accounts for 75% to 80% of neonatal morbidity and mortality.

This plan focuses on preterm infant care and the prevention of potential complicating events in specific systems.

ETIOLOGY AND PRECIPITATING FACTORS
• maternal problems
  □ disorders, such as hypertensive disease, toxemia, placenta previa, abruptio placentae, cervical incompetence, multiple gestation, malnutrition, and diabetes mellitus
  □ low socioeconomic status and no prenatal care
  □ preterm deliveries or induced abortion
  □ maternal use of any or all of the following: prescribed drugs, over-the-counter drugs, illegal drugs, alcohol, cigarettes, caffeine

PHYSICAL FINDINGS
Maternal history
• age under 16 years and educational background
• multiple gestation
• low socioeconomic status, no prenatal care, and poor nutrition
• possibly, genetic counseling

• previous preterm births and closely spaced pregnancies
• infections, such as TORCH, sexually transmitted diseases, or others
• conditions, such as toxemia, premature rupture of membranes, abruptio placentae, placenta previa, and prolapsed umbilical cord
• caffeine, cigarettes, alcohol, or prescribed, over-the-counter, or illegal drug use
• blood type, Rh factor, amniocentesis for lung profile, alpha fetoprotein with history of previous infants with neurologic defects

Infant status at birth
• gestational age usually 24 to 37 weeks, low birth weight, SGA, or large for gestational age
• weight usually less than 5 lb, 8 oz (2,500 g)
• thin, minimal subcutaneous fat deposits
• large head in proportion to body: circumference about 1¼″ (3 cm) larger than chest circumference
• possible visible physical anomalies
• Apgar score at 1 and 5 minutes: 0 to 3 indicates severe distress; 4 to 6, moderate distress; and 7 to 10, normal adjustment probable

Cardiovascular
• heart rate 120 to 160 beats/minute at apical site with regular rhythm
• at birth, possible murmur auscultated over base of heart or at third or fourth intercostal space at left sternal edge, indicating right-to-left shunt from pulmonary hypertension or atelectasis

Gastrointestinal
• protruding abdomen
• meconium passage usually within 12 hours
• weak sucking and diminished swallowing reflexes
• patent anus unless congenital abnormality present

Integumentary
• pallid, cyanotic, jaundiced, mottled, red, or bright pink skin
• little vernix caseosa, with lanugo over entire body
• thin, transparent appearance, both smooth and shiny
• generalized edema or localized edema in presenting part at delivery
• short nails; fine, fuzzy, scant, or no head hair
• possible petechiae or ecchymoses
• minimally creased soles and palms

Musculoskeletal
• ear cartilage poorly developed but soft and pliable
• fontanels and separation at suture lines present
• soft skull and rib bones
• relaxed state, inactive, or lethargic

Neurologic
• reflexes and movement to neurologic test meet with no resistance; reflex activity is only partly developed
• sucking, swallowing, gag reflex, and coughing may be weak or ineffectual
• absent or diminished neurologic signs
• eyes may be closed or fused before 25 to 26 gestational weeks
• unstable body temperature; usually hypothermic, ad ting to various environmental temperatures
ble tremors, twitching, and eye rolling; usually tran but may indicate neurologic abnormalities

Pulmonary
• respiratory rate ranging from 40 to 60 breaths/minute with short periods of apnea
• possible irregular respirations, with nasal flaring, grunting, and retractions (intercostal, suprasternal, substernal)
• possible audible fine crackles

Renal
• voiding occurring within 8 hours after birth
• possible inability to excrete solutes in urine

Reproductive
• girls: prominent clitoris with poorly developed labia majora
• boys: underdeveloped scrotum with minimal rugae and testes not down in scrotum, with inguinal hernia

BEHAVIORAL FINDINGS
• possible weak cry
• jitteriness
• inactivity

DIAGNOSTIC STUDIES
• X-ray studies of chest or other organs—to confir rule out suspected abnormalities
• Ultrasonography—to detect organ abnormalities

Laboratory data
• heelstick blood glucose levels (Chemstrip or Dextrostix testing)—to identify blood glucose decreases, followed by serum glucose test if values are less than 45 mg/dl, with second test for verification
• serum calcium level—to identify decreases that may lead to hypocalcemia
• bilirubin levels—to identify increases (because the preterm infant is more vulnerable to hyperbilirubinemia than the full-term infant); umbilical cord blood is tested
• complete blood count (CBC)—for hematocrit and hemoglobin decreases, red blood cell count decreases, platelet count decreases, white blood cell (WBC) count and differential abnormalities
• electrolyte levels—to determine potassium, sodium, and magnesium levels
• arterial blood gas (ABG) studies—to identify changes in pH, PO_2, PCO_2, or HCO_3, indicating acidosis
• blood type, Rh factor, and Coombs' test—to identify potential incompatibilities
• culture of blood, other body fluids, or drainage—to identify infectious agents, if any
• urinalysis for specific gravity and culture—to identify infection
• stool analysis—to identify occult blood (first stool usually is positive from blood swallowed during delivery)
• additional tests may be appropriate, depending on presenting signs and symptoms

---

Collaborative problem: *High risk for respiratory distress related to pulmonary immaturity with decreased surfactant production causing hypoxemia and acidosis*

GOAL: Maintain and maximize pulmonary function.

Interventions

1. Compile assessment data focusing on possible respiratory distress. Include data related to:

• maternal history of drug use or abnormal conditions during pregnancy or labor and delivery
• infant's condition at birth—Apgar score, need for resuscitation
• respiratory rate, depth, and ease; tachypnea with rate over 60 breaths/minute
• expiratory grunting, nasal flaring, or retractions with use of accessory muscles (intercostal, suprasternal, or substernal)

Rationales

1. Assessment data provide baseline information, permitting early interventions and a better prognosis if the infant should display respiratory distress signs (see Hyaline Membrane Disease—Respiratory Distress Syndrome [RDS I] plan, page 205, for complete care of respiratory distress in the preterm infant).

• Maternal conditions may predispose infant to respiratory distress.
• This provides data indicating respiratory distress at birth.
• Respiratory rate increases with respiratory distress as infant's need for oxygen increases.
• Respiratory distress signs appear as infant attempts to increase oxygen intake. They may also be present from meconium aspiration or diaphragmatic hernia.

Interventions

• cyanosis when breathing room air, decreased breath sounds.

2. Assess for apneic episodes lasting longer than 20 seconds, noting the following:
• bradycardia
• lethargy, position, and activity before, during, and after apneic episode (for example, while sleeping or feeding); side-lying, prone, or supine position; airway obstruction caused by mask (Bilimask) over nose
• abdominal distention
• skin temperature and mottling
• spontaneous return of breathing
• need for stimulation as well as type and amount
• episode's duration
• cause of apnea, such as cold stress, sepsis, respiratory failure, or preterm birth
• results of CBC with differential, blood culture, chest X-ray, and ABG studies, if performed.

3. Provide and monitor respiratory support as follows:

• Administer warm and humidified oxygen, with pulse oximeter or transcutaneous blood oxygen tension monitor in place. Check oxygen hourly. Reposition probe every 3 hours.

• Carefully suction nostrils and mouth for no more than 5 seconds.

• Maintain a neutral thermal environment.

• Position infant on abdomen or supine with a small pad beneath the shoulders or in a side-lying position with the head supported.

• Stimulate the infant by stroking feet, hands, and back and then trunk, face, arms, and legs with gentle motions, becoming more vigorous if needed.

4. Monitor serial ABG studies performed to identify respiratory or metabolic acidosis.

5. Prepare and administer pharmacologic therapy, such as theophylline I.V. Monitor blood levels every 1 to 2 days for toxicity (greater than 10 mcg/ml) or trough level (2 mcg/ml).

6. Additional individualized interventions: _____

Rationales

• These are later signs, as respiratory distress becomes severer.

2. Apneic episodes may occur because of hypoxia and carbon dioxide retention and decreased pH. Breathing cessation lasting less than 20 seconds is known as periodic breathing. Breathing that ceases for 20 to 30 seconds is apnea. Apnea may be a sign of such infant problems as sepsis, intracranial hemorrhage, RDS, cold stress, hypoglycemia, pneumonia, PDA, maternal oversedation, or other problems. Infants with apneic pauses lasting 15 seconds or more should be placed on an apnea monitor with alarms set to detect apneic episodes of 15 seconds (see Sepsis Neonatorum and Infectious Disorders plan, page 276, for procedure).

3. Respiratory support provides the infant with needed oxygen. Monitoring prevents oxygen toxicity.

• Oxygen administration supplements the infant's oxygen supply. Monitoring ensures the optimal oxygen level necessary for respiratory support. Changing probe postition prevents burns.

• Suctioning may be needed to maintain a patent airway if the infant is receiving mechanical ventilation.

• Temperature changes may contribute to apnea and increased oxygen consumption, which leads to decreased surfactant production.

• These positions facilitate breathing and chest expansion.

• Stimulating the central nervous system promotes spontaneous resumption of breathing during apneic episodes.

4. In the neonate, respiratory depression is reflected by ABG values; for example, PO_2 less than 50 mm Hg indicates hypoxia; PCO_2 more than 55 mm Hg indicates hypercapnia; pH value less than 7.30 indicates acidosis.

5. Theophylline is given for apnea. It increases ventilation through central stimulation, which causes bronchodilation. Monitoring these blood levels assures that therapeutic drug levels are maintained without toxicity.

6. Rationales: _____

Collaborative problem: *High risk for hypothermia or hyperthermia related to prematurity or changes in environmental temperatures*

GOAL: Maintain a neutral thermal environment.

Interventions

1. Maintain ambient nursery temperature of 77° F (25° C).

Rationales

1. Optimal room temperature minimizes heat loss.

Interventions

2. Assess infant's rectal temperature first and then axillary temperature every 2 hours or as needed.

3. Carry out appropriate warming procedure after infant's delivery.

4. Place the infant under radiant warmer or in incubator, if indicated.

5. Apply the temperature control (Servo-Control) probe over the abdomen; set heater output for 98.6° to 99.5° F (37° to 37.5° C); and maintain skin temperature of 96° to 97.7° F (35.6° to 36.5° C).

6. Avoid placing infant in external contact with sources of cold or heat. Also avoid exposure to cold or hot air. Institute measures to conserve body heat, such as keeping the infant dry and keeping the head covered.

7. Assess the infant for status changes that may indicate cold stress.

8. Additional individualized interventions: _____

Rationales

2. The preterm infant is susceptible to cold stress or temperature fluctuations because of decreased subcutaneous fat deposits, low metabolic reserves of substances needed for heat and energy, inability to shiver, and smaller ratio of body mass to surface area (see Hypothermia and Hyperthermia plan, page 229).

3. Warming conserves the infant's body heat and prevents temperature changes.

4. Radiant warmer or incubator ensures a neutral thermal environment, which helps the infant maintain body temperature and reduce oxygen consumption.

5. Apparatus controls infant's body temperature by turning on or off when the infant's temperature goes below or above a set point. The temperature setting depends on the infant's age and weight.

6. Avoiding exposure prevents potential hypothermic or hyperthermic responses. Measures to conserve body heat minimize heat loss through radiation, conduction, convection, and evaporation and prevent cold stress.

7. Cold stress increases oxygen and caloric needs, which may lead to hypoxia and acidosis (see Hypothermia and Hyperthermia plan, page 229).

8. Rationales: _____

Collaborative problem: *Nutritional deficiency related to inadequate stores of glycogen, iron, and calcium and to the depletion of these stores by the infant's higher metabolic rate and increased requirements, inadequate caloric intake, and loss of calories*

GOAL: Establish and maintain adequate caloric intake and the infant's overall nutritional status.

Interventions

1. Assess the infant's sucking and gag reflexes and swallowing ability. Begin oral feedings when the infant's condition is stable and respirations are controlled.

2. Assess and calculate the infant's caloric requirements.

3. Initiate breast-feeding or bottle-feeding 2 to 6 hours after birth. Begin with 3 to 5 ml per feeding every 3 hours. Increase as tolerated. Breast-feeding may be postponed until the infant demonstrates that it can feed by nipple and gain weight.

4. Weigh the infant daily, comparing weight with caloric intake, to determine appropriate intake amounts or the need for increasing that intake.

5. Provide dextrose 10% in water ($D_{10}W$) I.V. if infant does not feed orally.

Rationales

1. Immature reflexes, lethargy, or weakness may cause postponement of oral feedings.

2. To promote weight gain, the caloric requirement for preterm infants is about 120 to 150 cal/kg/24 hours when oral feedings are established.

3. Feedings should begin as soon as possible because the immature infant has not had the opportunity to build up stores of iron and glucose. Oral feedings may be tolerated by the stable preterm infant.

4. Daily weighing ensures adequate caloric intake as evidenced by weight gain (see Appendix 8: Fluid and Nutritional Needs in Infancy).

5. I.V. $D_{10}W$ supplies immediate fluid and glucose requirements to prevent hypoglycemia that can result from the preterm infant's depleted glucose stores.

Interventions	**Rationales**
6. Provide gavage feedings as appropriate.	6. Feeding by alternate route ensures nutritional intake if conditions prevent the infant from feeding orally (see Hyaline Membrane Disease — Respiratory Distress Syndrome [RDS I] plan, page 205, for gavage procedure and care).
7. Provide total parenteral nutrition (TPN) and intralipids as appropriate.	7. This alternative method feeding supplies nutritional requirements during a prolonged illness or after surgery (see Tracheoesophageal Fistula or Esophageal Atresia plan, page 297, for TPN procedure and care).
8. Monitor heelstick blood glucose levels, such as Chemstrip or Dextrostix; monitor serum for calcium, iron, and glucose levels.	8. Monitoring identifies low glucose, calcium, or iron levels that need replacement to prevent complications.
9. Additional individualized interventions: _____	9. Rationales: _____

Collaborative problem: *Fluid imbalance related to losses resulting from immaturity, radiant warmer, or phototherapy or from losses through skin or lungs*

GOAL: Maintain fluid and electrolyte balance.

Interventions	**Rationales**
1. Assess and calculate the infant's fluid requirements.	1. Careful assessment and calculation aid accurate administration of fluids. The infant's immature renal system affects its ability to concentrate urine and conserve fluid. In addition, more fluid is lost via the skin in the preterm infant than in the full-term infant during treatments (as much as 190%). (See Postoperative Care plan, page 257, for input-output procedure.)
2. Provide fluids of 150 to 180 ml/kg and up to 200 ml/kg, if needed. Fluids should not be withheld for very long.	2. This fulfills infant's fluid requirement. The amounts provided are based on needs or losses.
3. Weigh the infant daily.	3. Daily weight records reflect the infant's growth progress as well as fluid losses or gains.
4. Monitor and record the infant's fluid intake and output hourly. Compare amounts to identify imbalances. Include all sources of intake as well as output.	4. Comparing fluid intake and output prevents possibility of excess fluid losses.
5. Test the infant's urine for specific gravity and glycosuria.	5. The urine test provides information about potential dehydration or glycosuria.
6. Maintain a neutral thermal environment and dress the infant in proper clothing to protect the infant from additional fluid losses.	6. The preterm infant lacks insulating fat. Its thin skin with blood vessels close to the body surface increases the potential for fluid and heat loss through the skin.
7. Assess the infant for signs indicating increased fluid needs, such as: • increased body temperature • hypovolemic shock with decreased blood pressure and increased heart rate, diminished peripheral pulses, cool hands and feet, and skin mottling • sepsis • asphyxia and hypoxia.	7. The sick preterm infant needs careful hemodynamic monitoring because it is prone to cardiac dysrhythmias caused by immaturity of cardiac conduction tissue and autonomic nervous systems and by susceptibility to congenital heart defects other than PDA, which might occur secondary to prolonged exposure to decreased oxygen level.
8. Monitor potassium, sodium, and chloride levels; replace electrolytes and fluids (with $D_{10}W$ I.V.), if needed.	8. Electrolyte and fluid replacement maintains fluid and electrolyte balance (see Appendix 8: Fluid and Nutritional Needs in Infancy for requirements).

Interventions

9. Additional individualized interventions: _____

_____

Rationales

9. Rationales: _____

_____

Collaborative problem: *High risk for infection related to infant's immunologic immaturity and possible infection transmission from mother or health care personnel*

GOAL: Prevent infection.

Interventions

1. Assess for temperature fluctuations, lethargy, apnea, poor feeding, irritability, and jaundice.

2. Review maternal history, infant's condition at birth, and infection epidemics in nursery.

3. Obtain samples of blood and drainage from any source

4. Review CBC with WBC count and differential, platelet count, and immunoglobulins with WBCs less than 5,000 or greater than 25,000/mm³; absolute neutrophils less than 5,000; ratio of immature to mature neutrophils greater than 13; platelets less than 80,000/mm³; IgM increases.

5. Provide an environment that protects the infant from infection.
• Follow protocol for gown changes and handwashing before and between infant care.
• Follow protocol for isolating infants or excluding them from nursery.
• Follow meticulous sterile technique when caring for the infant and performing procedures.
• Follow protocol that protects the infant from contact with people who might transmit infection.
• Institute universal precautions as indicated.
• Instruct the parents how to prevent cross-contamination of infant and transmission of microorganisms.

6. Additional individualized interventions: _____

_____

Rationales

1. Identifying early signs of infection allows prompt treatment.

2. Infections may be transmitted perinatally by the mother or by hospital personnel.

3. Cultures identify microorganisms responsible for infection, making treatment choices possible.

4. The infant's immature defense systems at birth (with a deficiency in phagocytic and immune system activity and decreased inflammatory response) increase the potential for acquiring infection. This is a special concern for the compromised preterm infant. Review of laboratory data identifies actual or potential infection.

5. These actions prevent the transmission of infection to the infant (see Sepsis Neonatorum and Infectious Disorders plan, page 276, for complete care of infection in the preterm infant).

6. Rationales: _____

_____

Nursing diagnosis: *High risk for impaired skin integrity related to fragile, transparent immature skin*

GOAL: Maintain skin integrity.

Interventions

1. Assess the infant's skin for redness, irritation, rashes, and lesions and for breakdown in all pressure areas.

2. Assess I.V., electrode, and catheter sites or other insertion sites for signs of infection, skin breakdown, and extravasation of fluid.

Rationales

1. The preterm infant's skin is thinner and more fragile; capillaries are near the surface, and there is minimal subcutaneous fat to protect bony pressure areas.

2. The preterm infant is more likely to undergo invasive therapeutic procedures, which further expose skin to breakdown.

Interventions

3. Provide appropriate daily skin care. At the same time, protect the infant's skin from contact with cleansing agents, other solutions, and tapes.

4. Additional individualized interventions: _____

_____

Rationales

3. This action protects the skin by maintaining cleanliness and preventing loss of the protective bactericidal barrier or skin layer. (For more information on preterm infant skin care, see Skin Disorders plan, page 283.)

4. Rationales: _____

_____

Nursing diagnosis: Sensory-perceptual alteration: visual, auditory, kinesthetic, gustatory, tactile, and olfactory related to decreased or excessive stimulation of intensive care environment

GOAL: Ensure optimal sensory stimulation without sensory overload.

Interventions

1. Assess the infant's ability to respond to stimuli. Observe for:
• neurologic deficits
• alertness or inattention
• inappropriate response to noise, eye contact, or feeding and absent normal reflexes
• effects of medications on behavior.

2. Provide visual stimulation as follows:
• Dim bright lights.
• Suspend a black-and-white mobile with geometric shapes 7" to 9" from the infant's eyes.
• Hold the infant at eye level for eye contact; hold the infant upright on shoulder if possible.

3. Provide auditory stimulation as follows:
• Talk to the infant, using a low tone and voice inflections.
• Call the infant by name, speaking to the infant while giving care.
• Sing, play tapes, or turn on a radio.
• Avoid excessive noises and conversations around the infant.
• Reduce monitor noises if possible.

4. Provide tactile stimulation as follows:
• With warmed hands and fingers, stroke the infant gently from head to toe as well as all parts of the infant's body.
• Hold and caress the infant if appropriate.
• Give the infant a pacifier for sucking satisfaction.
• Touch the infant with articles of differing textures, such as cotton balls or smooth and napped cloth.
• Change the infant's position every other hour, if appropriate.
• Carry the infant in a strap-on carrier, if appropriate.

5. Provide gustatory stimulation by offering pacifier or feeding the infant breast or formula milk as indicated.

6. Provide rest and sleep periods that are uninterrupted by procedures.

7. Additional individualized interventions: _____

_____

Rationales

1. Assessment results suggest the types and amounts of sensory stimulation to provide or reduce.

2. The infant should be able to look at and respond to an object; too much visual stimulation may cause the infant to look away or sigh or cause respiratory changes.

3. Auditory responses, such as the infant turning its head toward the sounds, should occur; overstimulation may cause apnea, bradycardia, or minimal body response.

4. Tactile responses, such as motor activity, should be present appropriate to the infant's condition; overstimulation may cause hyperactivity or hypoactivity. Tactile deficiency may cause inappropriate crying spells or response only during procedures.

5. Gustatory responses, such as hand-to-mouth activity, feeding, and sucking pacifier, should occur.

6. Rest periods prevent overstimulation.

7. Rationales: _____

_____

Nursing diagnosis: *Knowledge deficit related to care of sick infant at home*

GOAL: Teach the parents and family about the infant's disease and follow-up care.

Interventions	Rationales
1. Inform the parents and family about: • disease process • care procedures • signs and symptoms of respiratory problems • follow-up care and therapy.	1. Learning about the infant's condition and tre[...] relieves family members' anxiety and allows th[...] prepare for the infant's discharge adequately.
2. Teach the parents and family about ordered treatments, such as: • home oxygen therapy • mechanical ventilation • chest physiotherapy • drug therapy • nutritional and fluid therapy • specialized monitoring, such as apnea or blood glucose monitoring.	2. Such teaching promotes family compliance and helps dispel their fears about equipment and procedures.
3. Have the parents and family give return demonstrations of all required procedures.	3. Return demonstrations boost family members' feelings of adequacy and independence and may alert the nurse to the need for more instruction.
4. Encourage the parents and family to participate in the infant's care.	4. Participation helps alleviate feelings of inadequacy and prepares family members to care for the infant at home.
5. Teach the parents and family how to balance activities with rest and how to evaluate the infant's tolerance for activities.	5. Stimulation of activity is crucial for normal infant growth and development, which may be delayed from prolonged hospitalization. Activity tolerance varies from one infant to the next.
6. Arrange for home health care follow-up.	6. Home health care provides the parents and family with continued support outside the hospital.
7. Additional individualized interventions: _____	7. Rationales: _____

ASSOCIATED PLANS

All plans for the full-term infant have applications relevant to the preterm infant, whose condition usually is compromised and who usually is vulnerable to the conditions listed in the Table of Contents. See the plan appropriate to the individual infant.

ADDITIONAL NURSING DIAGNOSES

• Altered family processes related to birth of high-risk infant
• Altered growth and development related to functional immaturity and prolonged environmental stress
• Altered parenting related to infant's need for intensive care nursery
• Anxiety (parental) related to vulnerability of small infant to illnesses
• Caregiver role strain related to infant's status and need for intensive care
• High risk for injury related to lack of cushioning from inadequate subcutaneous fat
• Impaired gas exchange related to pulmonary immaturity
• Ineffective breathing pattern related to respiratory and neurologic immaturity
• Ineffective individual coping (parental) related to stress of preterm birth
• Powerlessness (parental) related to health care environment and limited infant interaction

Sepsis Neonatorum and Infectious Disorders

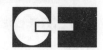

DEFINITION

Infectious diseases may occur in the infant before, during, and after birth. They may be acquired in the ascending genital tract, by intrauterine infection, or by transplacental inoculation. Postnatally, they may be acquired from nursery personnel or from equipment used during the infant's treatment and care. Nosocomial infections are hospital-acquired. Viral and protozoan infections are known as TORCH conditions, and include toxoplasmosis (TO), rubella (R), cytomegalovirus (C), and herpes I or II (H). The O of TO stands for other infections, such as syphilis, varicella, chlamydia, and group B streptococcus (see *Etiology of infection,* for mode of transmission to fetus or infant). A sexually transmitted group of diseases includes gonorrhea, herpes, chlamydia, and syphilis. Most common of the neonatal infections are pneumonia and septicemia; the most severe cases are caused by group B beta-hemolytic streptococci, with onset a few days after delivery. Infections caused by this organism are acquired in utero, by the ascending route, or by contact with infected tissue during birth.

The incidence of infection is higher in the preterm infant, indicating an association between the immature immune system, the infections, and the predisposing factors leading to infection. Like the adult, the infant defends itself against invasion by infectious agents with its intact skin and mucous membranes, by phagocytosis, by the inflammatory response, and by producing antibodies that act against a specific microorganism. However, because of immaturity, the preterm infant's defenses are deficient, limited, or reduced in their actions, leaving the infant more susceptible to infection.

This plan focuses on identifying potential or existing infectious states and caring for the infant with an infection.

PHYSICAL FINDINGS
Maternal history
• prenatal care, ethnicity, socioeconomic status
• premature rupture of membranes (PROM), dilatation of cervix 24 hours or more before delivery, or precipitous delivery
• birth outside of delivery or operating room
• history of or current sexually transmitted diseases, such as syphilis, herpes chlamydia, and gonorrhea
• infectious diseases, such as toxoplasmosis, rubella, cytomegalovirus, tuberculosis, hepatitis, or acquired immunodeficiency syndrome during pregnancy or at delivery
• amnionitis, maternal bleeding, or toxemia

Infant status at birth
• prematurity
• hypothermia or hypoglycemia from sepsis
• low Apgar score or use of resuscitation or invasive procedures

Cardiovascular
• pallor; mottling; cold, clammy skin with septic shock or delayed perfusion or refilling of nail beds
• hypotension
• tachycardia

Gastrointestinal
• feeding difficulty
• vomiting, diarrhea, or abdominal distention with sepsis or meningitis
• splenomegaly, hepatomegaly with toxoplasmosis, or hepatitis

Integumentary
• jaundice with meningitis, hepatitis, cytomegalovirus, toxoplasmosis, or sepsis neonatorum
• petechiae with cytomegalovirus
• pustules or lesions with herpes
• erythema with omphalitis (periumbilical)
• pustules, abscesses, or furuncles with streptococcal or staphylococcal septicemia
• maculopapular rash with toxoplasmosis

Neurologic
• low temperature (usually hypothermia, with sepsis)
• hypertonia or hypotonia with sepsis
• abnormal eye movements
• seizure activity

Pulmonary
• apnea, tachypnea, cyanosis with group B streptococcal disease causing sepsis, pneumonia, or meningitis

BEHAVIORAL FINDINGS
• lethargy
• irritability
• shrill cry

DIAGNOSTIC STUDIES
• chest X-ray—to show pulmonary changes or involvement
• skull X-ray and long bone and joint X-ray—to screen for TORCH or syphilis

Laboratory data

- complete blood count (CBC) — to identify white blood cell (WBC) count less than 5,000/mm^3 or greater than 25,000/mm^3; absolute neutrophils less than 5,000; ratio of immature to mature neutrophils greater than 0.13
- peripheral blood smear — to identify platelet count less than 80,000/mm^3, Döhle's inclusion bodies, and toxic granulation
- Gram stain of buffy coat of bacteria in association with blood culture positive for sepsis — to confirm sepsis
- gastric aspirate smear — to indicate intrauterine contamination by examining for WBC count and bacteria
- C-reactive protein levels — to indicate sepsis
- serum immunoglobulin studies — to identify increase of IgM

- enzyme-linked immunosorbent assay, Western blot, and CD4 levels — to identify presence of human immunodeficiency virus antibody and immune function (for more information, see Acquired Immunodeficiency Syndrome — Infant plan, page 134)
- serum glucose, calcium, and bilirubin studies — to detect abnormal increases or decreases
- blood culture from peripheral vein sample (two different sites) — to identify type of microorganism
- urine culture of specimen secured by suprapubic bladder aspiration — to identify type of microorganism
- cultures of fluid from ear, lesions, stool, drainage, suction aspirate, conjunctiva — to identify microorganism
- cerebrospinal fluid (CSF) studies (culture, protein, glucose, and cell count) — to identify abnormal levels or microorganisms

ETIOLOGY OF INFECTION

Infection	Causative Agent	Means of Transmission
VIRAL		
Acquired immunodeficiency syndrome	Human immunodeficiency virus	In utero via transplacental passage of virus, during labor and delivery through exposure to infected blood or vaginal secretions, and through breast milk
Cytomegalovirus	Cytomegalovirus	In utero, during birth, from contact with infected maternal cervical secretions, and in breast milk
Hepatitis	Hepatitis B virus	During birth or in breast milk
Herpes simplex	Herpes simplex virus type II	Genital tract during birth or in utero
Rubella	Rubella virus	In utero
PROTOZOAL		
Toxoplasmosis	*Toxoplasma gondii*	In utero
BACTERIAL		
Conjunctivitis	*Neisseria gonorrhoeae, Chlamydia trachomatis,* and *Staphylococcus* sp.	During birth (*N. gonorrhoeae* and *C. trachomatis*) or acquired postpartum (*Staphylococcus* sp.)
Diarrhea	*Escherichia coli, Salmonella* sp., *Shigella* sp., and *Staphylococcus* sp.	Acquired postpartum
Listeriosis	*Listeria monocytogenes*	In utero and during birth
Meningitis	Group B streptococci and *L. monocytogenes*	Acquired postpartum
Pneumonia	Group B streptococci, *E. coli, Pseudomonas aeruginosa,* and staphylococci resistant to penicillin	In utero (B streptococci and *E. coli*) or acquired postpartum (*P. aeruginosa* and penicillin-resistant staphylococci)
Septicemia	Group A or B streptococci (most often B), *E. coli,* and *P. aeruginosa*	In utero, during birth, or acquired postpartum
Syphilis	*Treponema pallidum*	In utero
Tuberculosis	*Mycobacterium tuberculosis*	In utero or acquired postpartum

Collaborative problem: *Infection related to transmission of infectious agent to infant before, during, or after birth (2 goals)*

GOAL 1: Recognize early the infant at risk for or with an infection.

Interventions

1. Assess infant for risk of infection; include the following:
• prematurity, small for gestational age, or large for gestational age
• low Apgar score
• surgery performed on infant
• epidemics of *Escherichia coli* or streptococcal infections in nursery
• invasive or resuscitative procedures.
Note: Review maternal history, assessing race, socioeconomic status, vaginal flora, PROM, illness, and infections.

2. Assess for early signs of infection, including:
• temperature instability (usually hypothermia)
• apnea
• jaundice
• poor feeding and sucking or abdominal distention
• lethargy or irritability.

3. Assess for system-related signs of infection, including:
• respiratory distress, apnea, tachypnea, cyanosis, shock (pallor, hypotension, and tachycardia) with group B streptococcal sepsis, pneumonia, or systemic infections from *Staphylococcus, E. coli, Klebsiella, Candida*, and others
• hypothermia, lethargy, hypertonia, hypotonia, jitteriness, bulging fontanels, abnormal eye movements, seizures with sepsis, or meningitis
• jaundice, petechiae, pustules, lesions, rash, or abscesses with TORCH
• difficulty feeding, vomiting, diarrhea, or weight loss with sepsis.

4. Review CBC with WBC and differential; platelet studies; immunoglobulin analysis; results of Gram stain of buffy coat; glucose, calcium, and bilirubin levels; and TORCH screen results.

5. Obtain samples, as needed, for cultures: blood, ear fluid, lesions, stool, drainage, eye, and gastric aspirate. Assist with obtaining urine specimen by suprapubic bladder aspiration and CSF by lumbar puncture. Send samples to laboratory for examination. Repeat as appropriate.

6. Review chest, skull, and long bone and joint X-rays.

7. Additional individualized interventions: _____

Rationales

1. The infant's immature defense system at birth, with a deficiency in phagocytic responses and in the immune system, decreases inflammatory response and increases susceptibility of infant to infection. The preterm infant is further compromised. Maternal involvement (both antepartum and intrapartum) always precedes infection.

2. Many early infection signs appear similar to those of other conditions. Unless early subtle signs are identified, infection might become difficult to manage. The infant may look well, but not do well.

3. Signs may or may not be related to a specific system but are manifested by the infection's effect on a system or organ. Similar signs may present themselves in infections involving different systems.

4. Infection and its cause may be determined by blood study results.

5. Cultures identify microorganisms and their sensitivity to antibiotics.

6. Results reveal changes caused by infection in these areas.

7. Rationales: _____

GOAL 2: Prevent and minimize infection and its effects.

Interventions

1. Provide a neutral thermal environment.

Rationales

1. This environment prevents temperature instability that further compromises infant.

Interventions

2. Provide for infant's fluid and nutritional needs by I.V. infusion, according to infant's weight, age, and condition.

3. Monitor vital signs continuously by transducer and other mechanical means.

4. Prepare and administer antibiotic and aminoglycoside therapy as follows:
• Calculate amount of drug needed per kilogram of body weight.
• Administer I.V. drugs at a proper rate regulated by infusion pump.
• Administer such antibiotics as penicillin G, ampicillin, or methicillin.
• Administer such aminoglycosides as gentamicin, kanamycin, or chloramphenicol.

5. Prepare and administer fresh frozen plasma I.V. as ordered.

6. Prepare and administer glucose, calcium, and electrolyte replacement therapy, as ordered.

7. Prepare for exchange transfusion with packed red blood cells, if indicated for sepsis.

8. Additional individualized interventions: _____

Rationales

2. This action supports fluid and electrolyte balance and nutritional status.

3. Monitoring vital signs ensures ongoing assessment data, indicating changes and facilitating early intervention.

4. Antibiotic and aminoglycoside therapy is given based on culture results that identify the infectious microorganism and its sensitivity. Antibiotics destroy bacteria by binding to cell wall, resulting in cell death, whereas aminoglycosides destroy bacteria by prohibiting protein synthesis, resulting in cell death.
   Antimicrobial therapy dosage depends on drug absorption, metabolism, and excretion, all of which vary according to infant's weight, gestational age, chronological age, and condition. Therapy is administered for up to 10 days (longer in meningitis) or until cultures are normal for 72 hours.

5. Fresh frozen plasma may be given for severe infection.

6. This action corrects abnormally low electrolyte levels associated with sepsis.

7. Transfusion may be needed for blood replacement in infant with sepsis.

8. Rationales: _____

Collaborative problem: *Nutritional deficiency related to poor feeding or feeding intolerance*

GOAL: Maintain nutritional needs of infant.

Interventions

1. Assess for feeding intolerance; include the following:
• weight loss
• vomiting or diarrhea
• abdominal distention or residual gastric contents before feeding with gavage
• poor sucking ability and poor swallowing reflex.

2. Initiate appropriate measures for nutritional needs as follows:

• Discontinue oral feedings and insert gastric tube, attaching it to suction or suction by hand.

• Provide dextrose 10% in water I.V., initially, and follow with total parenteral nutrition as appropriate. Or provide gavage feedings, if appropriate and needed.

• As condition improves, initiate oral feedings with breast milk if possible, although pumped breast milk, easily contaminated, may add to problem by overloading infant's gut with bacteria. If infant is too sick to breast-feed, use formula.

Rationales

1. Poor feeding and absorption as well as vomiting and diarrhea cause caloric loss and nutritional deficit.

2. Maintaining nutritional status enhances infant's ability to withstand infection.

• Gastric distention and mucus production occur with sepsis; decompression prevents aspiration.

• These measures provide nutritional needs during acute sepsis.

• Small quantities of formula or breast milk, with advancement as tolerated, provide essential nutrients; breast milk also provides IgA and IgC (immunoglobulins) and additional phagocytic cells needed to fight infection.

Interventions

• Continue increasing caloric intake until daily weight gain, as calculated, is achieved.

3. Additional individualized interventions: _____

_____

Rationales

• Increasing daily caloric intake ensures adequate nutrition.

3. Rationales: _____

_____

Collaborative problem: *Irregular respiratory effort related to apnea or periodic breathing*

GOAL: Maintain and support respiratory efforts and oxygenation.

Interventions

1. Assess respiratory changes; include tachypnea, nasal flaring, retractions, grunting, cyanosis, periodic breathing with apneic periods of more than 10 seconds, crackles.

2. Electronically monitor heart rate for tachycardia or bradycardia and blood pressure for changes. Monitor apnea with a thoracic impedance monitor as follows:
• Apply electrode jelly to electrodes and place on infant's chest.
• Plug in power and attach lead wires to electrodes.
• Adjust the system and set the alarms.
• Turn on monitor and readjust so that lights blink with each breath and heartbeat.
• If alarm sounds, check infant and confirm apnea by color and breathing.
• If infant is breathing and pink, readjust controls and electrodes. If infant is not breathing, wait 10 seconds and stimulate by a gentle shake, or a more vigorous one, slapping the soles.
• If apnea continues, begin resuscitation.

3. Provide warm, humidified oxygen therapy at minimal FIO_2 concentrations necessary to maintain energy expenditure and color.

4. Provide assistive or mechanical ventilation as appropriate.

5. Suction airway carefully, if appropriate.

6. Review arterial blood gas (ABG) studies as available or draw blood and monitor ABG levels as needed.

7. Organize infant care to prevent excessive handling.

8. Additional individualized interventions: _____

_____

Rationales

1. Early detection of irregularities ensures prompt treatment. These respiratory changes occur with pneumonia or other pulmonary infections.

2. Close monitoring permits observations of changes in condition as well as apneic periods that may cause brain damage. The thoracic impedance monitor detects changes caused by respiratory alterations and has an alarm to signal bradycardia.

3. Supplemental oxygen support may be needed with respiratory distress and decreased PO_2.

4. Respiratory support apparatus may be needed to sustain breathing.

5. Suctioning removes mucus from nasopharynx or endotracheal tubes.

6. ABG levels indicate acid-base balance and may suggest acidosis if PO_2 level is low, PCO_2 level is high, and pH value is low.

7. Handling increases the infant's energy expenditure and need for oxygen.

8. Rationales: _____

_____

Nursing diagnosis: *High risk for injury related to transmission of infection to infant by personnel*

GOAL: Prevent nosocomial infection.

Interventions

1. Institute universal precautions; follow institutional policy for excluding or removing from the nursery infants with diarrhea, draining infections, or viral infections.

2. Isolate infants (in an incubator) coming from outside the nursery until their blood, skin, and urine cultures are negative.

3. Exclude from the nursery or place in an isolation nursery infants whose mothers have an infection or a communicable disease.

4. Ensure that all personnel, relatives, and other caregivers are free of fever; respiratory or GI disorders; open, draining lesions or skin breaks; and any communicable disease before allowing them to enter nursery or care for infant.

5. Sterilize all equipment before use. Change all tubing, lines, and humidifiers or sterilize daily or according to hospital protocol.

6. Wash all cribs, incubators, and other apparatus with antiseptic solution once a week and after each use.

7. Clean and sterilize daily any equipment or sinks that become wet.

8. Use meticulous sterile technique in all procedures and in care of all catheters (umbilical, vein), I.V. lines, dressings, and in cord care.

9. Use handwashing techniques according to hospital protocol or as follows:
• Before entering nursery, wash hands to above the elbows for 2 minutes, using an antiseptic iodophor preparation or chlorhexidine (Hibiclens).
• Wash hands for 15 seconds before caring for another infant.
• Any physician, relative, or others who enter nursery briefly should wash hands and cover clothing with a clean gown.
• All nursing staff should wear short-sleeved gowns in the nursery.

10. Take samples for culture from equipment, supplies, and any possibly contaminated items in nursery.

11. Instruct visiting parents as follows:
• Touch only your own infant.
• Wash hands properly and dress in gown.
• Do not handle another infant's equipment or supplies or move things from one crib to another.

12. Additional individualized interventions: _____

Rationales

1. Using universal precautions minimizes the risk of infection transmission. Disease may be transmitted to and from healthy or sick infants if they are exposed to or cared for by same personnel.

2. This prevents cross-contamination with unknown microorganisms to other infants in nursery.

3. Infants may be delivered with a disease transmitted in utero or during delivery.

4. Contact with sick people creates a health hazard and encourages possible transmission of infections that might endanger all infants in the nursery.

5. Sterilization and frequent changes of equipment lines prevents spread of bacteria from objects to infants.

6. Washing maintains cleanliness and provides bacteriostatic action to reduce contaminants.

7. Dampness provides a good medium for microorganisms to thrive.

8. Any break in the first line of defense offers microorganisms the opportunity to enter and cause infection.

9. Hands are the principal mode of infection transmission and spread to infants.
• This is a general handwashing procedure. Individual hospital protocols may vary.

• Hands are considered contaminated after touching an infant or any materials in the nursery.
• All caregiving personnel are potential infection carriers. They should follow infection-preventing protocols.

• Wearing short sleeves allows for washing above the elbows.

10. Culturing identifies infection potential.

11. Attention to these details helps protect the infant in the nursery from infection through parents.

12. Rationales: _____

Nursing diagnosis: *Ineffective individual coping related to guilt and anxiety from transmitting infection to infant and possible serious consequences of the infection*

GOAL: Minimize parental guilt and support coping during crisis.

Interventions

1. Assess verbal and nonverbal expressions, feelings, and use of coping mechanisms.

2. Assist parents to verbalize concerns about sick infant, cause of infection, prolonged care, and possible poor prognosis.

3. Provide consistent and accurate information concerning infant's condition, progress, future care, and possible complications.

4. Encourage parents to visit and care for infant as appropriate.

5. Additional individualized interventions: _____

_____

Rationales

1. Assessment data enables caregiver to assist parents with identifying and developing effective coping strategies.

2. Verbalization helps to maintain a trusting, secure environment and acceptance of fears and concerns.

3. Information reduces parental anxiety caused by fear of the unknown and questions about whether infant is improving.

4. Visitation and touching promote bonding.

5. Rationales: _____

_____

ASSOCIATED PLANS
• Acquired Immunodeficiency Syndrome—Infant
• Acquired Immunodeficiency Syndrome—Maternal
• Anemia
• Birth Trauma
• Hyperbilirubinemia
• Hypocalcemia
• Hypoglycemia
• Hypothermia and Hyperthermia
• Intracranial Hemorrhage
• Necrotizing Enterocolitis
• Sexually Transmitted Diseases/TORCH
• Skin Disorders
• Vaginal and Urinary Infections

ADDITIONAL NURSING DIAGNOSES
• Altered growth and development related to illness and hospitalization
• High risk for altered parenting related to separation from infant as result of severe infection
• High risk for fluid volume deficit related to losses from vomiting and diarrhea
• Hyperthermia related to infectious process
• Hypothermia related to infectious process
• Ineffective airway clearance related to infection
• Knowledge deficit (parental) related to infection control

Skin Disorders

DEFINITION
Composed of three layers (dermis, epidermis, and sub-cutaneous tissue), the skin of a full-term infant is soft, wrinkled, and covered with vernix caseosa. A progressive color change occurs after birth, from ruddy to mottled tones that disappear with warming. In contrast, at birth, the preterm infant's skin is transparent, gelatinous, and smoother with less wrinkling than that of the full-term infant, and it is covered with noticeable lanugo. Because of its immaturity, the preterm infant's skin is more prone to vary in temperature and more vulnerable to infection and irritations.

Skin functions as the body's first line of defense against chemical, mechanical, and physical injuries. Usually, the full-term infant can maintain skin integrity, despite exposure to environmental factors. But the preterm infant has difficulty maintaining skin integrity, especially if adhesive materials, disinfectants, topical medications, phototherapy, or radiant warmers are used in the infant's care. Phototherapy and radiant warmers can threaten skin integrity by increasing insensible water loss. Use of topical substances can change the skin's pH, encouraging microorganism growth.

This plan focuses on care of the infant experiencing actual or potential skin disorders. Included is care to prevent skin impairment or breakdown during or because of therapeutic procedures.

ETIOLOGY AND PRECIPITATING FACTORS
• internal factors
  □ immature skin of preterm infant: fragile, transparent, and thin
  □ altered immunologic response (predisposing infant to infectious processes)
  □ impaired tissue perfusion
  □ poor skin turgor and general edema
  □ hypothermia or hyperthermia
  □ impaired nutrition and feedings
• external factors
  □ chemical: infiltrations of I.V. fluids, chemicals, or blood; topically applied medications, soaps, or lotions
  □ mechanical: adhesives (tapes and skin preparations), monitoring device electrodes, pressure from immobility or restraints, burns from electrodes that produce heat or from hot packs or an Isolette
  □ physical: immobility caused by medications; birth trauma; rough handling after birth; environmental irritants such as allergens; contact with irritants such as drainage, urine, or feces; breaks in skin integrity from surgical incisions, needle punctures, or gastric tubes

PHYSICAL FINDINGS
Maternal history
• difficult labor and delivery, forceps applied
• race and ethnicity
• family allergies
• infections

Infant status at birth
• prematurity, postmaturity, and gestational age—any of which affect texture, color, and condition of skin; lesions
• trauma during birth, forceps marks, edema, or lesions
• congenital anomalies requiring surgical intervention
• conditions requiring infusions or monitoring devices
• impaired thermoregulation

Integumentary
• ecchymoses anywhere on the body or petechiae on the head, face, or upper trunk caused by trauma, bleeding disorder, or infection
• erythema toxicum appearing 1 to 2 days after birth as a blotchy erythematous rash—small white papules surrounded by reddish areas
• subcutaneous fat necrosis appearing after birth as firm masses in the subcutaneous tissue, reddish purple and usually over bony prominences
• diaper dermatitis appearing as a red, excoriated area over buttocks, genitalia, and anal area, caused by urine, feces, or other irritants or allergy to diapers
• skin breaks or punctures from incisions, infusions, monitoring devices, or laboratory test procedures
• redness or irritation from pressure over bony prominences, from body excretions around stoma, or from adhesives
• edema or poor skin turgor; peeling, cracked, or dry skin
• thin and fragile skin in preterm infant; pale, thicker skin in postterm infant

DIAGNOSTIC STUDIES
Laboratory data
• culture of skin lesion—to identify infectious microorganisms
• bleeding and clotting times—to identify coagulation disorders (see Appendix 10: Normal Lab Values for the Newborn Infant).

Nursing diagnosis: *Impaired skin integrity related to disruption or breakdown of skin surface (2 goals)*

GOAL 1: Assess for skin abnormalities leading to skin impairment.

Interventions

1. Identify the infant at risk for skin breakdown, including:
• prematurity and gestational age
• poor feeding affecting hydration and nutrition
• trauma to skin during birth process
• use of monitoring devices, with electrodes and disks
• use of invasive devices, such as I.V. and total parenteral nutrition tubes, or monitors
• surgical procedures.

2. Assess infant's skin condition. Include:
• color and texture
• edema, turgor, and moisture
• temperature
• hematoma, petechiae, and bruising
• reddened areas, dermatitis and other rashes, abrasions, breaks, cracks, and irritations
• incisional sites or peristomal sites, such as gastrostomy, colostomy, or ileostomy.

3. Review the results of skin culture, if performed.

4. Additional individualized interventions: _____

Rationales

1. The infant's overall health status affects its ability to withstand factors that may alter skin integrity. The preterm infant is prone to skin impairment because of thin, fragile, and immature skin, which is more vulnerable to skin breakdown if trauma occurs from invasive procedures and devices.

2. An ongoing skin assessment provides information needed to carry out preventive measures to ensure skin integrity. Changes in skin integrity may be precipitated by humidity or temperature; trauma; contact with toxic substances, urine, feces, or drainage; fluid imbalances; bacterial colonization or invasive procedures.

3. Culture results identify infectious agents.

4. Rationales: _____

GOAL 2: Maintain skin integrity.

Interventions

1. Clean the infant's skin after birth, when body temperature has stabilized.

2. Provide safe skin care.

• Follow institutional policy regarding initial cleaning. Clean the infant's buttocks and perineum at each diaper change.
• Use warm water to bathe the infant during 1st week. Then give baths once or twice weekly, using a low-alkaline soap (Neutrogena, Aveeno, or Oilatum).

• Avoid perfumed lotions and creams.
• Use warm, sterile water if skin is irritated or excoriated.
• Apply emollient (Aquaphor) to cracks in skin.

• Provide oral care with moist, water-soaked gauze if oral intake is withheld.

Rationales

1. Vernix caseosa may have a protective function immediately after birth. Exposing or bathing preterm infant before body temperature is stable may lead to cold stress.

2. Safe skin care helps maintain skin integrity and promotes cleanliness and comfort.

• Substances other than water and mild-pH soap may irritate skin.

• Baths are limited initially to retain acid mantle (pH) of skin, which provides natural bactericidal action. Alkaline soaps change skin pH for about 1 hour and destroy acid mantle, predisposing infant to infection. Hexachlorophene (pHisoHex) may be used for initial bath to prevent bacterial colonization.
• Lotions and creams may be absorbed by skin.
• Sterile water prevents exposure to microorganisms.

• Emollients protect broken skin from bacterial exposure.

• Dry oral mucous membranes predispose mucosa to breakdown and injury from trauma.

Nursing diagnosis: *High risk for infection related to skin breakdown*

GOAL: Prevent or minimize risk for infection.

Interventions

1. Prevent skin damage as follows:

• Use tape and adhesive skin preparations minimally. To stop bleeding, apply pressure rather than an adhesive bandage, or use tape over a sterile dressing or gauze. When tape must be used, provide a buffer between the skin and the tape with a product like HolliHesive.

• Soften adhesives with water before removal.

• Use a transparent occlusive dressing, such as Op-Site, as a protective covering for pressure sites, burns, or excoriated and irritated areas.

• Use the lowest effective heat setting if transcutaneous electrodes must be used. For infants weighing less than 2.2. lb (1 kg), use needle electrodes; for infants weighing more than 2.2 lb, apply Syn-cor electrodes.

• Rotate position of electrode every 1 to 4 hours, depending on the infant's condition.

• Avoid using hot compresses for I.V. infiltration or to warm the infant's heels for blood testing.

• Assess I.V. sites hourly for infiltration and remove I.V. line if necessary.

• Reposition the infant every 2 hours, if appropriate. Perform range-of-motion exercises and gently massage pressure areas.

• Limit use of antiseptic solutions. If they must be applied, rinse the area with warm, water-soaked gauze after use.

• Use a water-type skin barrier when applying an ostomy pouch to skin exposed to irritating secretions or excretions.

• Change skin barrier every 4 days or only as necessary.

2. Provide a safe environment for the infant's skin.

• Place the preterm infant in a neutral thermal environment, such as an Isolette. Monitor temperature settings and exposure to cool-air current with Servo-Control probe.

• Observe the infant for signs of toxicity if topical medications are used.

Rationales

1. Delicate infant skin requires special care to prevent damage.

• Alternatives to using adhesive tape should be considered because tape removal may also remove the epidermal layer of skin, especially in preterm infants who have poor keratinization of skin. A porous adhesive skin barrier such as HolliHesive is used under the tape to secure I.V. armboards, umbilical artery catheters; endotracheal, gastrostomy, and chest tubes; nasal cannulas; and temperature probes.

• The infant's skin may be harmed by adhesive-remover substances. Rather than use them, adhesive tape can be softened in warm water, making removal safer and reducing the danger that skin will be removed with tape. Adhesives and electrodes should never be peeled off.

• Op-Site allows body moisture and air to permeate it. While the dressing covers damaged areas, it provides an environment for healing and protects against infectious agents.

• Low setting prevents thermal burns from heat-producing electrodes.

• Rotating the electrodes prevents thermal burn by limiting the time a particular area is exposed to heat.

• Hot compresses or other warming devices, especially at temperatures over 110° F (43.3° C), will burn the infant's fragile skin.

• I.V. infiltration may predispose infant's tissue to necrosis. I.V. calcium and anticonvulsants are particularly damaging to tissue.

• Sick infants may be unable to tolerate handling; however, those who can should be repositioned to prevent pressure on skin areas susceptible to breakdown. Range-of-motion exercises and gentle massages promote circulation.

• Antiseptic solutions may cause chemical burns, depending on the type and concentration of the agent and the skin's condition and maturity.

• Water-type barrier products, such as Stomahesive, HolliHesive, and Duoderm, protect the skin from damage caused by irritating enzymes; each can also be used on the skin where tape would be used.

• Minimizing changes will minimize skin damage.

2. Environmental factors may predispose the infant to skin damage.

• Having minimal subcutaneous fat and an immature skin thermoregulation mechanism places the preterm infant at risk for cold stress. A neutral thermal environment reduces that risk.

• Topical skin medications such as steroids, chlorophenols, and boric acid may be absorbed transdermally and cause adverse reactions in infants.

Interventions

• Monitor insensible water loss by measuring fluid intake and output and weight loss, especially loss produced by phototherapy or radiant warmers.

• Prevent infant contact with sharp objects, such as long fingernails and jewelry, when providing care.

3. Follow effective infection prevention procedures:

• Wash hands with antiseptic solution.

• Use aseptic technique to care for the umbilical cord, circumcision area, and other wound or skin break.

• Wear a clean gown when caring for the infant.

• Provide for infant's fluid and nutritional needs.

4. Additional individualized interventions: _____

_____

Rationales

• Preterm infants are especially prone to water loss because of their immature skin. Increased evaporation of the water from the skin occurs when the infant's body temperature rises; increased diffusion of water through the skin occurs with phototherapy and radiant warmers.

• Sharp objects, such as long fingernails and jewelry, can inadvertently damage infant skin and introduce infection.

3. The infant's skin is prone to bacterial colonization.

• Hands commonly carry microorganisms, which can be transferred to wound or skin break during care procedures.

• Handwashing and other aseptic techniques are essential for preventing infection.

• This prevents cross-contamination.

• Maintaining adequate hydration and nutrition helps the infant cope with the stress of infection. Hydration and nutritional deficiencies affect the skin and may indicate abnormal states.

4. Rationales: _____

_____

ASSOCIATED PLANS
• Birth Trauma
• Circumcision
• Hypothermia and Hyperthermia
• Inappropriate Size or Weight for Gestational Age, Large
• Inappropriate Size or Weight for Gestational Age, Small
• Postoperative Care

ADDITIONAL NURSING DIAGNOSES
• High risk for infection related to skin irritation, excoriation, and breakdown
• High risk for trauma related to skin's vulnerability
• Impaired tissue integrity related to immobility and poor peripheral perfusion
• Knowledge deficit (parental) related to peristomal care of skin or prevention of diaper dermatitis

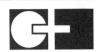

Spinal Cord Defects and Hydrocephalus

DEFINITION

Spinal cord defects include congenital neurologic abnormalities involving defective embryonic neural tube closure during the first trimester. The defects may be found in the cervical, thoracic, or sacral area but commonly occur in the lumbosacral area. Hydrocephalus, an excessive accumulation of cerebrospinal fluid (CSF) in the ventricles, often accompanies spinal cord defects, affecting about 90% of infants with myelomeningocele.

Spina bifida occulta, the incomplete closure of one or more vertebrae without protrusion of the cord or meninges, is the most common and least severe of the defects. Other forms of spina bifida, in which spinal contents protrude into an external sac through the incomplete closure, are considered more severe.

Meningocele is the protrusion of an external sac containing meninges and CSF with the spinal cord and nerve roots in their normal positions; myelocele is the protrusion of an external sac containing the spinal cord. Myelomeningocele is the protrusion of an external sac containing meninges, CSF, and a portion of the spinal cord or nerve roots; it is the most severe of the spinal cord defects and the one with the most serious long-term neurologic consequences.

Surgery may be performed early to close the protruding sac in meningocele, but repair of the sac in myelomeningocele may not reverse the neurologic deficit. Hydrocephalus may be surgically treated with a shunt to relieve pressure caused by fluid accumulation. The method of treatment depends on the type and extent of the defect, the infant's condition, associated defects, the family's desires, and the availability of and potential for rehabilitation. A multidisciplinary approach to the care of these infants is carried out by a team composed of nurses, a neurologist, a neurosurgeon, a pediatrician, an orthopedist, a urologist, and a physical therapist. The prognosis depends on the number and severity of abnormalities; those infants who are totally paralyzed below the defect have the poorest prognosis.

This plan focuses on care of the infant with a spinal cord defect, hydrocephalus, and other abnormalities and the prevention of associated complications before surgery.

ETIOLOGY AND PRECIPITATING FACTORS
Spinal cord defects
• genetic predisposition
• possibility of viruses, radiation, or other environmental factors

Hydrocephalus
• excessive production, inadequate reabsorption, or obstruction of circulating CSF through ventricles, preventing reabsorption

PHYSICAL FINDINGS
Maternal history
• other children with similar defect
• amniocentesis with increase in alpha-fetoprotein (AFP) levels in open neural tube defects; in closed defects (about 10% of cases), results are negative
• ethnic background of both parents (higher incidence in families of Irish descent)

Infant status at birth
• depression or dimple over defect area
• tuft of hair and soft fatty deposits over defect area
• port wine nevus over defect area
• sac protruding from spine
• other defects, such as hydrocephalus, talipes, hip dislocation, curvature of spine, and Arnold-Chiari syndrome (a form of hydrocephalus)

Gastrointestinal
• poor feeding if lethargic
• projectile vomiting with increasing intracranial pressure

Integumentary
• thin, shiny, fragile scalp skin; bulging fontanels; prominent scalp veins; possible enlarged head in hydrocephalus
• palpated depression over spinal defect area

Neurologic
• vary with level of defect
• flaccid or spastic paralysis of legs and trunk, fixed downward gaze in hydrocephalus, and setting-sun sign
• fever and nuchal rigidity with meningitis

BEHAVIORAL FINDINGS
• irritability
• lethargy

DIAGNOSTIC STUDIES
• analysis of AFP levels via amniocentesis—to reveal increase, possibly indicating neural tube defect
• maternal serum AFP levels—to detect increase, possibly indicating neural tube defect
• X-rays of spine, skull, hips, arms, and legs—to reveal bone defects, with separating fontanels in hydrocephalus
• cranial ultrasonography—to differentiate hydrocephalus from other conditions associated with increasing head size
• computed tomography scan—to reveal ventricular distention and intracranial lesions

• magnetic resonance imaging—to differentiate hydrocephalus from other conditions associated with increasing head size
• ventriculography in hydrocephalus with possible culture of CSF—to detect suspected infection

• transillumination—to reveal meningocele, but not myelomeningocele (may be performed during surgery), and to differentiate hydrocephalus from other conditions associated with increasing head size

---

Nursing diagnosis: *High risk for infection related to breakdown or rupture of protruding sac*

GOAL: Identify and minimize the risk of infection.

Interventions

1. Assess the infant for signs and symptoms of infection, including:
• restlessness and irritability
• excessive crying
• temperature increase
• changes in white blood cell count, differential, and platelet count
• increased sensitivity to light and noise
• breaks or abrasion of sac and leakage from sac.

2. Prevent exposure of sac to contaminants by:
• cleaning the area gently with warm, sterile normal saline solution
• covering the defect with sterile dressings moistened with sterile saline solution and changing the dressings every 2 hours
• covering the dressings with plastic wrap and placing a "myelo" apron between anus and defect
• positioning the infant in prone position to avoid contact with urine or feces. Do not position the infant on its back until repair heals.

3. Be prepared to administer prophylactic antibiotics if ordered, such as penicillin G, ampicillin, or methicillin, or aminoglycosides, such as kanamycin or gentamicin.

4. Additional individualized interventions: _____

Rationales

1. Early identification of infection allows for early treatment. These signs indicate possible infection. Sac rupture increases the infant's risk of contracting meningitis.

2. These actions maintain cleanliness and prevent the defect from coming into contact with microorganisms, urine, or feces.

3. Anti-infectives are administered to prevent central nervous system infection; their action is bactericidal because they inhibit protein biosynthesis of the bacterial cell wall.

4. Rationales: _____

Nursing diagnosis: *Impaired skin integrity related to irritation or abrasions*

GOAL: Minimize trauma to sac and skin and prevent skin breakdown.

Interventions

1. Assess the skin for irritation, redness, or breaks.

2. Keep the skin clean and dry. Wash sensitive and pressure areas gently, using warm water.

3. Place sheepskin and foam pad under the infant.

4. Apply lotion to knees, elbows, and other pressure areas, massaging gently.

Rationales

1. Assessment helps prevent continued deterioration by promoting immediate preventive treatment.

2. This prevents mechanical injury and promotes cleanliness.

3. Sheepskin and foam pad decrease pressure on skin.

4. Lotion protects these areas from rubbing against linens, and the massaging action promotes circulation.

Interventions

5. Handle the infant carefully without putting pressure on the defect or on the thin and fragile skin of the head.

6. Place the infant in a prone position supported by small pillows and sandbags or in a side-lying position, if allowed. Change position every 2 hours or as needed. Place a roll between the legs at hip level.

7. Support the enlarged head when moving or feeding the hydrocephalic infant.

8. Position the infant with a spinal cord defect on the abdomen when holding the infant on lap.

9. Dress the infant scantily, omitting diaper and shirt if placed over defect, and place the infant in an Isolette for a neutral thermal environment.

10. Additional individualized interventions: _____

_____

Rationales

5. Careful handling prevents the possibility of rupturing the sac or injuring the skin on the head.

6. This position prevents pressure on the sac or head. Raising the foot of the bed decreases pressure on the sac. Placing a roll at hip level maintains abduction of the legs.

7. Supporting the head prevents straining the infant's neck.

8. This position prevents pressure on the sac.

9. Dressing the infant lightly reduces pressure on the defect, and the Isolette maintains the infant's warmth without clothing that may irritate the sac.

10. Rationales: _____

_____

Collaborative problem: High risk for neurologic, musculoskeletal, or elimination impairment related to complications of spinal cord defect or hydrocephalus (2 goals)

GOAL 1: Recognize risk for complications.

Interventions

1. Assess the infant for signs and symptoms of neurologic complications:
- increasing head circumference measurements; bulging, full, or tense fontanels; lethargy and feeding difficulty; projectile or other vomiting
- irritability or nuchal rigidity
- variations in vital signs and temperature (taken every 2 hours)

- pupillary changes (assessed every 2 hours), including inequality and sluggish response to light.

2. Assess for musculoskeletal complications, such as:

- reduced movement of arms and legs, reduced response to stimulation, and muscle weakness
- talipes or hip displacement abnormalities.

3. Assess for urinary and bowel elimination complications, such as:
- continuous passage of stool, urinary retention

- urinary tract infection (by culture).

4. Additional individualized interventions: _____

_____

Rationales

1. Assessment data identify the infant at risk.

- These are signs of hydrocephalus; however, because of the latest developments in ultrasonography, few infants are born with gross hydrocephalus.
- These are indications of meningeal irritation.
- Increased temperature indicates infection. Blood pressure with widening pulse pressure changes indicates increased intracranial pressure. Bradycardia, with wild swings from tachycardia to bradycardia, indicates bradypnea.
- Pupillary changes indicate neurologic involvement and possibly increased intracranial pressure.

2. Assessment data identify the infant at risk for paralysis and congenital deformity.
- These signs indicate potential paralysis with motor or sensory involvement.
- These are common congenital defects associated with spina bifida.

3. These complications are associated with spinal cord defects.
- These signs indicate lack of control, not diarrhea, and lack of innervation to bladder and bowel.
- Culture identifies urinary tract infection.

4. Rationales: _____

_____

GOAL 2: Minimize the effects of complications caused by the spinal cord defect.

Interventions

1. Perform passive range-of-motion exercises every 4 hours or as needed and muscle-stretching exercises.

2. Perform the exercises carefully while supporting the arms and legs properly.

3. Position the hips in slight to moderate abduction.

4. Perform the procedures for hip dislocation or talipes if present.

5. Help the infant empty its bladder every 2 hours by applying slight pressure to the suprapubic area (Credé's maneuver) from the umbilicus to the symphysis pubis.

6. After bowel elimination, gently clean and apply petrolatum to the infant's perianal area.

7. Devise a comfortable position for feeding, facing the infant when possible.

8. Caress, fondle, and speak to the infant.

9. Additional individualized interventions: _____

_____

Rationales

1. These exercises prevent contractures and muscle weakness.

2. Support prevents injury to fragile bones.

3. This position prevents hip dislocation.

4. Immediate serial casting, splinting, or another intervention may be needed (see Talipes Deformity plan, page 293, and Hip Dysplasia plan, page 201).

5. Assistance prevents urinary retention by releasing residual urine retained in the neurogenic bladder; this technique may also liberate stool.

6. These actions prevent excoriation of the perianal area and skin breakdown.

7. Facing the infant while feeding provides adequate intake and stimulation by eye contact.

8. Stroking and talking to the infant provide stimulation by touch and sound.

9. Rationales: _____

_____

Nursing diagnosis: *Anxiety (parental) related to defect in infant and potential defects in future children*

GOAL: Minimize parental anxiety.

Interventions

1. Offer referral to genetic counselor.

2. Review family history. Answer questions honestly and accurately or refer parents to physician for information.

3. Help parents adjust to shock related to their infant's defect, and aid them in grieving over having an infant with an anomaly.

4. Refer parents and family to local associations and support groups.

5. Additional individualized interventions: _____

_____

Rationales

1. Information may reduce parents' fear of unknown. Tests can be performed to detect neural tube defects early in pregnancy and options presented.

2. Open discussion increases parental knowledge about condition and reduces potential for recurrence.

3. Adjustment to physical and emotional aspects of the infant's condition promotes parent-infant interaction.

4. Such referrals allow family members to share their feelings with others in similar situations, which helps them work through anxieties and fears.

5. Rationales: _____

_____

Nursing diagnosis: *Ineffective family coping related to guilt, emotional conflict, and fear about the infant's immediate and long-term care*

GOAL: Promote the environment necessary for the parents to start adapting to the crisis and to begin the grieving process.

Interventions

1. Encourage and allow parents to express feelings and fears about infant care, about what others might say, and about loss of the "perfect child."

2. Allow the parents to see and hold the infant as soon after birth as possible, after the obstetrician has informed them of the defect.

3. Reinforce the normal and healthy aspects of the infant when interacting with the parents.

4. Handle the infant in a caring manner, and instruct the parents how to hold and cuddle the infant, being careful to avoid placing pressure on sac and supporting the infant on the side or abdomen.

5. Allow the parents to visit the infant when desired, and encourage them to participate in infant's care.

6. Encourage the parents to participate in support groups, such as the Spina Bifida Association of America.

7. Additional individualized interventions: _____

Rationales

1. The birth of a child with a congenital defect precipitates a major family crisis, and the parents and family must mourn the loss of the "perfect child" that they had expected.

2. Delay in seeing the infant may heighten parental anxiety and sadness, causing unrealistic expectations. Important bonding takes place as soon after birth as possible and with continued close contact between the infant and its parents.

3. This reinforcement helps reduce the parents' chronic sorrow and anger.

4. These actions promote bonding and the infant's normal social and emotional development.

5. Open visitation promotes a flexible, secure environment for the development of a parent-infant relationship.

6. Group involvement offers the parents a support system and a positive view of the treatment outcome.

7. Rationales: _____

Nursing diagnosis: *Knowledge deficit (parental) related to long-term care of child*

GOAL: Promote parental understanding of the infant's defect and care.

Interventions

1. Assess parental and family understanding of spina bifida, hydrocephalus, or other deformity if present.

2. Provide information regarding:

• infant's condition

• defect's etiology, occurrence, and type

• infant's immediate needs and care

• surgery to insert a shunt, if infant is hydrocephalic, or to correct myelomeningocele, if infant has spina bifida

• infant's potential and long-term problems with myelomeningocele, such as paralysis with motor and sensory deficits, renal disorders, bowel and bladder training, mental retardation, and pulmonary infections (if relevant).

Rationales

1. Assessment reveals the need and readiness for information, the kind of information needed, and previous misinformation.

2. Information maximizes parental understanding of the defect and the potential care.

• This information allays parental anxiety about the seriousness of the infant's condition.

• This action assists in resolving the parents' guilt feelings about the infant's abnormality.

• This clarifies the reasons for the infant's treatment regimen while in the hospital.

• All decisions regarding medical and surgical interventions are made with family input after discussing the treatment's potential success.

• Care of the infant with long-term care needs is aimed at improving the quality of life for the infant and family, with careful attention to resource use.

Interventions

3. Teach parents about ordered procedures and treatments, such as range-of-motion exercises, shunt care, skin care, positioning, handling, and feeding.

4. Allow the parents to ask as many questions as they like; answer them honestly and patiently. Encourage family participation in care.

5. Arrange for home health care follow-up.

6. Additional individualized interventions: _____

Rationales

3. Proper instruction aids compliance and helps dispel parents' fears.

4. Questions may indicate that adaptation is taking place and that the parents' interest in caring for the infant is increasing. Participation helps to alleviate feelings of inadequacy and prepares for home care.

5. Home health care follow-up offers parents continued support outside the hospital.

6. Rationales: _____

Nursing diagnosis: *High risk for altered parenting related to lack of attachment and bonding opportunities because of intensive care and surgery performed in another hospital*

GOAL: Promote parent-child interactions and bonding.

Interventions

1. Encourage the parents to visit, provide care, and touch the infant.

2. Provide time for the parents to be alone with the infant.

3. Provide support when the parents hold the infant.

4. Accept parental reactions without showing anger or shock or withdrawing from the situation.

5. Explain the need to transfer the infant to a different facility for special procedures if this is indicated. Allow the father to accompany the infant if the mother is still hospitalized (see Appendix 11: Transporting an Infant to Another Hospital).

6. Give anticipatory guidance in caring for the infant. Explain that the family may feel chronic sorrow if the infant has severe anomalies.

7. Additional individualized interventions: _____

Rationales

1. Visitation and infant contact promote bonding.

2. Time spent with the infant enhances bonding.

3. The parents may be afraid of injuring the infant.

4. Parents need time to overcome probable shock.

5. Understanding the need for the transfer and having the opportunity to accompany the infant prevent parental feelings of abandoning the infant and not knowing where and when they can be with their infant.

6. This adds to parental understanding that sorrow is a normal feeling that may persist.

7. Rationales: _____

ASSOCIATED PLANS
• Hip Dysplasia
• Skin Disorders
• Talipes Deformity

ADDITIONAL NURSING DIAGNOSES
• Altered growth and development related to neurologic impairment
• Dysfunctional grieving (parental) related to loss of perfect child

• High risk for injury related to protruding sac
• Impaired home maintenance management (parental) related to care of infant with defect and cost of long-term habilitation
• Impaired tissue integrity related to spinal cord defect
• Knowledge deficit (parental) related to prevention and care of complications associated with defect
• Total incontinence related to bladder and bowel involvement from spinal cord defect

Talipes Deformity

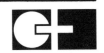

DEFINITION

Talipes deformity, also known as clubfoot, is a congenital deformity of the muscles and bones of one or both feet. Common types of talipes include:
- talipes varus, in which the foot is bent inward (inversion)
- talipes valgus, in which the foot is bent outward (eversion)
- talipes calcaneus, in which the toes are higher than the heel (dorsiflexion)
- talipes equinus, in which the toes are lower than the heel (plantar flexion).

Combinations of these malformations also may ocur; the most common is talipes equinovarus, in which the foot is abducted, turned inward and downward, with a shortened Achilles tendon. Some deformities can be manipulated into a correct position; true clubfoot cannot.

Treatment begins shortly after birth. It varies from serial casting to splinting to corrective shoes, depending on the severity and type of the deformity. Surgical correction may be needed at a later date. The prognosis is based on early detection and initiation and consistent application of corrective measures.

Found in 1 in 1,000 live births, this abnormality commonly occurs with other congenital defects. It is thought to result from familial tendencies; it is twice as common in boys as in girls. When unilateral, talipes usually occurs on the right side.

This plan focuses on the care of the infant at the beginning of the first stage of treatment, immediately after birth.

ETIOLOGY AND PRECIPITATING FACTORS
- cause unknown
- may be genetic because familial tendency exists
- may result from position of fetus in utero or from lack of movement or activity in utero
- may result from arrested development during early fetal stage

PHYSICAL FINDINGS
Family history
- other members of family with clubfoot

Infant status at birth
- exaggerated attitudes or positioning of feet
- other congenital abnormalities, especially spinal cord defects
- obvious deformity of feet with or without a decrease in the degree of manipulation allowed

DIAGNOSTIC STUDIES
- X-rays—to reveal abnormality of talus and calcaneus and ladderlike appearance of metatarsals

---

Collaborative problem: *Physiologic injury related to failure to provide appropriate care, leading to complications (2 goals)*

GOAL 1: Recognize the abnormality of the feet and the rationale for treatment.

Interventions

1. Assess the infant's feet as follows:
- Check position, turning, and flexion of foot and toes.
- Note how easily each foot moves.

2. Be aware of proposed medical treatment, such as:

- changing of serial plaster casting until defect is corrected, starting with adduction deformity (most common therapy)

- Denis Browne splint in infants less than 1 year old

- shoes fixed to metal crossbar.

3. Prepare and assist in the application of a cast or splint, holding the feet in the correct position.

Rationales

1. Early recognition and treatment produce the best results because cartilage and muscles are supple and the feet are more malleable at birth.

2. Medical treatment varies with deformity's type and severity.

- Plaster casting, used in first-stage correction, accommodates the infant's rapid growth; second-stage correction focuses on inversion, and the third-stage focuses on plantar flexion.

- The infant's feet are fastened to two padded metal plates with tape and then connected to a metal crossbar that can be adjusted to permit rotation, eversion, and dorsiflexion of feet.

- This device fixes shoes to allow adjustment of feet to a desired position.

3. Correctly positioned feet during cast application are essential for good results.

Interventions	Rationales
4. Additional individualized interventions: _____	4. Rationales: _____

GOAL 2: Prevent circulatory impairment.

Interventions	Rationales
1. Assess for signs of circulatory impairment in the legs, including: • tightness of cast or splint • coolness, duskiness, and motion of toes every 1 to 2 hours if casts are applied • edema of toes • capillary refill of toes.	1. Assessment provides for interventions to prevent complications. • Pressure impairs circulation to tissues. • The space between the cast and skin should be wide enough so that a finger can be inserted. • Edema is a sign of decreased circulation. • Decreased capillary refill time indicates impaired circulation.
2. Elevate casted feet on pillows.	2. Elevation assists with venous return and reduces edema.
3. Additional individualized interventions: _____	3. Rationales: _____

Nursing diagnosis: *High risk for impaired skin integrity related to casting or splinting*

GOAL: Maintain skin integrity.

Interventions	Rationales
1. Assess the infant's skin for: • cleanliness and dryness under or around cast or splint • redness, excoriation, abrasions, pallor, paresthesias, pulselessness, and pinprick sensitivity • cast-related irritation from rough edges touching skin.	1. Assessment data suggest measures to prevent skin irritation and breakdown.
2. Protect skin with foam rubber padding and petal the cast edges.	2. Foam rubber padding and petaling prevent rough edges from irritating skin.
3. Turn infant every 2 hours during the day and every 4 hours at night.	3. Change of position relieves pressure on the area.
4. Wash and dry skin thoroughly under the splint and around the cast.	4. These actions maintain cleanliness and dryness. Oils and powders are not advised.
5. Additional individualized interventions: _____	5. Rationales: _____

Nursing diagnosis: *Ineffective family coping: compromised related to situational crisis of infant with congenital deformity and probability of long-term therapy*

GOAL: Promote parental understanding of the infant's defect and parental coping skills.

Interventions	Rationales
1. Encourage and allow parents to express fears about caring for the infant, need for long-term care and rehabilitation, and possible future surgical correction.	1. Parents may feel disappointment because of the abnormality and future effect on the child's appearance and function.

Interventions

2. Inform family about the abnormality and allow them to see and hold the infant as soon as possible after birth. Encourage them to hold and cuddle the infant regardless of the cast.

3. Assist the parents to identify necessary coping skills and available support systems.

4. Assess the family's understanding of the talipes deformity.

5. Assure the family that the abnormality can be corrected with appropriate treatment.

6. Provide information regarding:

• infant's condition

• etiology, prevalence, and nature of the abnormality

• infant's long-term needs, such as serial casting with the foot held in position for several days or weeks, followed by maintaining alignment of feet with night splints as well as exercise and orthopedic shoes

• possible surgery to correct deformity in the infant

• importance of immediate and ongoing therapy and orthopedic supervision until child's growth is completed.

7. Additional individualized interventions: _____

_____

Rationales

2. Parental involvement with the child promotes bonding and a normal parent-child relationship.

3. This enables parents to determine the need for assistance in adapting to the new situation.

4. Assessment reveals parental need for information, kind of information needed, and past misinformation.

5. This should reassure the family and help them cope with the crisis.

6. Increased knowledge enhances the parents' understanding of the defect.
• Information about the infant's condition allays potential anxiety.
• Information helps the parents resolve guilt feelings about the abnormality.
• Information prepares the family for long-term correctional care (usually for 3 months but longer in certain cases). The cast may be completely changed or wedged (Kite method) to change its shape when needed. The Denis Browne splint may be used to promote correction and strengthen the foot muscles.
• Resistant clubfoot, which usually is the result of recurrent neglected deformities, may need surgical correction.
• Long-term therapy is needed to ensure correction of the abnormality, and time and patience are needed for permanent correction.

7. Rationales: _____

_____

Nursing diagnosis: *Knowledge deficit (parental) related to care of infant with cast or splint device*

GOAL: Provide appropriate information regarding infant care.

Interventions

1. Identify parents' knowledge and their interest, readiness, and ability to learn.

2. Inform the parents that the treatment may be long and requires patience.

3. Encourage the parents to fondle, hold, and cuddle the infant, regardless of the cast.

4. Provide splint device or cast care instructions. Cast care instructions include the following:
• Elevate infant's feet on pillows after casts are reapplied.
• Check infant's toes for warmth, color, movement, sensation, and edema every 1 to 2 hours after each new cast application.

Rationales

1. Assessment provides base for a teaching plan commensurate with parents' needs and abilities.

2. Restrictive movement may make the infant irritable at first, but the infant eventually will adjust.

3. This facilitates developmental progress and stimulation.

4. Teaching ensures safe infant care and prevents skin or circulatory complications.
• Elevating the feet promotes venous return and prevents edema.
• These are indications of circulatory impairment that should be reported to the physician.

Interventions

• Protect skin by petaling cast edges or padding them with adhesive tape or foam rubber; check for irritation every 2 to 4 hours.

• Protect the cast from urine or other wetness while bathing, covering the cast with a plastic bag and securing the bag with rubber bands.

5. Inform parents of the importance of keeping appointments with orthopedist for cast changes or evaluations.

6. Allow time for questions, clarifications, and demonstrations of cast care techniques, as needed.

7. Refer parents to community agencies and home health care.

8. Additional individualized interventions: _____

Rationales

• These measures prevent skin irritation or breakdown from the cast's rough edges.

• Wetness softens cast, impairing its corrective effect.

5. Ongoing therapy is necessary for successful correction.

6. Discussions and demonstrations reinforce parents' learning and reduce their anxiety.

7. These referrals provide continued support and enhance compliance with follow-up care.

8. Rationales: _____

ASSOCIATED PLANS
• Hip Dysplasia
• Preoperative Care
• Skin Disorders
• Spinal Cord Defects and Hydrocephalus

ADDITIONAL NURSING DIAGNOSES
• Altered growth and development related to effects of long-term therapy, stimulation deficiencies
• High risk for altered parenting related to lack of knowledge, lack of support from significant other, or unrealistic expectations for infant
• High risk for peripheral neurovascular dysfunction related to ill-fitting cast or splint device
• Impaired physical mobility related to casting and splinting

Tracheoesophageal Fistula or Esophageal Atresia

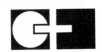

DEFINITION

Tracheoesophageal fistula (TEF) is an abnormal congenital opening between the trachea and the esophagus with or without an associated esophageal interruption. The most common of the abnormalities is atresia of a segment of the esophagus involving an upper blind pouch and the lower portion connected to the stomach. A fistula connects the trachea to the lower portion of the esophagus.

An esophageal atresia without tracheal involvement or a fistula that connects an otherwise normal trachea and esophagus (H-type fistula) may also occur. At birth, this defect may be associated with congenital heart disease, GI disorders, skeletal defects, or neurologic disorders.

All these defects are repaired surgically by transthoracic extrapleural fistula ligation and end-to-end esophageal anastomosis, depending on the length of the proximal and distal ends of the esophagus and if tolerance for the surgery is confirmed. If not, GI decompression is advocated by a gastrostomy tube inserted under local anesthesia. Feeding by total parenteral nutrition (TPN) may be indicated until surgery is performed. The survival rate is about 97% for full-term infants and about 50% for preterm infants; pneumonia, septicemia, and other anomalies are the usual cause of death.

This plan focuses on care of the infant before surgery and preventing complications while maintaining pulmonary and nutritional status.

ETIOLOGY AND PRECIPITATING FACTORS
• defective separation of trachea and esophagus and incomplete fusing of trachea after this separation during the 4th and 5th weeks of gestation.

PHYSICAL FINDINGS
Maternal history
• polyhydramnios

Infant status at birth
• prematurity and small size for gestational age
• low Apgar score and cyanosis
• inability to pass catheter into stomach
• congenital anomalies

Gastrointestinal
• pooling of secretions with excessive drooling from mouth
• difficulty feeding with regurgitation of feedings
• excessive gastric air and gastric distention caused by air from lungs traveling to stomach via fistula

Pulmonary
• respiratory distress and tachypnea if secretions are aspirated
• coughing, choking, sneezing, or cyanosis during feeding

DIAGNOSTIC STUDIES
• chest X-ray —to reveal pneumonia, atelectasis in upper lobe of right lung, blind pouch filled with air, and excessive gastric air; after attempt to pass radiopaque catheter from nares through esophagus into stomach, X-ray may show tube ending or coiling in upper esophageal pouch
• contrast studies with bronchoscopy or barium X-ray— to detect TEF (performed with caution because aspiration of contrast medium can cause chemical pneumonia)

Laboratory data
• white blood cell count and differential for neutrophils and platelets—to determine pneumonitis
• serum glucose level—to ensure adequate glucose level
• arterial blood gas values—to determine pH, oxygen, and carbon dioxide levels with respiratory distress
• cultures—to identify infectious organisms

Collaborative problem: *High risk for respiratory distress related to excessive secretions in mouth and blind pouch or aspiration of secretions and feedings (3 goals)*

GOAL 1: Identify airway obstruction and potential for aspiration.

Interventions

1. Assess for respiratory distress, including:
• respiratory rate and ease, use of accessory muscles, nasal flaring, retractions, and grunting
• cyanosis, mottling, or pallor
• choking and coughing
• regurgitation of feedings through mouth and nose
• amount of secretions.

Rationales

1. Assessment determines presence of the anomaly. The signs noted indicate respiratory problems and possible aspiration (swallowed secretions or feedings entering the esophageal pouch and then being aspirated into the trachea). The normal respiratory rate for a neonate infant is 40 to 60 breaths/minute.

Interventions

2. Additional individualized interventions: _____

Rationales

2. Rationales: _____

GOAL 2: Maintain patent airway and support lung expansion.

Interventions

1. Have suctioning and intubation equipment, oxygen, and resuscitation bag on hand at all times.

2. Perform oral, nasal, and endotracheal suctioning every 1 to 2 hours or more frequently if needed.

3. Withhold oral food and fluids.

4. Insert #10 Replogle tube into the blind pouch, then attach it to low intermittent suction according to physician's order, and monitor output.

5. Position infant on abdomen or side, as tolerated, with head elevated 20 to 40 degrees. Reposition infant every 2 hours if feasible. Position infant with head down if defect involves blind pouch at each end only or fistula from trachea to upper esophageal segment.

6. If gastrostomy tube is inserted for decompression, attach it to straight drainage to check patency.

7. Institute comfort measures to prevent crying.

8. Additional individualized interventions: _____

Rationales

1. Emergency apparatus should be on hand in case aspiration causes respiratory difficulty.

2. Suctioning clears secretions from oropharynx area and maintains patent airway.

3. This prevents aspiration of feedings.

4. The tube provides continuous removal of secretions from the pouch if the infant has esophageal atresia.

5. Abdominal or side position prevents aspiration of mucus or stomach contents and reduces gastric reflux. It also allows for better lung expansion and breathing pattern. Head-down positioning for infants with these forms of the defect reduces risk of aspiration.

6. Gastrostomy is performed to decompress the stomach and prevent gastric reflux through fistula into trachea and lungs.

7. Crying increases the amount of air swallowed through the fistula, worsens gastric distention, and increases the risk of gastric reflux.

8. Rationales: _____

GOAL 3: Prevent complications of chemical pneumonitis and atelectasis caused by aspiration.

Interventions

1. Assess for respiratory complications. Include:
• increased respiratory rate and effort
• increased heart rate
• severe retractions and nasal flaring
• cyanosis
• diminished breath sounds
• arterial or capillary blood gas values showing low oxygen level
• serial X-ray findings
• culture results indicating infection.

2. Continue ventilatory assistance if present.

3. Prepare and administer antibiotic by route ordered.

4. Use sterile technique for all care, treatments, and procedures, including sterile solutions for irrigations, dressings, and suctioning equipment.

5. Additional individualized interventions: _____

Rationales

1. These are signs of respiratory distress and complications involving the lungs. Early assessment promotes prompt treatment.

2. Assistance ensures respiratory stability.

3. This is preventive therapy for possible aspiration pneumonitis.

4. Sterile technique is a preventive measure to reduce the possibility of introducing pathologic organisms.

5. Rationales: _____

Collaborative problem: *Altered nutrition: less than body requirements related to inability to take oral feedings and withholding of food and fluids*

GOAL: Establish and maintain adequate nutrition.

Interventions	Rationales
1. Calculate caloric requirements according to infant's weight and age.	1. This ensures optimal caloric intake for weight gain.
2. Weigh infant daily or as needed and report loss greater than 50 g/24 hours (depending on infant's birth weight).	2. This is a good gauge of whether nutritional needs are being met.
3. Test for glucose levels by heelstick, such as Chemstrip, every 1 to 2 hours or as needed.	3. Glucose stores are limited and quickly used up in the infant, causing potential for hypoglycemia.
4. Administer and monitor peripheral parenternal nutrition with infusion-control device. Amount depends on infant's size and condition.	4. Peripheral parenteral nutrition is a short-term treatment providing up to 2,500 kcal/day used to maintain infant's glucose and fluid needs when food and water are withheld. Solutions of glucose less than 12% are given peripherally. Using an infusion-control device minimizes the risk of infusing too much solution too quickly.
5. Administer and monitor TPN if indicated (see *Comparing types of parenteral nutrition,* page 301). Follow these guildlines:	5. TPN may be administered to meet the infant's nutritional needs for a prolonged period; it can provide up to 4,000 kcal/day if necessary if infant does not meet criteria for surgery. TPN satisfies the infant's caloric, protein, carbohydrate, intralipid, mineral, and vitamin requirements. The total volume of the infusion solution varies; calculations are done daily, based on infant's weight, use of radiant warmer and phototherapy, and other factors. Fungal or bacterial infection or sepsis is a complication of TPN because the high glucose content of the solution provides a good medium for bacterial growth.
• Carry out all aspects of procedure with strict aseptic technique. Also, ensure that fluids are prepared in pharmacy under strict sterile conditions, using a laminar flow hood.	• Sterile technique prevents the entry of microorganisms or contamination of highly concentrated solutions, which provide an excellent medium for bacterial growth.
• Position and restrain infant.	• This prevents displacement of catheter.
• Prepare umbilical artery catheter (UAC) or central vein for infusion with intralipids administered through a separate line.	• Because TPN solutions are hyperosmotic, large central veins are used to rapidly dilute the solutions. UAC may be used for infusion of TPN and intralipids. Silicone or Silastic catheters with single or multiple lumens are used.
• Prime I.V. tubing and filter with glucose solution, removing all bubbles. Do not use a filter to administer intralipids.	• This prevents air embolism. Filters are not used with intralipids because intalipid molecules cannot pass through a filter.
• Label the solution with the time marked on tape.	• This assists monitoring amount infused over a specific period and prevents overinfusion of hyperosmolar solution.
• Assist with passing the catheter through the vein after the area is anesthetized with a local injection.	• This prevents possible catheter displacement.
• Use infusion-control device with pressure alarm to regulate rate of infusion.	• This ensures infusion of correct amount of fluid at correct rate, minimizing risk of fluid overload.
• Tape all connections to prevent disconnection; clamp lines when connections are open.	• This prevents hemorrhage or air embolism.
• Monitor as follows: □ Change filter, dressings, and connecting tubing daily. □ Clean infusion site daily, using antiseptic solution as ordered.	• Monitoring administration is vital to prevent complications such as local skin irritation, hyperglycemia or hypoglycemia, metabolic acidosis, hemorrhage, pulmonary embolism, and infection.

Interventions

□ Use transparent occlusive dressings, such as Op-Site, for dressings and to secure line.
□ Culture filter fluid as policy dictates.
□ Check infusion rate, patency of tubing, and site for infiltration every hour.
□ Record all vital information and changes regarding TPN on flow sheet.

6. When TPN is discontinued, gradually wean infant while increasing oral or enteral feedings.

7. Administer and monitor gastrostomy tube feedings, when indicated, as follows:

• Secure the tube after placement.

• Aspirate the tube before each feeding, and measure for residual stomach contents greater than 2 ml.

• Start with small, dilute feeding amounts and increase as tolerated (volume and osmolality).

• Assess abdominal girth every 2 hours and observe for diarrhea.

• Allow for feedings by gravity.

• Ensure initial feeding of 4 to 5 ml every 4 hours for neonate.

• Provide pacifier for infant to suck on.

8. Provide mouth care every 2 hours.

9. Review daily, or according to hospital policy, results of the following tests: serum glucose, electrolytes, blood urea nitrogen, serum glutamic-oxaloacetic transaminase (SGOT [aspartate aminotransferase, AST]), serum glutamic-pyruvic transaminase (SGPT [alanine aminotransferase, ALT]), and hematocrit levels; prothrombin time and partial thromboplastin time, osmolality; urine for glucose, osmolality, and specific gravity; and weekly serum ammonia and triglyceride levels.

10. Additional individualized interventions: _____

Rationales

6. This intervention maintains glucose level, prevents rapid shifts in fluid balance, and helps evaluate the infant's ability to tolerate the feeding.

7. Feedings through a gastrostomy tube may be ordered until the defect can be surgically corrected.

• This prevents tube dislodgment.

• With residual contents, withhold feedings to prevent distention.

• This allows for feedings to be gradually increased as tolerated, preventing fluid imbalances.

• Increased abdominal girth and diarrhea indicate distention and are caused by overfeeding and osmolality imbalances.

• Pressure exerted to instill feedings may cause gastric perforation.

• This is optimal amount of feeding for neonate.

• Pacifier provides oral stimulation for tube-fed infant.

8. This prevents mucosal drying that occurs with parenteral and enteral feedings.

9. This is done to monitor effects of nutritional support. Monitoring of lipid infusion and hepatic and renal function is necessary, as is monitoring of other changes that typically occur with TPN.

10. Rationales: _____

Nursing diagnosis: High risk for fluid volume deficit related to fluid loss through indwelling tube and food and fluid being withheld

GOAL: Establish and maintain fluid and electrolyte balance.

Interventions

1. Calculate fluid requirements daily.

2. Weigh infant every day or as infant's condition permits.

3. Maintain accurate fluid intake and output records every hour.

Rationales

1. Fluid needs vary according to individual infant weight and fluid losses from various routes.

2. Weight gains and losses reflect fluid gains and losses and help determine the infant's fluid needs.

3. Hourly assessment ensures optimal fluid balance by indicating need for fluid replacement.

COMPARING TYPES OF PARENTERAL NUTRITION

Parenteral nutrition is a specialized feeding method used to provide nutrients and maintain fluid and electrolyte balance in patients who cannot eat normally. The solution is delivered via a peripheral or central vein. Infants who may be candidates for parenteral nutrition include those whose

GI tract cannot be used and those whose high metabolic needs cannot be met by oral or enteral feedings.

Types of parenteral nutrition include peripheral and total. The chart below compares these types.

Method	Indications	Nutrient Solutions
Peripheral parenteral nutrition Administered through a peripheral vein	• Short-term therapy in patients requiring 2,500 kcal/day or less • Adjunct to oral or enteral feedings	• Dextrose 5% in water • Dextrose 10% in water • Amino acid solution • Protein hydrolysates • Fat emulsions
Total parenteral nutrition Administered through a large central vein	• Long-term therapy in patients requiring more than 2,500 kcal/day (provides up to 4,000 kcal/day)	• Admixtures of dextrose in water (20% to 50%) and crystalline amino acids • Fat emulsions • Total nutrient admixtures (lipids premixed with dextrose and crystalline amino acids)

Interventions

4. Monitor urine output every hour, and report if less than 3 ml/kg/hour.

5. Monitor I.V. fluids for rate, amount, and site infiltration.

6. Monitor urine specific gravity at each voiding.

7. Additional individualized interventions: _____

Rationales

4. Adequate urine output should be 3 ml/kg/hour, with a specific gravity of 1.005 to 1.020. Low urine output and increased specific gravity are caused by low fluid intake.

5. I.V. fluids provide an adequate method to replace fluids. Fluid replacement is calculated and monitored to provide adequate daily fluid amount per infant's body weight and to prevent hypervolemia.

6. These measures provide data related to possible inadequate fluid intake.

7. Rationales: _____

Nursing diagnosis: *Impaired skin integrity related to irritation at stomal site because of secretions*

GOAL: Maintain skin integrity around stomal site.

Interventions

1. Assess gastrostomy or esophagostomy stoma for redness, excoriation, or other changes.

2. Provide sterile technique when caring for stoma.

3. Apply protective covering around stoma, such as skin barrier powder (Op-Site or HolliHesive), or keep stoma clean and exposed to air.

4. Keep area clean and dry.

5. Additional individualized interventions: _____

Rationales

1. These changes indicate that inflammation and skin breakdown may be present, destroying the body's first line of defense and allowing for infection.

2. This prevents contact with contaminants.

3. These preparations protect skin from irritants. If powder is used, keep it well away from tracheostomy site if present.

4. This helps maintain skin integrity and prevent irritation and excoriation.

5. Rationales: _____

Nursing diagnosis: *Anxiety (parental) related to impending surgery and threat of child's death*

GOAL: Minimize parental anxiety.

Interventions

1. Allow and encourage parental expression of feelings and fears about the loss of the "perfect child."

2. Reinforce the infant's normal and healthy aspects and the possibility that surgery will correct the defect, leaving no visible effects.

3. Provide accurate information regarding:
• infant's condition
• defect's etiology, occurrence, and type
• special procedures and equipment
• preparation for surgery and care after surgery.

4. Additional individualized interventions: _____

_____

Rationales

1. This promotes a trusting relationship and a secure environment to decrease parental anxiety.

2. Positive reinforcement helps to reduce parental stress and sadness and to increase positive feelings about surgical correction.

3. Information reduces parental anxiety and maximizes understanding. (See Preoperative Care, page 263, and Postoperative Care, page 257, for more information.)

4. Rationales: _____

_____

Nursing diagnosis: *Ineffective family coping: compromised related to guilt and emotional conflict caused by crisis associated with infant's defect and postponement of surgery*

GOAL: Promote understanding and support parental coping mechanisms.

Interventions

1. Assess verbal and nonverbal expressions of anxiety and use of coping mechanisms.

2. Assist parents to verbalize feelings about loss of the "perfect child," prolonged intensive-care nursery care, and changes in infant's appearance because of gastrostomy tube feedings or other treatments.

3. Provide consistent and accurate information concerning infant's condition.

4. Encourage parents to hold and care for infant.

5. Additional individualized interventions: _____

_____

Rationales

1. Assessment helps to identify and develop constructive coping strategies.

2. This helps to maintain a trusting, secure environment and shows your acceptance of parents' concerns and fears.

3. Being familiar with the infant's progress and condition helps parents cope.

4. Parental involvement promotes bonding.

5. Rationales: _____

_____

ASSOCIATED PLANS
• Hyaline Membrane Disease—Respiratory Distress Syndrome (RDS I)
• Necrotizing Enterocolitis
• Postoperative Care
• Preoperative Care
• Skin Disorders

ADDITIONAL NURSING DIAGNOSES
• Altered family processes related to guilt associated with infant's defect
• Dysfunctional grieving (parental) related to loss of the perfect child
• High risk for altered parenting related to interruption in bonding process
• High risk for aspiration related to TEF
• High risk for infection related to aspiration of secretions, feedings
• Impaired gas exchange related to aspiration
• Ineffective breathing pattern related to pulmonary scar tissue, chronic lung damage
• Ineffective infant feeding pattern related to TEF
• Knowledge deficit (parental) related to lack of information

Transient Tachypnea (RDS II)

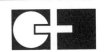

DEFINITION

Also called retained lung fluid, wet lung, or respiratory distress syndrome type II, transient tachypnea of the newborn develops at birth or shortly afterward and lasts from a few hours to 2 to 4 days. It affects full-term infants and preterm infants of 34 to 37 weeks' gestation born by cesarean birth. Fluid remaining in the lungs affects breathing because reabsorption is delayed by the lymphatics, which are engorged in their attempt to reabsorb the fluid as fast as possible. This results in a splinting of the lung, preventing effective ventilation.

The prognosis is good because the condition usually runs its course in about 1 to 4 days without any resultant chronic lung disorder.

This plan focuses on care of the infant who is at risk for retaining or who has retained lung fluid after birth.

ETIOLOGY AND PRECIPITATING FACTORS

• retention of fetal lung fluid because of delayed or slowed reabsorption
• aspiration of large amounts of amniotic fluid from perinatal stress or asphyxia, large-for-gestational-age infant of diabetic mother, or difficult transition of breech birth
• cesarean birth in which infant is not subject to vaginal squeeze during delivery that helps remove pulmonary fluid and does not experience the stress alarm initiated by labor to begin lung fluid reabsorption because birth is imminent

PHYSICAL FINDINGS
Maternal history
• perinatal conditions or diseases requiring cesarean birth

• difficulty during delivery
• diabetes mellitus

Infant status at birth
• full-term or preterm status
• Apgar score indicating respiratory difficulty
• presentation at birth
• cesarean birth

Integumentary
• skin duskiness
• possible central cyanosis

Pulmonary
• persistently high respiratory rate and tachypnea
• possible chest retractions and nasal flaring
• possible expiratory grunt from trying to eject trapped alveolar air
• possible cyanosis when breathing room air

DIAGNOSTIC STUDIES
• chest X-ray—to reveal hyperinflation, fluid in fissures, costophrenic angles, and flattened diaphragm; patches of collapse may be seen

Laboratory data
• arterial blood gas (ABG) studies—to possibly reveal pH slightly decreased with PCO_2 slightly elevated, but both within normal ranges (see Appendix 10: Normal Lab Values for the Newborn Infant).

Collaborative problem: *High risk for respiratory deficiency related to obstruction (2 goals)*

GOAL 1: Identify signs and symptoms of respiratory distress and deviations from desired functioning.

Interventions

1. Assess the infant for changes or difficulty in breathing, including:
• respiratory rate, depth, and ease
• central cyanosis and dusky skin
• grunting, nasal flaring, and retractions
• secretions in airway.

2. Monitor ABG results and pulse oximetry or transcutaneous monitoring sensor (if used) for oxygen level.

Rationales

1. Early identification of changes permits differentiation from more serious respiratory distress disorders and allows for appropriate treatment. Normal respiratory rate for full-term infant is 40 to 60 breaths/minute.

2. Monitoring results alert the nurse to changes. Results should fall within normal limits with oxygen at optimal level.

Interventions	Rationales
3. Review chest X-ray.	3. X-ray study reveals fluid in lungs and rules out pneumothorax.
4. Additional individualized interventions: _____	4. Rationales: _____

GOAL 2: Ensure patent airway and support respiratory efforts.

Interventions	Rationales
1. Elevate the head of the bed slightly and position the infant with its head supported when side-lying or with a shoulder roll if in a prone or supine position. Avoid hyperextending the head. Lowering the head and elevating the feet may be advised.	1. These positions are optimal for maintaining ease of breathing and for maximizing lung expansion. Lowering head facilitates drainage of secretions. The infant's condition determines best position.
2. Change the infant's position from side to side every 2 hours.	2. Side-lying position prevents aspiration.
3. Maintain a neutral thermal environment.	3. This conserves energy and minimizes oxygen demand.
4. Suction secretions from nasopharynx as needed or if advocated.	4. Suctioning ensures that airway is free of obstruction caused by mucus, although it may be too far down for the catheter to reach; it may be more feasible to wait for the lymphatics to do the job of absorption if secretions are too deep for removal with catheter and suctioning.
5. Administer warmed, humidified oxygen at 35% to 40% or less by hood, mask, or other method.	5. Oxygen delivery maintains normal PO_2 and pink skin color with minimal respiratory effort (see Hyaline Membrane Disease — Respiratory Distress Syndrome [RDS I] plan, page 205, for various methods).
6. If the infant's respiratory status does not improve or if it further deteriorates (possibly from fatigue), provide continuous positive airway pressure (CPAP) or other mechanical ventilation as ordered.	6. CPAP or a brief period of mechanical ventilation may be indicated to maintain airway patency.
7. If a transcutaneous PO_2 sensor is used, calibrate it according to manufacturer's directions and rotate the sensor position every 3 to 4 hours. Apply and monitor the pulse oximeter if one is used to measure oxygen levels. Correlate settings with ABG values.	7. This monitoring ensures safe use of apparatus and accurate readings. A pulse oximeter is preferred because it gauges oxygen saturation by fiberoptic light without producing heat that might burn the skin.
8. If a transcutaneous PO_2 sensor is used, place the high and low alarms in the ON position and watch for causes of abnormal readings.	8. These alarms alert staff to high or low oxygen levels administered to infant.
9. Additional individualized interventions: _____	9. Rationales: _____

Nursing diagnosis: *Knowledge deficit (parental) related to the infant's condition, treatment, and ability to overcome temporary respiratory distress*

GOAL: Provide information regarding the infant's status and progress.

Interventions	Rationales
1. Identify the parents' knowledge needs, interest in learning, and learning readiness and capability.	1. This assessment provides the basis of a teaching plan that matches the parents' needs and abilities.

Interventions	Rationales
2. Inform the parents about the following: • cause of the infant's condition • treatment being given • special procedures and equipment • progress and prognosis.	2. Information reduces parents' anxiety and concerns regarding their sick infant.
3. Reassure the parents about their ability to care for the infant.	3. Encouragement shows your support of the parents' ability to care for the infant after discharge.
4. Allow for the parents' questions and clarify aspects of care as needed.	4. Addressing the parents' questions and concerns provides reinforcement of learning while decreasing their anxiety about caring for the infant.
5. Refer the parents to home health care services as appropriate.	5. Referral to home health care services provides the family with continued support.
6. Additional individualized interventions: _____	6. Rationales: _____

ASSOCIATED PLANS
• Cesarean Section Birth
• Hyaline Membrane Disease — Respiratory Distress Syndrome (RDS I)
• Pregnancy Complicated by Diabetes Mellitus

ADDITIONAL NURSING DIAGNOSES
• Anxiety (parental) related to unknown potential for complications
• High risk for altered parenting related to lack of knowledge, unrealistic expectations for infant
• High risk for infection related to retained lung fluid
• Ineffective airway clearance related to retained lung fluid
• Ineffective family coping: compromised related to fear, guilt over condition of infant, admission to special care unit

APPENDICES

1. NANDA Taxonomy of Nursing Diagnoses   307
2. Selected Daily Dietary Allowances — Maternal 309
3. Selected Substances and Fetal Abnormalities   310
4. Aspects of Psychological Care — Maternal   312
5. Preparing for Nonemergency Surgery   317
6. Selected Methods of Family Planning   318
7. The Family and Home Assessment   321
8. Fluid and Nutritional Needs in Infancy   322
9. Assessing Vital Signs in the Infant   323
10. Normal Lab Values for the Newborn Infant   324
11. Transporting an Infant to Another Hospital   327
12. Parent Teaching Guides   328
    How to Bathe Your Infant   328
    Breast-feeding the Infant   330
    Bottle-feeding the Infant   333
    How to Hold the Infant   333
    Postpartum Exercises   334
13. 1993 CDC Revised Classification System
    for HIV Infection/AIDS Surveillance Case
    Definition   336
14. CDC Guidelines for Preventing HIV
    Transmission in Health Care Settings   337

Selected References   338

Index   339

APPENDIX 1

NANDA Taxonomy of Nursing Diagnoses

The currently accepted classification system for nursing diagnoses is that of the North American Nursing Diagnosis Association (NANDA), as shown in *NANDA Nursing Diagnoses: Definitions and Classification 1992-1993*. It is organized around nine human response patterns: exchanging, communicating, relating, valuing, choosing, moving, perceiving, knowing, and feeling.

The complete taxonomic structure is listed here. The series of numbers before each diagnosis is its classification number, used to determine the placement of the diagnosis within the taxonomy. The number of digits delineates the level of abstraction of the nursing diagnosis (more specific diagnoses are assigned longer numbers).

Pattern 1. Exchanging (Mutual giving and receiving)
1.1.2.1	Altered nutrition: More than body requirements
1.1.2.2	Altered nutrition: Less than body requirements
1.1.2.3	Altered nutrition: Potential for more than body requirements
1.2.1.1	High risk for infection
1.2.2.1	High risk for altered body temperature
1.2.2.2	Hypothermia
1.2.2.3	Hyperthermia
1.2.2.4	Ineffective thermoregulation
1.2.3.1	Dysreflexia
1.3.1.1	Constipation
1.3.1.1.1	Perceived constipation
1.3.1.1.2	Colonic constipation
1.3.1.2	Diarrhea
1.3.1.3	Bowel incontinence
1.3.2	Altered urinary elimination
1.3.2.1.1	Stress incontinence
1.3.2.1.2	Reflex incontinence
1.3.2.1.3	Urge incontinence
1.3.2.1.4	Functional incontinence
1.3.2.1.5	Total incontinence
1.3.2.2	Urinary retention
1.4.1.1	Altered (specify type) tissue perfusion (renal, cerebral, cardiopulmonary, gastrointestinal, peripheral)
1.4.1.2.1	Fluid volume excess
1.4.1.2.2.1	Fluid volume deficit
1.4.1.2.2.2	High risk for fluid volume deficit
1.4.2.1	Decreased cardiac output
1.5.1.1	Impaired gas exchange
1.5.1.2	Ineffective airway clearance
1.5.1.3	Ineffective breathing pattern
1.5.1.3.1	Inability to sustain spontaneous ventilation
1.5.1.3.2	Dysfunctional ventilatory weaning response
1.6.1	High risk for injury
1.6.1.1	High risk for suffocation
1.6.1.2	High risk for poisoning
1.6.1.3	High risk for trauma
1.6.1.4	High risk for aspiration
1.6.1.5	High risk for disuse syndrome
1.6.2	Altered protection
1.6.2.1	Impaired tissue integrity
1.6.2.1.1	Altered oral mucous membrane
1.6.2.1.2.1	Impaired skin integrity
1.6.2.1.2.2	High risk for impaired skin integrity

Pattern 2. Communicating (Sending messages)
2.1.1.1	Impaired verbal communication

Pattern 3. Relating (Establishing bonds)
3.1.1	Impaired social interaction
3.1.2	Social isolation
3.2.1	Altered role performance
3.2.1.1.1	Altered parenting
3.2.1.1.2	High risk for altered parenting
3.2.1.2.1	Sexual dysfunction
3.2.2	Altered family processes
3.2.2.1	Caregiver role strain
3.2.2.2	High risk for caregiver role strain
3.2.3.1	Parental role conflict
3.3	Altered sexuality patterns

Pattern 4. Valuing (Assigning relative worth)
4.1.1	Spiritual distress (distress of the human spirit)

Pattern 5. Choosing (Selecting alternatives)
5.1.1.1	Ineffective individual coping
5.1.1.1.1	Impaired adjustment
5.1.1.1.2	Defensive coping
5.1.1.1.3	Ineffective denial
5.1.2.1.1	Ineffective family coping: Disabling
5.1.2.1.2	Ineffective family coping: Compromised
5.1.2.2	Family coping: Potential for growth
5.2.1	Ineffective management of therapeutic regimen (individual)
5.2.1.1	Noncompliance (specify)
5.3.1.1	Decisional conflict (specify)
5.4	Health-seeking behaviors (specify)

Pattern 6. Moving (Involving activity)
6.1.1.1	Impaired physical mobility
6.1.1.1.1	High risk for peripheral neurovascular dysfunction
6.1.1.2	Activity intolerance
6.1.1.2.1	Fatigue
6.1.1.3	High risk for activity intolerance
6.2.1	Sleep pattern disturbance
6.3.1.1	Diversional activity deficit
6.4.1.1	Impaired home maintenance management
6.4.2	Altered health maintenance
6.5.1	Feeding self-care deficit
6.5.1.1	Impaired swallowing
6.5.1.2	Ineffective breast-feeding
6.5.1.2.1	Interrupted breast-feeding
6.5.1.3	Effective breast-feeding
6.5.1.4	Ineffective infant feeding pattern
6.5.2	Bathing or hygiene self-care deficit
6.5.3	Dressing or grooming self-care deficit
6.5.4	Toileting self-care deficit
6.6	Altered growth and development
6.7	Relocation stress syndrome

Pattern 7. Perceiving (Receiving information)
7.1.1	Body image disturbance
7.1.2	Self-esteem disturbance
7.1.2.1	Chronic low self-esteem
7.1.2.2	Situational low self-esteem
7.1.3	Personal identity disturbance
7.2	Sensory or perceptual alterations (specify visual, auditory, kinesthetic, gustatory, tactile, olfactory)
7.2.1.1	Unilateral neglect
7.3.1	Hopelessness
7.3.2	Powerlessness

Pattern 8. Knowing (Associating meaning with information)
8.1.1	Knowledge deficit (specify)
8.3	Altered thought processes

(continued)

NANDA Taxonomy of Nursing Diagnoses *(continued)*

Pattern 9. Feeling (Being subjectively aware of information)

9.1.1	Pain
9.1.1.1	Chronic pain
9.2.1.1	Dysfunctional grieving
9.2.1.2	Anticipatory grieving
9.2.2	High risk for violence: Self-directed or directed at others
9.2.2.1	High risk for self-mutilation
9.2.3	Post-trauma response
9.2.3.1	Rape-trauma syndrome
9.2.3.1.1	Rape-trauma syndrome: Compound reaction
9.2.3.1.2	Rape-trauma syndrome: Silent reaction
9.3.1	Anxiety
9.3.2	Fear

APPENDIX 2

Selected Daily Dietary Allowances — Maternal

The following chart shows selected daily dietary allowances for pregnant, lactating, and nonpregnant women.

Nutrient	Pregnant women	Lactating women		Nonpregnant women		
		Months 1 through 6	Months 7 through 12	Ages 15 to 18	Ages 19 to 24	Ages 25 to 50
Calcium	1,200 mg	1,200 mg	1,200 mg	1,200 mg	1,200 mg	800 mg
Folate	400 mcg	280 mcg	260 mcg	180 mcg	180 mcg	180 mcg
Iodine	175 mcg	200 mcg	200 mcg	150 mcg	150 mcg	150 mcg
Iron	30 mg	15 mg	15 mg	15 mg	15 mg	15 mg
Magnesium	320 mg	355 mg	340 mg	300 mg	280 mg	280 mg
Niacin	17 mg NE*	20 mg NE	20 mg NE	15 mg NE	15 mg NE	15 mg NE
Phosphorus	1,200 mg	1,200 mg	1,200 mg	1,200 mg	1,200 mg	800 mg
Protein	60 g	65 g	62 g	44 g	46 g	50 g
Riboflavin	1.6 mg	1.8 mg	1.7 mg	1.3 mg	1.3 mg	1.3 mg
Selenium	65 mcg	75 mcg	75 mcg	50 mcg	55 mcg	55 mcg
Thiamine	1.5 mg	1.6 mg	1.6 mg	1.1 mg	1.1 mg	1.1 mg
Vitamin A	800 mcg RE†	1,300 mcg RE	1,200 mcg RE	800 mcg RE	800 mcg RE	800 mcg RE
Vitamin B$_6$	2.2 mg	2.1 mg	2.1 mg	1.5 mg	1.6 mg	1.6 mg
Vitamin B$_{12}$	2.2 mcg	2.6 mcg	2.6 mcg	2.0 mcg	2.0 mcg	2.0 mcg
Vitamin C	70 mg	95 mg	90 mg	60 mg	60 mg	60 mg
Vitamin D	10 mcg	10 mcg	10 mcg	10 mcg	5 mcg	5 mcg
Vitamin E	10 mg TE‡	12 mg TE	11 mg TE	8 mg TE	8 mg TE	8 mg TE
Zinc	15 mg	19 mg	16 mg	12 mg	12 mg	12 mg*

*NE: niacin equivalent
†RE: retinol equivalent
‡TE: tocopherol equivalent
Adapted with permission from *Recommended Dietary Allowances,* 10th ed. Washington, D.C.: National Academy of Sciences, 1989.

APPENDIX 3

Selected Substances and Fetal Abnormalities

All drugs used by the gravida are potentially teratogenic and drugs crossing the placental barrier may affect the fetus. A correlation does not necessarily exist between maternal reaction to a drug and fetal response to a drug. Any drug use (over-the-counter or prescribed) should be discussed with the physician and decided by the risk-benefit ratio. The following list includes drugs taken by the gravida and their reported effects on the fetus.

Chemical substance use by the patient may adversely affect the fetus, either directly or indirectly. Fetal effects depend largely on gestational age, drug potency, and dosage. Maternal drug reaction and fetal response do not necessarily correlate. Food and Drug Administration drug category ratings assist in determining the risk-benefit ratio.

Before using any chemical substance, the patient should consult the physician. This chart shows the fetal effects of selected substances used by pregnant women.

Maternal drug or substance	Reported effects on fetus
alcohol	hypoglycemia; fetal alcohol syndrome; cardiac anomalies; craniofacial anomalies; prenatal and postnatal growth retardation; brain, spinal, and cardiac defects; mental retardation and other neurobehavioral abnormalities
amphetamines	thrombocytopenia, transposition of the great vessels, cleft palate
anesthetics	
conduction anesthesia	acidosis, bradycardia, convulsions, death, hypotension, myocardial depression
general anesthesia	chromosomal anomalies, methemoglobinemia, respiratory depression
local anesthesia (paracervical)	acidosis, bradycardia, convulsions, myocardial and neurologic depression
antacids	anomalies, electrolyte imbalances
aspirin	hemorrhage, premature closing of ductus arteriosus, prolonged gestation
barbiturates	withdrawal symptoms, increased anomalies, diminished sucking, diminished serum bilirubin levels, neonatal bleeding
chlorothiazide	thrombocytopenia, sodium and water depletion
cocaine	cardiac, central nervous system, and genitourinary anomalies; dysmorphic features, skeletal defects; atresias; small-for-gestational-age status; neurobehavioral abnormalities
corticosteroids	accelerated fetal lung maturation, adrenal suppression, increased incidence of fetal anomalies and death
diazepam	withdrawal symptoms, anomalies, hypothermia
insulin	hypoglycemia, skeletal defects, death
lysergic acid diethylamide (LSD)	chromosomal damage
magnesium sulfate	hypermagnesemia, CNS depression, peripheral neuromuscular blockage
nicotine	low birth weight, stillbirth

Maternal drug or substance	**Reported effects on fetus**
morphine, heroin, and methadone	intrauterine growth retardation (IUGR), withdrawal symptoms, respiratory depression, death
phenytoin	patent ductus arteriosus, pulmonary atresia, cleft lip, cleft palate or gum, syndactyly, polydactyly, diaphragmatic hernia, microencephaly, anencephaly
radioactive iodine	abnormal thyroid function, hypothyroidism, thyroid destruction
reserpine	anomalies, bradycardia, hypothermia, lethargy, respiratory difficulties from nasal congestion, increased secretions

APPENDIX 4

Aspects of Psychological Care – Maternal

Pregnancy and parenthood require many maternal psychological as well as physiologic adjustments. The diagnoses, goals, and nursing interventions and rationales presented here will help to plan health care related to potential problems arising from maternal anxiety, stress, depression, grief, deprivation, undeveloped parenting skills, and self-concept disturbances. These nursing diagnoses and interventions complement the maternal health care plans in this book.

Nursing diagnosis: *Anxiety related to pregnancy and its outcome*

GOAL: Reduce maternal anxiety level.

Interventions

1. Determine maternal anxiety level; consider the following:
• mild symptoms (increased alertness, ability to recognize threatening feelings and to learn and comprehend)
• moderate symptoms (periodic inattention, decreased ability to communicate or learn, and need for direction)
• severe symptoms (severely impaired ability to perceive and communicate details and inability to learn)
• panic (distorted perception, inability to communicate or function in everyday living and to learn).

2. Assess behavioral changes associated with anxiety, including irritability and restlessness; rapid speech, repetitive statements and questions, and quivering voice; hand wringing and hand tremors; insomnia, tension, and apprehension; inability to maintain eye contact; inability to concentrate and retain information and a short attention span; inability to communicate and reduced intellectual functioning.

3. Assess physiologic changes associated with anxiety, including increased blood pressure and pulse and respiratory rates; palpitations; perspiration and cold, clammy hands; nausea and vomiting; headache and dizziness; tremors; dry mouth; and dilated pupils.

4. Provide calm, accepting environment for maternal expression of feelings and concerns.

5. Acknowledge the mother's anxiety. Assist her to identify her symptoms and describe how she is experiencing anxiety.

6. Assist the mother to identify source of stressors during perinatal period.

7. Assist and support the mother to identify and use coping mechanisms that help decrease anxiety (talking, crying, walking, or keeping busy, for example).

8. Inform the mother of all procedures and expectations, presenting accurate information and answering her questions.

9. Allow the mother to participate in all decisions.

10. Suggest and teach relaxation techniques if appropriate.

11. Additional individualized interventions: _____

Rationales

1. Anxiety levels may range from mild to panic, with each level accompanied by behavioral and physiologic symptoms. Anxiety is a generalized feeling or tension related to a perceived threat.

2. Behavioral changes become apparent during anxiety states; they increase in severity as anxiety increases.

3. Anxiety stimulates the autonomic nervous system, causing physiologic responses.

4. An accepting, peaceful, nonthreatening environment encourages the mother to externalize her feelings and fears and to identify these emotions and their causes. Accepting the mother's feelings validates them, allowing her to discuss them without fear of ridicule or rejection.

5. Recognizing the behavioral and physiologic manifestations of anxiety defines and validates the anxiety level and, consequently, the steps to reduce it.

6. Discussion of stressors helps to identify and resolve anxiety.

7. Coping mechanisms temporarily help protect or distance a person from a real or perceived threat.

8. Information reduces the mother's fear of the unknown.

9. The mother's participation in all decisions helps her maintain control over her own care and well-being.

10. These techniques may help to relieve anxiety.

11. Rationales: _____

Nursing diagnosis: *Ineffective individual coping related to stress or potential complications of perinatal period and to life changes because of this crisis*

GOAL: Develop and support maternal coping skills.

Interventions	Rationales
1. Assess maternal internal and external stressors and use of coping skills, including current stressors and concerns; ability to cope and use coping mechanisms; illness or physical limits to coping ability; ability to accept assistance with coping; and existing support systems.	1. Effective coping requires the ability to identify and manage stressors by solving problems and adapting to change. Pregnancy is a situational crisis that creates the need for increased coping abilities and adaptation.
2. Assist the mother to identify effective coping skills or new behaviors or techniques.	2. As the mother uses coping skills effectively, her feelings of autonomy and her ability to cope with stressors will increase.
3. Suggest and initiate problem-solving development by: • role playing • improving sending and receiving skills by communication • openly discussing alternative solutions • developing alternative coping strategies.	3. These techniques increase the mother's problem-solving ability, needed to deal more effectively with crises.
4. Support the mother's helpful coping behaviors and existing or possible support systems.	4. This supports the mother's continued success in using effective coping behaviors and existing support systems. It may also encourage her to develop a broader support base if familiar supports are ineffective.
5. Assist the mother to develop goals and define ways and methods to achieve them.	5. This encourages independence and positive results in dealing with pregnancy-related stress.
6. Additional individualized interventions: _____	6. Rationales: _____

Collaborative problem: *High risk for postpartum depression related to physiologic and psychological stresses of pregnancy*

GOAL: Identify and reduce potential for "maternity blues," or postpartum depression.

Interventions	Rationales
1. Assess factors predisposing the mother to postpartum mental illness, such as: • family history of postpartum depression • previous depression or psychiatric problem during pregnancy • maternal doubt regarding competence to care for infant • few or no support systems • disinterest in infant • fatigue and overwhelmed feeling • marital problems, family crisis • preoccupation with discomfort and physical problems • low self-esteem.	1. Postpartum emotional changes may be transitory; responses can range from maternity blues (30% to 80% of all childbirths) to psychosis (1% to 2%). Role changes and increased responsibilities cause stress for the new mother adapting to physiologic changes that occur post partum.
2. Observe for responses indicating maternity blues, such as: • mood swings • tearful and weepy behavior • "let down" and depressed feelings • quiet, passive, discouraged feelings • poor concentration and despondency.	2. This condition usually occurs and subsides within the 1st week after delivery (although the symptoms may be prolonged). However, in rare instances, maternity blues may develop into depressive psychosis.
3. Allow the mother to express her feelings and questions. Maintain a supportive and nonjudgmental attitude.	3. This provides an atmosphere of trust in which the mother can vent and deal with feelings of inadequacy or other concerns.
4. Reassure the mother about her abilities to care for her infant and her coping abilities.	4. The mother may be concerned about her ability to care for her infant and her coping abilities.
5. Inform the mother that feeling "let down" is normal after delivery. Protect her privacy so she can cry and vent her feelings.	5. This allows the mother to feel that this response is normal and will pass.

Interventions

6. Include the mother in all planning and activities related to her infant's care.

7. Suggest referral or follow-up visits if depressed feelings are unresolved.

8. Additional individualized interventions: _____

_____

Rationales

6. This instills self-confidence in the mother as she begins parenting.

7. Counseling may prevent postpartum psychosis.

8. Rationales: _____

_____

Nursing diagnosis: *Dysfunctional grieving related to infant death or malformation*

GOAL: Support emotional reactions and work toward resolution of grieving.

Interventions

1. Stay with the parents when the physician informs them of the infant's death or malformation. Ensure their privacy.

2. In case of infant's death, call clergy, if requested.

3. Answer questions or give information in simple terms.

4. Remain present and listen; minimize speaking to allow the parents to express their feelings, cry, or show anger, guilt, or other feelings. Use touch to show your support.

5. Prepare the infant for viewing by parents. Stay in the room if they request it.

6. If the infant has a physical malformation, allow the parents to see the infant as soon as possible after being informed.

7. Assess parental responses to loss (death or the "perfect child"), including:
• crying, rage, or silence
• anger at God or themselves
• hostility toward staff
• expression of denial or feelings of guilt
• somatic symptoms, such as shortness of breath, sighing, choking feeling, emptiness in stomach, tightness in throat, and insomnia
• disinterest in activities
• inability to communicate
• ability or inability to vent anger and guilt feelings.

8. Assess for pathologic responses to grieving, such as:
• total denial of the loss
• hostility or cheerfulness with friends and relatives
• psychosomatic disorders or symptoms of illness of the deceased
• deep depression
• loss of social interactions and relationships.

9. Inform the parents about the feelings they can expect throughout the normal grieving process. Emphasize their need to express these feelings. Include that time and understanding assist in resolution of grief.

Rationales

1. The care provider's presence provides support and shows concern and acceptance of parent's feelings. Quiet and privacy allow the parents to express their feelings without fear of judgment or embarrassment.

2. Religious rites and clerical presence support parents' grieving.

3. The parents' grief may preclude them from processing information until the initial shock of loss passes. More information may be given later, as appropriate.

4. Using therapeutic communication techniques demonstrates support, caring, and concern.

5. This offers the parents the opportunity for contact with infant by holding and touching or by taking mementoes, such as the crib card or identification band. These actions help the parents eliminate denial and allow them to feel the reality of death.

6. Seeing the infant helps the parents overcome inaccurate images or denial of the infant's abnormality.

7. Grief, a normal process after loss, causes significant emotional pain as well as physical reactions. Initial shock and disbelief give way to denial, which buffers the impact of the loss and allows the parents time to seek ways to respond to the devastating event. Later, when reality cannot be denied, the parents will experience feelings of guilt, anger, and helplessness. Somatic symptoms are common. As the grieving process continues, depression occurs as a response to the loss as well as to the fear and anxiety. The grieving parents eventually reach a state of restitution, which results in gradual acceptance, recovery, and normalcy.

8. Some parents react to grief with pathologic distortions because of their unsuccessful movement through the grieving process.

9. This relieves parents of feeling additional stress about their behavior during the grieving process.

Interventions

10. Offer information about support groups, booklets that may be helpful as appropriate, and psychiatric counseling with pathologic mourning.

11. Call the parents the day after infant's death and send a card.

12. Offer information about the autopsy conference in case the parents want to attend.

13. Suggest meeting with the physician after discharge in 3 to 4 months.

14. Additional individualized interventions: _____

Rationales

10. Support groups, self-help materials, and counseling provide additional support, if needed, especially for parents of infants who have congenital anomalies and who may need continual support over a long period.

11. Consolation and caring are shown to parents.

12. This helps them understand the infant's illness and cause of death.

13. The physician can assess the parents' grieving process and special needs.

14. Rationales: _____

Nursing diagnosis: *Altered health maintenance related to lack of material resources and support system*

GOAL: Establish and support prenatal care.

Interventions

1. Assess factors associated with lack of prenatal care:
• low socioeconomic status
• health beliefs and practices
• personal strengths and reliability
• scarcity of clinics and low-cost or free prenatal care
• use of drugs or alcohol
• lack of supportive family or paternal relationships.

2. Assist the mother to define and clarify prenatal needs.

3. Inform the mother about resources available for prenatal care.

4. Support the decision to contact an agency for care.

5. Monitor ongoing management of prenatal care by mother.

6. Additional individualized interventions: _____

Rationales

1. Ideally, all potential mothers should receive prenatal care starting at 6 to 8 weeks of pregnancy and continuing to the expected date of confinement. Physical examination, measurements, weight gains, nutritional and activity instruction, vital signs, and laboratory tests are monitored to prevent perinatal complications and injury to the fetus or infant. Most preterm births and infants born with complications occur in mothers who have not had prenatal care.

2. Some pregnant women are unaware of the need for prenatal care, especially if they are young or in their teenage years.

3. This information is not always readily available or the mother is not always informed about health care agencies.

4. Supporting the mother's effort to seek adequate, affordable care helps to establish and maintain maternal-infant health.

5. Periodic contact shows interest and support in mother's ability to maintain health.

6. Rationales: _____

Nursing diagnosis: *High risk for altered parenting related to knowledge deficit in infant care and inadequate role identity*

GOAL: Promote parental role identification and practice in infant care.

Interventions

1. Assess parent teaching needs in infant care; including:
• parity and infant care experience
• stated knowledge deficit
• parental expectations related to self and infant
• perceptions of parenting and behaviors
• role priorities as stated
• learning readiness
• education and communication level.

Rationales

1. The teaching plan is based on data collected from parents about their perceptions, experiences, interests, and education levels.

Interventions	**Rationales**
2. Provide demonstrations and return demonstrations in infant care as follows: • bathing the infant, sponge and tub baths • dressing the infant • caring for cord and circumcision areas • holding the infant • feeding the infant • preparing the infant's feedings.	2. Knowledge base is necessary for effective parenting and role identity. Return demonstrations give the parents hands-on experience and increases parental comfort level in providing infant care (see Appendix 13: Parent Teaching Guides).
3. Provide information about parenting groups.	3. These groups help new parents explore their expectations, behaviors, and roles.
4. Provide referrals or follow-ups as needed for Visiting Nurse Association, physician, and clinic visits.	4. Medical and nursing attention supports well-baby care after discharge.
5. Provide a positive learning environment, encourage the parents to ask questions, and clarify information for them.	5. These approaches and actions facilitate and reinforce parental learning.
6. Additional individualized interventions: _____	6. Rationales: _____

Nursing diagnosis: *Body image disturbance related to temporary, pregnancy-induced changes in appearance*

GOAL: Promote adaptation to change in appearance during pregnancy.

Interventions	**Rationales**
1. Assess maternal feelings concerning change in appearance, including: • expression of how mother sees herself • verbalization of adaptability to changes • unkempt appearance and inability to maintain self-care • withdrawal or hostility.	1. Society places great importance on appearances. Changes in body shape and size, although gradual, need to be accepted by mother as normal during pregnancy.
2. Assist mother to develop goals and actions to preserve self-esteem and self-image; include: • clothing selection • becoming and easy-to-care-for hair style • appropriate weight gain • attractive accessories • moderate cosmetic use.	2. Attractive appearance during pregnancy helps preserve a positive self-image and prevents possible negative reactions from others.
3. Accept mother as an individual with individual needs during her pregnancy.	3. This attitude promotes a trusting relationship.
4. Stress positive features of pregnancy, downplay negative ones.	4. This helps promote a positive maternal attitude.
5. Additional individualized interventions: _____	5. Rationales: _____

APPENDIX 5

Preparing for Nonemergency Surgery

When a pregnant woman has nonemergency, acute but nonemergency, or scheduled surgery—for instance, for ectopic pregnancy, spontaneous abortion, or cesarean section—nursing care proceeds according to general preoperative guidelines, which are reviewed below.

• Obtain a full maternal health history, including data on gynecologic and obstetric histories, gestational age, expected date of confinement, outstanding medical problems, and drug allergies. Perform a physical assessment. Obtain fetal heart sounds, if applicable.

• Review the results of complete blood count, electrolyte analysis, blood typing and crossmatching, and radiographic and electrocardiographic studies. Report abnormalities to the primary physician. Make sure ordered blood is available.

• Determine the extent of the mother's knowledge of the surgical procedure and of anesthesia. Witness an informed consent before administering preoperative medication.

• Withhold food and fluids.

• Inform the mother of what she can expect postoperatively. Discuss:
   □ when the infant can be seen (if surgery is to be a cesarean section)
   □ length of time in recovery room
   □ availability of pain medication
   □ pulmonary hygiene measures, for example, turning, coughing, deep-breathing, spirometry. Demonstrate these exercises for the patient and have her return the demonstration, if her condition permits.
   □ circulatory hygiene measures, for example, leg exercise and progressive ambulation
   □ I.V. apparatus, abdominal dressing, perineal pad, and indwelling catheter.

• Establish where family members can be contacted and inform them of the patient's progress.

• Contact clergy, if the patient requests.

• Prepare the operative site. Assist with morning care, toilet. Catheterize, and start an I.V. infusion as indicated. Remove the patient's nail polish, jewelry, or prosthetic devices. If the patient wants to wear her wedding band during surgery, tape or tie it to her hand. Attach (and note placement of) religious articles to the patient's hospital gown if she desires. Apply thromboembolic stockings, as indicated.

• Record vital signs, reporting unexpected findings to primary physician and to the operating room staff.

• Administer preoperative medications, as ordered. Thereafter, the patient should remain in bed. Ensure that both side rails are raised and that the call device is within the patient's reach.

• Document all activities and findings.

APPENDIX 6

Selected Methods of Family Planning

The following chart highlights selected family planning methods that commonly are available and chosen by patients seen in the maternal health care setting.

Method and examples	How the method works	Advantages	Disadvantages
Natural family planning methods: cervical mucus rhythm, basal body temperature rhythm, calendar rhythm, symptothermal, fertility awareness	Couple abstains from sexual intercourse during fertile period	• Require no devices, prescriptions, or use of medication • Morally acceptable to people whose religious beliefs forbid use of mechanical or chemical contraception	• Require high degree of motivation and training • Limit sexual spontaneity • May require protracted periods of sexual abstinence • Require observation and record-keeping associated with menstrual cycle • Rhythm method has highest incidence of failure (pregnancy)
Withdrawal before ejaculation (coitus interruptus)	Prevents deposition of semen in vagina	• Requires no devices, preparations, prescriptions, or use of medication	• Effectiveness depends on correct and consistent use, which is influenced by age, education, degree of motivation, and training and experience in contraceptive use • Requires absolute cooperation of and control by partners; is associated with high level of sexual frustration for both partners • Seminal fluid remaining on vulva may cause fertilization
Barrier methods: male and female condoms; diaphragm; cervical cap; spermicides — sponge with spermicidal agents, spermicidal foams, gels, creams, and suppositories	Mechanical barriers (condom, cap, and diaphragm) prevent sperm penetration; spermicides immobilize or chemically destroy sperm	• Except for diaphragm and cap, barrier methods require no prescriptions or ingestion of systemic medications • May protect against sexually transmitted diseases; (STDs); male latex condoms are highly effective against transmission of human immunodeficiency virus • Sponge is effective for up to 24 hours	• Condom application requires interruption of foreplay; new condom must be applied for each intercourse; some partners report diminished sensations; condoms have limited storage life; female condoms have high failure rate • Diaphragms may develop tears or holes; require fitting initially and again after childbirth or abortion; should be used with spermicidal agent; should remain in place at least 8 hours after intercourse; to apply diaphragm, user must be comfortable handling genital area • Cervical cap must be fitted; may remain in place up to 48 hours; should be used with spermicide • Spermicidal agents are messy and may cause local irritation in either partner; multiple coitus necessitates repeated application of spermicidal agent; incorrect or inconsistent use is associated with high failure rate

Method and Examples	How the Method Works	Advantages	Disadvantages
Hormonal contraceptives: estrogen and progestin combination (the pill) or progestinal agent alone (the minipill); subdermal implants of levonorgestrel	Inhibit ovulation, impair sperm transport, render endometrium inhospitable to implantation of fertilized ovum	• Most effective reversible method of birth control • Separate use from sexual activity • Regulate irregular menstrual cycles • Are associated with reduced incidence of menstrual blood loss, anemia, dysmenorrhea, premenstrual symptoms, functional ovarian cysts, endometrial and ovarian cancers, salpingitis, pelvic inflammatory disease (PID), various benign breast diseases, toxic shock syndrome, and rheumatoid arthritis	• May be morally unacceptable to people who believe life begins at conception • Necessitate comprehensive physical assessment and annual cervical cytologic examination • Cause metabolic changes that may lead to cardiovascular diseases, especially deep-vein thrombosis and pulmonary embolism • May lead to range of adverse metabolic effects many of which are estrogen-dose related • Not recommended for women over age 40 with systemic or chronic disease • Absolute contraindications for oral contraceptives include known or suspected pregnancy, undiagnosed genital bleeding, thromboembolic disorders, hyperlipidemia, uncontrolled hypertension, diabetes mellitus with vascular changes, coronary artery disease, cerebrovascular accident, estrogen-dependent breast or endometrial carcinoma, and liver dysfunction or tumors • Relative contraindications for oral contraceptives include heavy cigarette smoking and history of migraine or vascular headaches, varicose veins, cardiac or renal disease or dysfunction, gestational diabetes or prediabetes, depression, sickle cell disease, and cholestatic disease during pregnancy • Require ingesting medication 21 or 28 days per month; missed doses may necessitate use of backup barrier contraceptive • May lead to multiple drug interactions • Associated with nutritional deficiencies, cervical mucorrhea, vaginitis, and weight gain • Progestinal agents cause fewer adverse effects but are associated with increased failure rate, ectopic pregnancy, and irregular bleeding • Subdermal implants require subcutaneous insertion of six polysiloxone capsules into upper arm; replacement after maximum 5-year cycle may be difficult because of local fibrosis

(continued)

APPENDICES

Selected Methods of Family Planning *(continued)*

Method and Examples	How the Method Works	Advantages	Disadvantages
Intrauterine devices (IUDs): chemically inert devices, copper or progesterone-impregnated devices	Cause intrauterine inflammatory response that is toxic to sperm and fertilized ovum	• Second only to oral contraceptives as most effective reversible birth control method; effectiveness measured in years; copper IUD is effective for 6 to 8 years • Separate use from sexual activity • Affect genital tract only • Require no motivation or learning • Inexpensive	• May be expelled; extrauterine expulsion may result in penetration or perforation of adjacent structures • Pregnancy may occur with device in utero • Contraindicated in known or suspected pregnancy, uterine bleeding, PID, and cervical or uterine cancer • Relative contraindications include nulliparous status, high risk for STD, history of ectopic pregnancy or fallopian tube reconstructive surgery, endometriosis, uterine leiomyoma, impaired coagulation, valvular heart disease, and Wilson's disease • May cause cramping, ulceration, pain, and increased bleeding during or between menstrual periods; contribute to pelvic infection; increase risk of spontaneous abortion and ectopic pregnancy • Uterine perforation or interruption of pregnancy may occur during insertion • Progesterone-releasing IUD must be changed yearly
Sterilization; tubal ligation	Terminates fertility by means of surgical transection of oviduct by occlusion, ligation, partial excision, or fulguration	• One-time procedure that may be performed on outpatient basis • Essentially 100% effective and should be considered permanent; virtual infallibility may provide psychological comfort and security	• Coagulation burns of adjacent structures may occur during surgery • Mortality (although low) is associated with use of general anesthesia • Unacceptable to certain religious, political, and professional groups • Surgical reversal is expensive and has success rate of 50% to 80%

APPENDIX 7

The Family and Home Assessment

To ensure that the maternal-infant health plans and teaching relate to the patient's life situation, the following factors should be included in the database.

THE FAMILY

• Composition: names, ages, genders, family or birth order, relationships, race, ethnicity, religion, and education

• Type: single parent, nuclear, extended, cohabitational, divorced, merged (includes divorce and remarriage), stepfamilies, foster families

• Control: autocratic, patriarchal, matriarchal, democratic, or laissez-faire

• Developmental stage (according to Duvall):
  ☐ marriage
  ☐ early childbearing
  ☐ families with preschool children
  ☐ families with school-aged children
  ☐ families with teenagers
  ☐ launching-center families
  ☐ families of middle years
  ☐ families in retirement or old age

• Roles (singly or in combination): provider, nurturer, decision maker, problem solver, tradition or value setter, or health supervisor

• Health of members: current wellness level; acute or chronic illness; congenital defects; accident, surgery, immunization, and mental health histories

• Health values: health values and conflicts, role of prophylaxis, nutritional status, exercise, work or school, recreation, type of health provider sought (medical specialist physician, general practitioner, doctor of osteopathy, chiropractor, nurse practitioner, free clinics, government-sponsored services, herbalists, or other nonmedical, traditional practitioners)

• Significance of community: work, school, neighbors, church-community members, professional or trade groups, and self-help or resource groups

• Preparation (for infant and family): child preparation classes—for infant, selves, siblings, or other family members

THE HOME

• Type of dwelling: single or multifamily, adequacy of facilities, living conditions including environmental hazards

• Finances: incomes; insurance; budget for rent, food, utilities, transportation, clothing, health care, insurance, education, and recreation

• Occupation: professional, managerial, clerical, skilled trade, manual laborer, or other

• Educational level: advanced degrees or college, high school, or grade school level completed

APPENDIX 8

Fluid and Nutritional Needs in Infancy

Infant fluid-electrolyte and nutritional-caloric needs depend on the infant's weight and gestational age because these determine GI capacity and metabolic rates and capabilities.

FLUID AND ELECTROLYTE REQUIREMENTS
Fluid and electrolyte requirements vary with each infant. Factors that usually increase the infant's fluid-electrolyte requirements include insensible water loss, phototherapy, radiant warming, abnormal losses preoperatively and postoperatively, vomiting and diarrhea, and labile body or ambient temperatures.

In general, the healthy full-term infant (40 weeks' gestation) requires about 100 ml/kg/day. Sodium, potassium, and chloride requirements for the full-term infant are sodium, 2 mEq/kg/day; potassium, 2 mEq/kg/day; and chloride, 2 to 4 mEq/kg/day.

Smaller and less mature, the preterm infant has a greater proportion of body weight as water and needs up to 200 ml/kg/day of fluid. Sodium needs range from 3 to 4 mEq/kg/day; potassium and chloride needs vary.

NUTRITIONAL AND CALORIC NEEDS
The goal of nutritional intake is to supply metabolic requirements for growth and for replacement of losses through urine, feces, sweat, and tissue breakdown.

The full-term infant needs 100 to 120 kcal/kg/day. Both full-term and preterm infants need proteins, carbohydrates, and fats as follows:
• protein: 2.5 to 4 g/kg/day (10% to 15% of caloric intake)
• carbohydrates: 10 to 15 g/kg/day (45% to 55% of caloric intake)
• fats: 5 to 7 g/kg/day (40% to 50% of caloric intake).

Note: To gain 1 g of weight, the infant must store 2 to 3 calories from nutrients composed of about 60% to 80% water, 30% protein, and the rest fat. A low-birth-weight infant must store 20 to 40 calories daily to maintain growth. (See *Nutritional and caloric content of milk and formulas* and *Proposed schedule for feeding low-birth-weight infants,* for more information).

NUTRITIONAL AND CALORIC CONTENT OF MILK AND FORMULAS

Milk product	kcal/dl	Protein (g/dl)	Carbohydrate (g/dl)	Fat (g/dl)
Breast milk	67	1.2	7.0	3.8
Cow's milk	67	3.3	4.8	3.7
Enfamil	67	1.5	7.0	3.7
Pregestimil	67	2.2	8.8	2.8
Premature	67 to 100	2.8	9.0	3.7
Similac PM	67	1.5	7.2	3.4
SMA	67	1.5	7.2	3.6

PROPOSED SCHEDULE FOR FEEDING LOW-BIRTH-WEIGHT INFANT

Infant weight	First feeding	Formula feeding
2 lb, 7 oz to 3 lb, 2 oz (1,250 to 1,500 g)	5% to 10% glucose (3 ml); follow with 5 ml in 2 to 3 hours	5 ml every 2 to 3 hours; increase 1 ml every other feeding up to 10 to 15 ml
3 lb, 2 oz to 4 lb, 3 oz (1,500 to 2,000 g)	5% to 10% glucose (5 ml); follow with 8 ml in 2 to 3 hours	8 ml every 2 to 3 hours; increase 1 ml every other feeding up to 15 ml
2,000 g or more	5% glucose (15 ml); repeat if tolerated	15 ml every 3 hours; increase 5 ml every other feeding up to 30 ml

APPENDIX 9

Assessing Vital Signs in the Infant

ASSESSING VITAL SIGNS IN THE INFANT

This guide to assessing the newborn infant's vital signs—presents normal ranges for body temperature, heart and respiratory rates, and blood pressure. In a preterm infant, weight and gestational age affect vital signs; therefore, normal ranges vary from one preterm infant to the next.

Measurement	Normal values	Nursing implications
Temperature Fetus: 99.7° to 100.0° F (37.6° to 37.7° C)	Full-term infant: • 97.7° to 98.6° F (36.5° to 37.0° C) axillary • 96° to 99.5° F (35.5° to 37.5° C) rectally Preterm infant: • temperature varies with weight and gestational age	• Measure temperature when infant is admitted to the nursery; follow institutional policy regarding type of temperature to take. • Continue to monitor temperature frequently, and notify the physician if the temperature drops below 97.5° F (36.4° C). • Institute measures to conserve body heat, such as keeping the infant's head covered and keeping the infant's dry
Heart rate	• Fetus: 110 to 160 beats per minute • Full-term infant: 120 to 160 beats per minute (apical) • Preterm infant: 130 to 170 beats per minute (apical)	• Take the infant's heart rate at the apical site and count for one full minute using an appropriate sixed stethoscope • Monitor for bradycardia (less than 120- beats per minute) or tachycardia (more than 160 to 170 beats per minute) • Keep in mind that infant crying or activity will increase the heart rate and that sleep may decrease the heart rate to less than 100 beats per minute in some full-term infants
Respiratory rate	• Full-term infant: 40 to 60 breaths per minute • Preterm infant: respiratory rate varies with gestational age and infant's condition	• Count the breaths for one full minute by observing the rise and fall of the abdomen; auscultate with a stethoscope • Monitor for tachypnea (more than 60 breaths per minute • Keep in mind that crying or activity will increase the infant's respiratory rate

Blood pressure	• Full-term: 60 to 80 mm Hg systolic; 40 to 50 mm Hg diastolic
	• Preterm infant: blood pressure range varies depending on gestational age
		• Use a blood pressure cuff that is appropriately sized because the wrong sized cuff can affect the reading
		• Consider using the following devices to measure an infant's blood pressure:
		  □ *Doppler instrument* (to reflect changes in ultrasound frequency caused by blood movement translated to audible sound by a transducer in the cuff)
		  □ *Transducer device* (connected to the umbilical artery catheter to directly measure blood pressure in newborn infants)
		  □ *Dinamap blood pressure device* (to electronically measure blood pressure)
		  □ Keep in mind that crying, activity, and sleep may cause blood pressure fluctuations

APPENDIX 10
Normal Lab Values for the Newborn Infant

This chart shows laboratory tests that may be ordered for the newborn infant, with normal ranges when available. Because test results for the preterm infant usually reflect weight and gestational age, preterm infant ranges vary with the infant.

Test	Normal range: Full-term infant	Normal range: Preterm infant
Blood		
Acid phosphatase	7.4 to 19.4 units/liter	-
Albumin	3.6 to 5.4 g/dl	3.1 to 4.2 g/dl
Alkaline phosphatase	40 to 300 units/liter (1 week)	134 to 308 units/liter
Alpha-fetoprotein	up to 10 mg/liter, with none detected after 21 days	-
Ammonia	90 to 150 mcg/dl	-
Amylase	0 to 1,000 IU/hour	-
Bicarbonate	20 to 26 mmol/L	18 to 26 mmol/L
Bilirubin, direct	less than 0.5 mg/dl	less than 0.5 mg/dl
Bilirubin, total	less than 2.8 mg/dl (cord blood)	less than 2.8 mg/dl (cord blood)
0 to 1 day	2 to 6 mg/dl (peripheral blood)	1 to 6 mg/dl (peripheral blood)
1 to 2 days	6 to 7 mg/dl (peripheral blood)	6 to 8 mg/dl (peripheral blood)
3 to 5 days	4 to 6 mg/dl (peripheral blood)	10 to 12 mg/dl (peripheral blood)
Bleeding time	2 minutes	
Arterial blood gases		
pH	7.35 to 7.45	-
$PaCO_2$	35 to 45 mm Hg	-
PaO_2	50 to 90 mm Hg	-
Venous blood gases		
pH	7.32 to 7.42	-
PCO_2	41 to 51 mm Hg	-
PO_2	20 to 49 mm Hg	-
Calcium, ionized	2.5 to 5.0 mg/dl	2.5 to 5.0 mg/dl
Calcium, total	7 to 12 mg/dl	6 to 10 mg/dl
Chloride	95 to 110 mEq/liter	100 to 117 mEq/liter
Clotting time (2 tube)	5 to 8 minutes	-
Creatine phosphokinase	10 to 300 IU/liter	-
Creatinine	0.3 to 1.0 mg/dl	1.3 mg/dl

Test	Normal range: full-term infant	Normal range: preterm infant
Blood (continued)		
Digoxin level	greater than 2 ng/ml possible; greater than 30 ng/ml probable	-
Fibrinogen	0.18 to 0.38 g/dl	-
Glucose	30 to 125 mg/dl	20 to 125 mg/dl
Glutamyltransferase	14 to 331 units/liter	52 to 233 units/liter
Hematocrit	52% to 58%	45% to 55%
	53% (cord blood)	-
Hemoglobin	17.0 to 18.4 g/dl	15 to 17 g/dl
	16.8 g/dl (cord blood)	-
Immunoglobulins, total	660 to 1,439 mg/dl	-
IgG	398 to 1,244 mg/dl	-
IgM	5 to 30 mg/dl	-
IgA	0 to 2.2 mg/dl	-
Iron	100 to 250 mcg/dl	-
Iron-binding capacity	100 to 400 mcg/dl	-
Lactic dehydrogenase	357 to 953 IU/liter	-
Magnesium	1.5 to 2.5 mEq/liter	-
Osmolality	270 to 294 mOsm/kg H_2O	-
Partial thromboplastin time	40 to 80 seconds	-
Phenobarbital level	15 to 40 mcg/dl	-
Phosphorus	5.0 to 7.8 mg/dl (birth)	5.6 to 8.0 mg/dl (birth)
	4.9 to 8.9 mg/dl (7 days)	6.1 to 11.7 mg/dl (7 days)
Platelets	100,000 to 300,000/mm³;	120,000 to 180,000/mm³
Potassium	4.5 to 6.8 mEq/liter	3.9 to 6.0 mEq/liter
Protein, total	4.6 to 7.4 g/dl	4.3 to 7.6 g/dl
Prothrombin time	12 to 21 seconds	-
Red blood cell count	5.1 to 5.8 (1,000,000/mm³)	4.4 (1,000,000/mm³)
Reticulocytes	3% to 7% (cord blood)	up to 10%
Sodium	136 to 143 mEq/liter	-
Theophylline level	5 to 10 µg/ml	-
Thyroid stimulating hormone	less than 7 microunits/ml	-
Thyroxine (T_4)	10.2 to 19.0 mcg/dl	7.5 to 15.5 mcg/dl

(continued)

Normal Lab Values for the Newborn Infant *(continued)*

Test	Normal range: full-term infant	Normal range: preterm infant
Blood *(continued)*		
Transaminase		
glutamic-oxaloacetic (aspartate)	24 to 81 units/liter	–
glutamic-pyruvic (alanine)	10 to 33 units/liter	–
Triglycerides	36 to 233 mg/dl	–
Urea nitrogen (BUN)	5 to 25 mg/dl	3.1 to 25.5 mg/dl
White blood cell (WBC) count	18,000/mm³	10,000 to 20,000/mm³
eosinophils-basophils	3%	–
immature WBCs	10%	16%
lymphocytes	30%	33%
monocytes	5%	4%
neutrophils	45%	47%
Urine		
Casts, WBC	present 1st 2 to 4 days	–
Osmolality	50 to 600 mOsm/kg	–
pH	5 to 7	–
Phenylketonuria (PKU)	no color change	–
Protein	present 1st 2 to 4 days	–
Specific gravity	1.006 to 1.008	–
Cerebrospinal fluid		
Calcium	4.2 to 5.4 mg/dl	–
Cell count	0 to 15 WBC/mm³; 0 to 500 RBC/mm³	–
Chloride	110 to 120 mg/liter	–
Glucose	32 to 62 mg/dl	–
pH	7.33 to 7.42	–
Pressure	50 to 80 mm Hg	–
Protein	32 to 148 mg/dl	–
Sodium	130 to 165 mg/liter	–
Specific gravity	1.007 to 1.009	–

APPENDIX 11

Transporting an Infant to Another Hospital

Transporting a sick infant to a hospital providing neonatal intensive care services requires an optimal and safe environment and continuing care by a physician or nurse during transit. A mobile intensive care van or, if appropriate, a helicopter or airplane may be used.

Members of the transport team, directed by a physician (neonatologist), include a nurse from the intensive care nursery (ICN), and possibly a respiratory therapist and a paramedic or emergency medical technician. Nurses with special expertise in neonatal care also may serve as group leader. Experienced teams are essential to ensuring appropriate, continuous care for the high-risk infant because he usually is very small, sick, and unstable, and his condition is unpredictable.

To ensure appropriate care, the receiving hospital recruits the transport team.

THE WELL-EQUIPPED MOBILE UNIT
The infant carrier should have the following equipment:
• Transport incubator—both battery-operated and electrically powered (can be plugged into the vehicle to ensure a heating source)
• Oxygen source equipped with transcutaneous skin electrode or oximeter (oxygen source should have a 3-hour capability)
• Transport ventilator and standby ventilation system (manual)
• Monitors to measure heart rate, blood pressure, and core and skin temperatures
• Plastic hood for oxygen administration
• Emergency respiratory equipment (laryngoscope, endotracheal tubes and adapter, Ambu-bag, airways, and masks)
• Suction equipment with catheter and tubing
• Sterile syringes and needles, lancets, and scalp needles
• Catheters and feeding tubes
• Gloves, connectors, stopcocks, and needle caps
• Ampules of sterile water, saline solutions
• Ampules or vials of such medications as heparin, sodium bicarbonate, 50% glucose, calcium gluconate, phenobarbital, and adrenalin
• Chemstrips, alcohol sponges, and specimen collection tubes
• Scissors, tape, and miscellaneous items
• Flow sheets, record sheets.

HOW THE TRANSPORT PROCEEDS
The transport proceeds as follows:
• A physician requests transfer of the infant believed to need special care.
• A physician controller receives the call, decides which hospital can accept the infant, and then notifies the transport team.
• The controller notifies the receiving ICN and relays the information needed for the ICN to prepare equipment and plan care for the sick infant.
• Instructed by the leader, the transport team prepares the vehicle with appropriate equipment and medications. The team makes sure that all necessary equipment is aboard and functioning properly,
• The physician controller requests the referring physician to send the following articles and information with the infant:
  □ duplicated copies of mother's and infant's records
  □ blood sample from mother (10 ml clotted blood)
  □ X-rays and specimens
  □ cord blood sample (10 ml clotted blood)
  □ signed transfer consent form with a written order from the physician for the transfer
  □ names of the infant, parents, and physician and the parents' address and telephone number.
• The referring physician informs the parents of transport and why it is necessary. They are allowed to see and touch their infant in the transport incubator.

• The physician controller may ask the referring physician to facilitate transfer by:
  □ providing increased oxygen if needed, intubating infant to ensure a patent airway if appropriate, and suctioning the endotracheal tube if indicated
  □ inserting gastric tube and suctioning to empty stomach
  □ starting I.V. infusion or ensuring that existing I.V. line is patent and in place
  □ testing blood glucose level with Chemstrip
  □ maintaining infant temperature and color
  □ administering therapy for heart failure, seizures, or other conditions
  □ monitoring and recording vital signs and arterial blood gas values
  □ placing an identification bracelet on the infant.
• Records of all procedures, medications, complications, and conditions before and during transit are given to the receiving hospital; a completed form is given to the staff at the receiving hospital.
• The receiving hospital staff (transport team) hastens to pick up the infant, accompanying and caring for him en route. When the infant arrives, the receiving hospital admits him to the ICN and notifies the referring physician of the diagnosis and other information when the infant's condition stabilizes.
• The receiving hospital staff and referring physician keep the parents informed.

PROBLEMS ENCOUNTERED IN TRANSPORT
One reason for using an experienced transport team is to ensure that problems encountered en route to the ICN do not interrupt infant care. Some difficult travel situations include:
• bad weather or climate variations, causing problems with maintaining a neutral thermal environment
• noise, vibrations, stops and starts, mechanical problems
• high altitudes requiring more oxygen
• long distances, taking valuable time to transport infant to special-care source
• faulty equipment, causing unexpected failure or malfunction
• inadequate planning and preparation for transport.

PARENTAL CONSIDERATIONS
• Transport of a sick infant to another hospital increases parental fears and stress over separation from infant.
• Parents feel guilt and anxiety associated with the illness of their infant and a sense of helplessness when faced with the infant's transfer.
• Inform parents of plans for the transfer as soon as possible.
• Clearly and accurately tell them why and where the infant will receive special care.
• Allow both parents to see and touch the infant before transport. If possible, give them an instant photo (Polaroid) of the infant.
• Allow a flexible visiting and phoning policy, especially for the father, who is probably visiting the mother and infant at separate hospitals and informing the mother about the infant.
• Allow the mother to visit the infant as soon as possible. This familiarizes her with the ICN and the infant and promotes bonding.
• Inform the parents about their infant's new hospital. Give them concise and accurate directions to get there. Allow the father to follow the transport van.
• Encourage the parents to ask questions and express their concerns.
• Inform the parents of available support groups or offer them a brochure or other printed matter, if appropriate.
• Prepare the parents for the infant's return to the original hospital nursery, which will require them to readapt to a new staff and set of rules.

APPENDIX 12

Parent Teaching Guides

HOW TO BATHE YOUR INFANT

Now that you've brought your infant home, you'll want to keep him clean by giving him sponge or tub baths. How often you bathe him is up to you. If the weather's warm, you may want to bathe him daily and sponge him off every few hours. In cold weather, however, you may reduce the number of baths to one every 2nd or 3rd day. Why? Because the heating system in your home probably keeps the humidity low; by reducing the number of baths, you protect the infant from itchy, dry skin.

No matter which type of bath you give your infant, never leave him unattended in the water, even for a few seconds. If you turn away to reach for soap or powder, always hold your infant firmly with one hand. If the telephone or doorbell rings, wrap him in a towel and bring him with you.

Before bathing your infant, review these helpful guidelines:
• Give him a sponge bath the first 3 or 4 weeks after his birth, until his belly button heals. If he's been circumcised, wait until the circumcision heals, too. Then you can begin tub bathing.

• Set a regular time for his bath; for instance, after his morning feeding and bowel movement.
• Establish a regular place to bathe him. Select a spot that's warm, away from drafts, and at a comfortable height for you.
• Keep bath supplies together in a tray or basket so you won't have to search for them.
• Place the bath supplies within easy reach.
• Test the water temperature by placing a few drops on the crook of your arm; the water should be comfortably warm but not hot.
• Give your infant time to get used to tub baths. If he doesn't like being placed in water, soap him on a towel outside the tub, and put him in the tub only to rinse him. (This home care aid shows you how.) Chances are, he'll soon begin to enjoy the water.
• Use your hands or a soft cloth and mild, unscented soap to bathe your infant. Start with his face, using warm water only. Using soap, bathe his head

from front to back; scrub it well, using your fingertips. Soap and rinse his head at least three times a week, and just rinse it the other days.
• Wash only the outer areas of your infant's ears. When you do, use a soft cloth or cotton ball rather than a cotton-tipped stick. Never insert anything in his ears.
• Wipe eyes from inner to outer direction using a cotton ball and warm water.
• Clean genitalia with cotton balls or wash cloth and warm water.
• Take special care when holding your infant. Remember, he'll be slippery when he's wet and soapy.
• After completing the bath, don't rub a lot of infant oil on his skin; it may clog his pores. You can prevent chafing by using lotion, cream, or infant powder. If you use powder, apply it lightly.
• Dress the infant in a loose shirt, diaper, and other clothing as weather dictates. A cotton receiving blanket may also be used.

Giving a sponge bath

1 Before you start bathing your infant, make sure the room and bath water are comfortably warm. Gather unscented soap and two towels (or a towel and soft cloth). Also place a clean diaper nearby. Sit on a low chair and lay a towel across your lap. Then, as you support your infant under his shoulders, undress him except for his diaper.

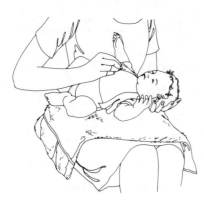

2 Next, take the other towel (or the cloth) and lay it across his legs and stomach to keep him warm. Wet the top end of the towel and gently wipe his face.

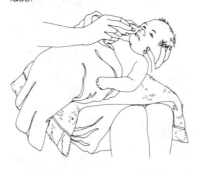

3 Then, soap his neck, chest, arms, and hands. Make sure you wash between all his skin folds. Now, again dampen the top end of the towel and rinse his neck, chest, arms, and hands. Make sure you remove any soap trapped in his skin folds, too. Then, take a dry area of the towel and lightly pat him dry. Be gentle—remember, his skin is delicate.

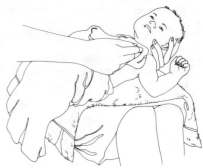

4 To bathe your infant's back, gently but firmly support his head with your hand and turn him on his side. Make sure you pat him dry after washing and rinsing him.

5 Then, remove the diaper. Soap and rinse his abdomen, buttocks, genitals, legs, and feet. Dab gently around his belly button, if it hasn't healed yet. Again, pat him dry.

6 After you finish bathing your infant, you may want to apply powder or cornstarch around his genitals and buttocks before putting on a clean diaper. Then, dress him immediately, so he doesn't become chilled.

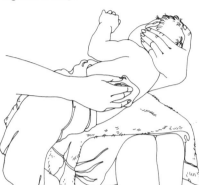

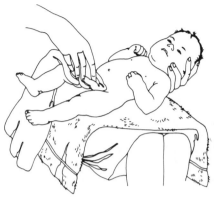

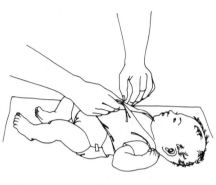

Giving a tub bath and shampoo

To give your infant a tub bath and shampoo, you'll need a tub or basin of warm water, soap, shampoo, a large towel, and a soft cloth.
Remember: You can shampoo the infant's head anytime, but don't place him in a tub of water until his belly button and circumcision have healed.

1 First, lay the towel on a secure surface and place your infant on it. Next, wash and rinse his face with the moistened cloth, and then shampoo his hair.

2 To rinse your infant's hair, hold him in a *football carry* over the tub, as shown. Take care to securely support his head with your hand. Wet the cloth and gently wipe the shampoo from his hair. Then, immediately dry his face and hair with an end of the towel.

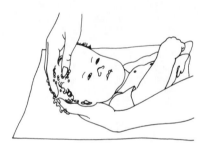

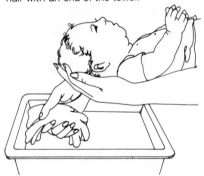

3 Now, take off your infant's shirt and soap his neck, chest, arms, hands, and back, as you would for a sponge bath. Then, remove his diaper and soap his abdomen, buttocks, genitals, legs, and feet. Make sure you wash between his toes.

4 Carefully lift your infant by holding his ankles together and gently soap all the skin folds in his diaper area.

5 Then, with one hand supporting your infant's head and your other hand holding his feet and ankles, place him in the tub to rinse him. Keep him in a sitting position, as shown here.

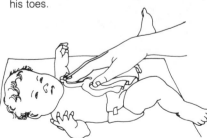

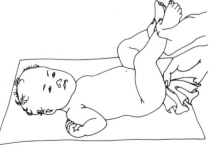

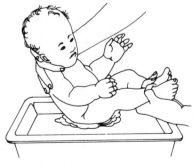

Giving a tub bath and shampoo *(continued)*

6 As you continue to support his head, take the wet cloth and thoroughly rinse his body.

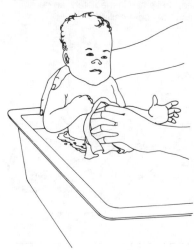

7 When you finish rinsing him, *carefully* lift him out of the tub and immediately wrap him in the towel to keep him warm. Next, pat him dry. Apply powder or cornstarch around his genitals and on his buttocks, if you want. Then, put a clean diaper on him and dress him quickly.

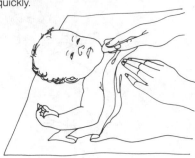

BREAST-FEEDING THE INFANT

As you begin breast-feeding, remember that many substances are eliminated from your body through breast milk. Some common ones include alcohol, barbiturates, bromides, cathartics or laxatives, diuretics, narcotics, oral contraceptives, anticonvulsants, radioactive isotopes (used for tests), steroids, sulfonamides, and tetracycline. Consult your physician about the effects of any prescribed medication or over-the-counter drug.

1 First, thoroughly wash and dry your hands before each feeding.
Remember, stress interferes with the let-down reflex, so do your best to relax. Select a position for breast-feeding: either sitting or side-lying. If you choose a side-lying position, make sure your back is comfortably supported and the arm closer to the bed is raised. Hold the infant between your arm and side, as shown, so the infant's head is level with your breast. Support the infant with your arm.

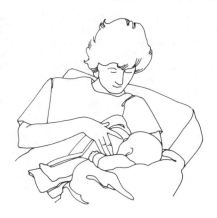

2 If you decide to sit up, select a comfortable chair and support your feet with a stool. Hold the infant on your lap at breast level, as shown, so the infant doesn't stretch the breast while feeding. (You can place the infant on a pillow for support and height, if necessary.)

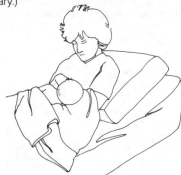

3 If you had a cesarean section—or if you gave birth to twins and want to nurse them simultaneously—use the football carry (see page 333). Place the infant alongside you on a pillow, as shown here.
Give the infant time to become accustomed to the position and to look for the breast. Remember, don't rush. Tension will inhibit both you and your infant.

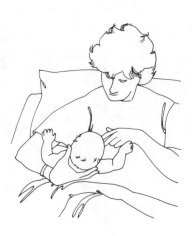

4 Now, stimulate the infant's rooting reflex. Use the second and third fingers of your free hand to hold the nipple just above the areola. Brush the nipple against the infant's cheek. In response, the infant will turn toward your breast. (Don't touch the infant's cheek or head with your supporting arm, because the infant may turn *toward* the arm and *away* from the breast.)

5 Make sure your infant has the entire nipple and most or all of the areola in his mouth. Otherwise, the infant won't be able to adequately compress the milk ducts and will have difficulty expressing milk.

When the infant is feeding properly, you'll see his jaws moving up and down rhythmically and he will swallow regularly. If he is having difficulty, make sure the nipple's on top of his tongue—not beneath it.

6 Also make sure the breast doesn't press against his nose, obstructing his breathing. If it does, gently depress the breast with your fingers, as shown here.

Offer the infant both breasts at each feeding and alternate the breast he begins feeding with. Encourage the infant to empty the first breast and then to continue as long as possible with the second.

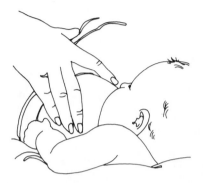
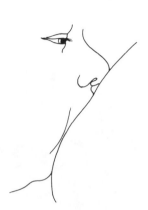
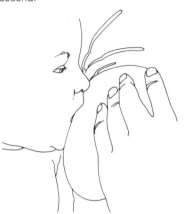

7 To avoid nipple soreness, limit feeding to 7 minutes for each breast and gradually increase the time.

To remove the infant from the first breast, break the suction by gently inserting a fingertip into the infant's mouth, as shown.

8 You can also break suction by gently pressing down on your breast until the infant's grip is broken, or by gently pulling down the infant's chin, as shown here. *Important:* Use one of these techniques when removing the infant from the breast. Otherwise, the nipple may be injured.

9 Before encouraging the infant to take the other breast, you'll want to burp (bubble) him. Sit the infant upright and support the head or chin. Place a diaper, blanket, or towel nearby, because the infant may burp up fluid as well as gas. Then, gently pat or stroke the infant's back. Pounding and other forceful motions aren't necessary and may hurt the infant.

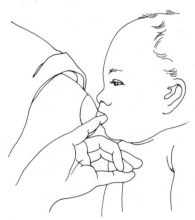
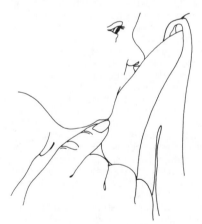
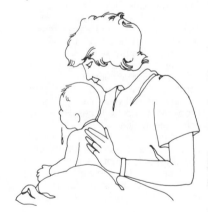

Breast-feeding the infant *(continued)*

10 Alternately, you may hold the infant upright against your shoulder and rub the infant's back. (Make sure to protect your shoulder with a diaper, blanket, or towel.) Or, position the infant prone over your knees, as shown here, and gently rub his back.

Note: A breast-fed infant probably won't swallow as much air as a bottle-fed infant. As a result, he probably won't burp as much.

11 Now, reposition the infant at your other breast. When the infant's satisfied, burp him again. (Keep in mind that several feeding patterns exist. You'll want to accommodate the infant's preferences.)

Hint: Put a safety pin on your bra strap to remind you which breast to start with at the next feeding.

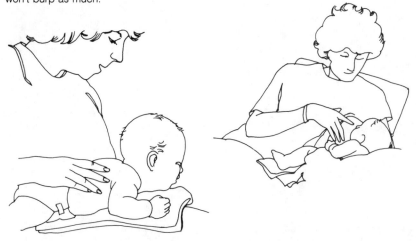

Some do's and dont's for breast-feeding

As young as he is, a newborn infant has a personality of his own. As a result, breast-feeding may not go smoothly at first. You may become anxious and frustrated—and stress, as you know, can inhibit milk flow and compound the problem.

Remember, breast-feeding is a new experience for you and your infant. You'll need several weeks to become acquainted with your infant's unique problems and preferences. Here are some helpful tips:

• Don't try to nurse the infant when he's drowsy. Instead, spend a few minutes playing with him, until he seems alert.
• Arouse the infant's interest in nursing by manually expressing a few drops of milk before encouraging him to take the nipple. Tasting the milk tends to stimulate his sucking reflex.
• If the infant has difficulty grasping the nipple, try rolling your nipple between your fingers first. Or, try applying a breast shield. It'll help draw out the nipple, which may be flattened because of breast engorgement. But don't use this device routinely, because it prevents the infant from completely compressing the milk ducts and emptying the breast.
• If your infant needs supplemental feedings or fluid, breast-feed him *before* you give him the supplement. This way, he won't lose interest in breast-feeding.
• If your breasts are sore, use the breathing and relaxation techniques you learned for delivery. They may reduce pain while you breast-feed.
• If milk flows quickly from your breast, the infant may have difficulty swallowing fast enough. To help prevent him from choking, sit him in a more upright position. Or, if he wishes, let him stop and rest periodically while nursing.
• Once the infant begins to nurse, don't touch his head. You may distract him from nursing.
• If, despite all your efforts, the infant won't feed, don't panic. He will let you know when he's hungry by crying. Plan to feed him as soon as he tells you he's hungry. If you let the infant set his own schedule, you'll have fewer problems feeding him.

BOTTLE-FEEDING THE INFANT

1. Thoroughly wash your hands before feeding the infant.
2. Seat yourself comfortably in a chair with arms.
3. Hold the infant in the crook of your arm. Hold the bottle in the hand of your other arm. Hold the infant with his head slightly elevated to decrease the chance of aspiration or choking. The formula should be at room temperature.
4. Always hold the infant for feedings. Do not prop the bottle with your infant in a supine position.
5. Insert the nipple in the infant's mouth, holding the bottle at an angle and maintaining milk in the nipple so the infant will swallow formula, not air.
6. Maintain your infant's ease of sucking by making sure nipple hole is properly sized.
7. Allow your infant to take about half of the feeding, then remove the bottle to burp or bubble him; resume feeding and burp your infant at the end of feeding. Burp the infant more often if infant swallows a large amount of air or has been crying vigorously.
8. Burp the infant by holding him on your shoulder or placing him on your lap in a sitting position with support. Stroke or pat his back.
9. Stop feeding when the infant no longer sucks. Refrain from overfeeding because this causes regurgitation and possible abdominal cramping.
10. Gently wipe the infant's mouth and place him in bed on his side or stomach.

HOW TO HOLD THE INFANT

• You won't hurt your infant by holding him firmly. His bones are flexible. They won't break when he is carried.
• But remember, his neck muscles are weak and his head must be supported with a hand or an arm.
• Here are some ways to hold him.

Vertical hold

First, place a towel on your shoulder to protect your clothing. Remove any sharp objects from shirt pockets before holding the infant. Then, support the infant against your shoulder, placing one hand under his buttocks and supporting his head with your other hand. You may use this hold for walking or talking to your infant because he is positioned close enough to hear your voice.

Horizontal hold

Support the baby's head in the crook of the arm and place the other arm under the buttocks. This hold is excellent for rocking and comforting the baby.

Football carry

Lay the infant along your forearm, supporting the infant's head with your hand and his side with your hip. This frees your other hand, for example, to answer the telephone.

Note: If you had a cesarean section, you may use this hold to breast-feed your infant.

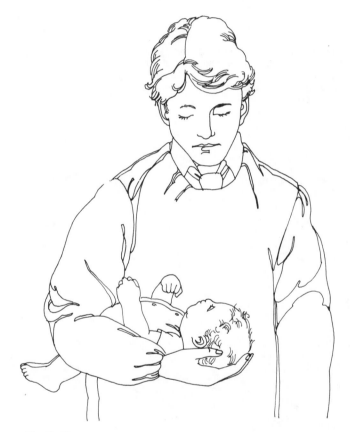

Football carry

POSTPARTUM EXERCISES

After giving birth, you should maintain a regular exercise program to regain your strength, promote healing, and restore your figure. Discuss an appropriate regimen with your physican before you leave the hospital. Use the exercises shown in this aid as a guide. Begin with the first exercise, and add a new one every day or so, as you become stronger. Perform each exercise five times twice a day. Or, follow these special directions from your nurse, nurse midwife, or doctor:_____

_____

1 First, lie flat on your back, with your knees slightly bent, as shown. Breathe in deeply, so your chest rises. Then, slowly exhale and tightly pull in your abdominal muscles. Hold these muscles tight while counting to five; then relax.

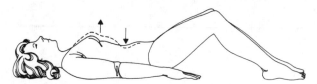

2 While lying in the same position, raise your head. As you do, try to keep the rest of your body still. Bring your head as close as possible to your chest; then, slowly return to starting position.

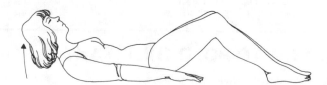

3 For this exercise, lie on your back, with your legs apart and knees slightly bent. Stretch your arms straight out from your shoulders. Then, slowly raise them, until your hands meet directly above your chest. Without bending your elbows, lower your arms to starting position.

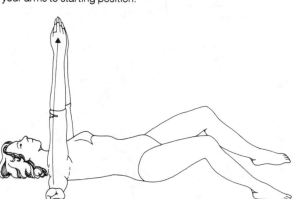

4 Next, again lie flat with your legs straight. Raise your head and slightly bend one knee. Using your opposite hand, reach toward this knee, but don't touch it. Return to starting position and repeat with your other leg and hand.

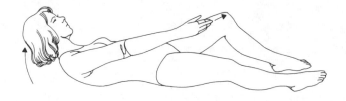

5 Now, bend one knee. Bring your knee toward your chin and your heel toward your buttock. Return to starting position and repeat with your other leg.

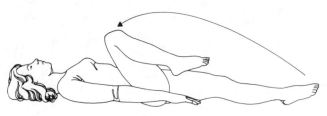

6 Lie flat, with your arms at your sides. Bend one knee toward your chin, and then straighten your leg until it's perpendicular to the floor, as shown. Lower this leg and repeat with your other leg.

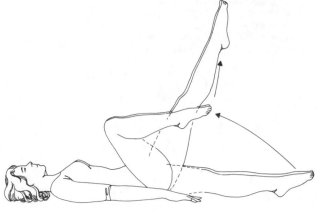

7 Now, sit upright, with your knees bent and feet flat on the floor. Clasp your hands behind your head and lean back at about a 45-degree angle to the floor, as shown. Hold this position for several seconds; then, sit upright again.

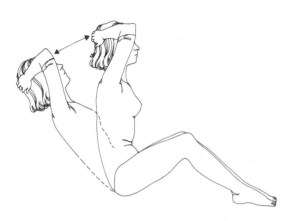

8 For the next exercise, lie flat, as you did for exercise number 6. This time bend *both* knees toward your chin, and then straighten them, until your legs are perpendicular to the floor. Lower your legs.

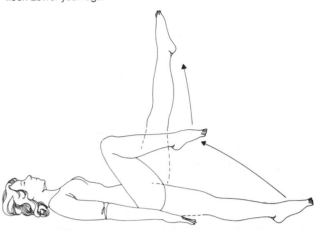

9 Now, lie with your knees bent and your feet flat on the floor, close to your buttocks. Keep your feet apart. Raise your buttocks slightly off the floor. As you raise your buttocks, tighten them and push your lower back down. Hold this position for several seconds; then, return to starting position.

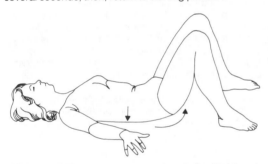

10 Repeat exercise number 9, this time raising your head and tightening your abdominal muscles as you lift your buttocks.

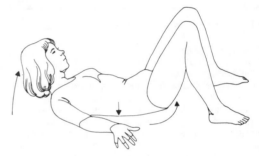

11 Finally, rest on your elbows and knees, as shown here, with your arms and legs perpendicular to your body. Hump your back upward (see arrow), tighten your buttocks, and draw in your abdomen. Then, relax and take a deep breath.

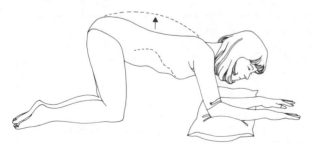

APPENDIX 13

1993 CDC Revised Classification System for HIV Infection/AIDS Surveillance Case Definition

In 1993, the Centers for Disease Control and Prevention (CDC) revised its system for classifying adults and adolescents with human immunodeficiency virus (HIV) infection and expanded the AIDS surveillance case definition for adults and adolescents.

The new HIV classification system has three clinical categories, which are based on the patient's clinical condition and CD4 T-lymphocyte count. Each clinical category has three subdivisions, resulting in a matrix of nine mutually exclusive subcategories. (See the table below.) To determine the clinical category, the patient's lowest accurate CD4 count (not necessarily the most recent count) should be used.

CD4 LYMPHOCYTE COUNT	CATEGORY A: Patient is asymptomatic, with acute primary HIV or persistent generalized lymphadenopathy	CATEGORY B: Patient is symptomatic, but lacking conditions seen in categories A and C	CATEGORY C: Patient has one or more AIDS-indicator conditions
≥500/μl	A1	B1	C1
200 to 499/μl	A2	B2	C2
<200/μl	A3	B3	C3

Category B conditions must meet at least one of the following criteria:
• must not be listed in category C
• must be attributable to HIV infection or indicative of a defect in cell-mediated immunity or
• must have a clinical course or require management that is complicated by HIV disease.

Examples of category B conditions include bacillary angiomatosis; oropharyngeal candidiasis; vulvovaginal candidiasis that is persistent or frequent or that responds poorly to therapy; moderate or severe cervical dysplasia or cervical carcinoma in situ; constitutional symptoms, such as fever (38.5° C or higher) or diarrhea lasting more than 1 month; oral hairy leukoplakia; herpes zoster (shingles) involving at least two distinct episodes or more than one dermatome; idiopathic thrombocytopenic purpura; listeriosis; pelvic inflammatory disease, especially if complicated by tubo-ovarian abscess; and peripheral neuropathy. A patient who has been treated for a category B condition retains category B status even when asymptomatic.

Category C conditions (what the CDC defines as AIDS-indicator conditions) include those listed in the AIDS surveillance case definition (see below).

1993 CDC AIDS SURVEILLANCE CASE DEFINITION

The conditions listed below are AIDS-indicator conditions, which place the patient in category C of the 1993 CDC HIV classification system.

• Candidiasis of bronchi, trachea, or lungs
• Candidiasis, esophageal
• Cervical cancer, invasive*
• Coccidioidomycosis, disseminated or extrapulmonary
• Cryptococcosis, extrapulmonary
• Cryptosporidiosis, chronic intestinal (more than 1 month's duration)
• Cytomegalovirus disease (affecting organs other than the liver, spleen, or lymph nodes)
• Cytomegalovirus retinitis (with loss of vision)
• Encephalopathy, HIV-related
• Herpes simplex: chronic ulcer(s) (more than 1 month's duration); or herpetic bronchitis, pneumonitis, or esophagitis
• Histoplasmosis, disseminated or extrapulmonary
• Isosporiasis, chronic intestinal (more than 1 month's duration)

• Kaposi's sarcoma
• Lymphoma, Burkitt's (or its equivalent)
• Lymphoma, immunoblastic (or its equivalent)
• Lymphoma, primary, of brain
• *Mycobacterium avium* complex or *M. kansasii*, disseminated or extrapulmonary
• *Mycobacterium tuberculosis* (any site—pulmonary* or extrapulmonary)
• *Mycobacterium*, other species or unidentified species, disseminated or extrapulmonary
• *Pneumocystis carinii* pneumonia
• Pneumonia, recurrent*
• Progressive multifocal leukoencephalopathy
• *Salmonella* septicemia, recurrent
• Toxoplasmosis of brain
• HIV wasting syndrome

*Added in 1993 expansion of AIDS surveillance case definition.

Centers for Disease Control. "1993 Revised Classification System for HIV Infection and Expanded Surveillance Case Definition for AIDS Among Adolescents and Adults," *Morbidity and Mortality Weekly Report* 41(RR-17), December 18, 1992.

APPENDIX 14

CDC Guidelines for Preventing HIV Transmission in Health Care Settings

UNIVERSAL PRECAUTIONS FOR BLOOD AND BODY FLUID

All health care workers routinely should use appropriate barrier precautions to prevent skin and mucous membrane exposure when contact with blood or other body fluids of any patient is anticipated.

Universal precautions apply to blood and other body fluids containing visible blood, semen, vaginal secretions, cerebrospinal fluid, synovial fluid, pleural fluid, peritoneal fluid, pericardial fluid, and amniotic fluid. Universal precautions do *not* apply to feces, nasal secretions, sputum, sweat, tears, urine, and vomitus—unless these contain visible blood. Although universal precautions—also do not apply to saliva or breast milk, special precautions are recommended for some health care workers. For instance, dental workers should use infection control precautions and wear gloves during oral examination and treatment to avoid contact with patients' saliva; health care workers with frequent exposure to breast milk (such as those who work in breast milk banks) may wear gloves.

Gloves should be worn for touching blood and body fluids, mucous membranes, or nonintact skin of all patients; for handling items or surfaces soiled with blood or body fluids; and for performing venipuncture and other vascular access procedures. Gloves should be changed after contact with each patient. Masks and protective eyewear or face shields should be worn during procedures that are likely to generate droplets of blood or other body fluids to prevent exposure of mucous membranes of the mouth, nose, and eyes. Gowns or aprons should be worn during procedures that are likely to generate splashes of blood or other body fluids.

Hands and other skin surfaces should be washed immediately and thoroughly if contaminated with blood or other body fluids. Hands should be washed immediately after gloves are removed.

All health care workers should take precautions to prevent injuries caused by needles, scalpels, and other sharp instruments or devices during procedures; when cleaning used instruments; during disposal of used needles; and when handling sharp instruments after procedures. To prevent needlestick injuries, needles should not be recapped, purposely bent or broken by hand, removed from disposable syringes, or otherwise manipulated by hand. After they are used, disposable syringes and needles, scalpel blades, and other sharp items should be placed in puncture-resistant containers for disposal; these containers should be located as close as practical to the use area. Large-bore reusable needles should be placed in a puncture-resistant container for transport to the reprocessing area.

Although saliva has not been implicated in HIV transmission, to minimize the need for emergency mouth-to-mouth resuscitation, mouthpieces, resuscitation bags, or other ventilation devices should be available for use in areas in which the need for resuscitation is predictable.

Health care workers who have exudative lesions or weeping dermatitis should refrain from all direct patient care and from handling patient-care equipment until the condition resolves.

The universal blood and body fluid precautions named here, combined with the following precautions, should be the minimum precautions for all invasive procedures, including vaginal or cesarean delivery or any other invasive obstetric procedure during which bleeding may occur.

PRECAUTIONS FOR INVASIVE PROCEDURES

All health care workers who participate in invasive procedures must routinely use appropriate barrier precautions to prevent skin and mucous membrane contact with blood and other body fluids of all patients. Gloves and surgical masks must be worn for all invasive procedures. Protective eyewear or face shields should be worn for all procedures that commonly result in the generation of droplets, splashing of blood or other body fluids, or the generation of bone chips. Gowns or aprons made of materials that provide an effective barrier should be worn during invasive procedures that are likely to result in the splashing of blood or other body fluids. All health care workers who perform or assist in vaginal or cesarean deliveries should wear gloves and gowns when handling the placenta or the infant until blood and amniotic fluid have been removed from the infant's skin and should wear gloves during postdelivery care of the umbilical cord.

If a glove is torn or a needlestick or other injury occurs, the glove should be removed and a new glove used as promptly as patient safety permits; the needle or instrument involved in the incident should also be removed from the sterile field.

Source: U.S. Department of Health and Human Services, Centers for Disease Control. *Guidelines for Prevention of Transmission of HIV and HBV to Health-Care and Public-Safety Workers.* February 1989, and U.S. Department of Labor, Occupational Safety and Health Administration. *Occupational Exposure to Bloodborne Pathogens: Final Rule.* Washington, D.C.: Government Printing Office, December 1991.

APPENDICES

SELECTED REFERENCES

Anderson, K.N., et al. (eds.) *Mosby's Medical Nursing and Allied Health Dictionary,* 4th ed. St. Louis: Mosby, 1994.

Avery, G.B. *Neonatology, Pathophysiology and Management of the Newborn,* 4th ed. Philadelphia: J.B. Lippincott Co., 1984.

Bates, B. *A Guide to Physical Examination,* 5th ed. Philadelphia: J.B. Lippincott Co., 1991.

Berkow, R., ed. *The Merck Manual,* 16th ed. Rahway, N.J.: Merck Sharp & Dohme Research Laboratories, 1992.

Bobak, I.M. *Maternity and Gynecologic Care: The Nurse and the Family,* 5th ed. St. Louis: Mosby, 1993.

Carpenito, L.J. *Nursing Diagnosis: Application to Clinical Practice,* 5th ed. Philadelphia: J.B. Lippincott Co., 1993.

Cashore, W., and Stern, L. "Neonatal Hyperbilirubinemia," *Neonatal Network* 29, October 1982.

Centers for Disease Control. "1993 Revised Classification System for HIV Infection and Expanded Surveillance Case Definition for AIDS Among Adolescents and Adults," *Morbidity and Mortality Weekly Report* 41(RR-17), December 18, 1992.

Centers for Disease Control. "Recommendations for Preventing Transmission of Human Immunodeficiency Virus and Hepatitis B Virus to Patients during Exposure-Prone Invasive Procedures," *Morbidity and Mortality Weekly Report* 40(RR-8), July 12, 1991.

Centers for Disease Control. "Update: Barrier Protection Against HIV Infection and Other Sexually Transmitted Diseases," *Morbidity and Mortality Weekly Report* 42(30), August 6, 1993.

Cohn, J. A. "Human Immunodeficiency Virus and AIDS 1993 Update," *Journal of Nurse-Midwifery* 38(2), March/April 1993.

Cunningham, F.G., et al. *Williams Obstetrics,* 19th ed. E. Norwalk, Conn: Appleton and Lange, 1993.

DeFerrari, E., et al. "Nurse-Midwifery Management of Women with Human Immunodeficiency Virus Disease," *Journal of Nurse-Midwifery* 38(2), March/April 1993.

DeVita, V.T., et al. *AIDS—Etiology, Diagnosis, Treatment and Prevention.* 3rd ed. Philadelphia: J.B. Lippincott Co., 1992.

Doenges, M.E., et al. *Maternal/Newborn and Gynecologic Care Plans: Standards for Planning Patient Care,* 2nd ed. Philadelphia: F.A. Davis Co., 1993.

Dunn, N. "Nursing Practice in Neonatal Transport," *Neonatal Network* 1:5, April 1983.

Gabbe, S.G., et al. *Obstetrics: Normal and Problem Pregnancies,* 2nd ed. New York: Churchill Livingstone, 1991.

Green, M.L., and Harry, J. *Nutrition in Contemporary Nursing Practice.* New York: John Wiley & Sons, 1981.

Gulanick, M., et al. *Nursing Care Plans, Nursing Diagnosis and Intervention,* 3rd ed. St. Louis: Mosby, 1994.

Hazinski, M.F. "Congenital Heart Disease in the Neonate, Part I," *Neonatal Network* 1(4), February 1983.

Hazinski, M.F. "Congenital Heart Disease in the Neonate, Part II," *Neonatal Network* 1(5), April 1983.

Hazinski, M.F. "Congenital Heart Disease in the Neonate, Part III," *Neonatal Network* 1(6), June 1983.

Hunter, D. "Bilirubin and the Neonate," *Neonatal Network* 1(6), June 1983.

Jaffe, M.S., and Melson, K.A. *Laboratory and Diagnostic Cards, Clinical Implications and Teaching.* St. Louis: Mosby, 1988.

Johanson, B.C., et al. *Standards for Critical Care,* 2nd ed. St. Louis: Mosby, 1985.

Joint Advisory Notice, Departments of Labor and Health and Human Services, HBV/HIV, *Federal Register,* 52(210):41818-41823, October 30, 1987.

Judd, J. "Assessing the Newborn from Head to Toe," *Nursing85* 15(12):34-41, December 1985.

Kim, M.J., et al. *Pocket Guide to Nursing Diagnoses,* 5th ed. St. Louis: Mosby, 1993.

Klaus, M.H., and Fanaroff, A.A. *Care of the High-Risk Neonate,* 4th ed. Philadelphia: W.B. Saunders Co., 1993.

Korones, S.B. *High-Risk Newborn Infants: The Basis for Intensive Nursing Care,* 4th ed. St. Louis: Mosby, 1986.

Kuller, J.M. "Skin Development and Function, Part I," *Neonatal Network* 3(3), December 1984.

Loebl, S., and Spratto, G. *The Nurse's Drug Handbook,* 6th ed. Albany, N.Y.: DELMAR, 1991.

Minkoff, H. (ed.). "HIV Disease in Pregnancy," *OB/GYN Clinics of North America* 17(3), September 1990.

Minkoff, H., and De Hovitz, J. "Care of Women Infected with the Human Immunodeficiency Virus," *Journal of the American Medical Association* 266(16), October 20/30, 1991.

Nze, R., et al. "Supporting the Mother and Infant at Risk for Aids," *Nursing87* 17(11):44-47, November 1987.

Olds, S.B., et al. *Maternal-Newborn Nursing: A Family Centered Approach,* 4th ed. Menlo Park, Calif.: Addison-Wesley Publishing Co., 1992.

Policar, M. "Clinical Manifestations of HIV Infection in Women," *Clinical Advances in the Treatment of Infections* 1(2):1-3, August 8, 1987.

Simpkin, P., "The Impact of Sexual Abuse on the Childbearing Woman and New Mother," presentation, 9th Annual Perinatal Conference, El Paso, Tex., May 28, 1993.

Thomas, C.F., ed. *Taber's Cyclopedic Medical Dictionary,* 17th ed. Philadelphia: F.A. Davis Co., 1993.

Whaley, L.F., and Wong, D.L. *Nursing Care of Infants and Children,* 4th ed. St. Louis: Mosby, 1994.

INDEX

A

Abortion, 14-19
  anxiety related to, 18-19
  fluid volume deficit and, 16
  infection and, 17
  maternal injury and, 17-18
  pain and, 18
  prevention of, 15
  signs of, 13
  spiritual distress and, 19
  types of, 14
Abruptio placentae, 20-23
  fear related to, 23
  fetal injury and, 23
  fluid volume deficit and, 21-22
  pain related to, 22
Acquired immunodeficiency syndrome
  infant, 134-138
    criteria for, 134
    parental fear related to, 137
    perinatal transmission of, 135-136
    postnatal transmission of, 136-137
  maternal, 24-29
    coping and, 29
    identifying, 25
    knowledge deficit and, 28-29
    populations at risk for, 25-28
    prophylaxis for, 25, 26
    symptoms of, 27-28
    transmission of, 24, 26, 28-29
Activity intolerance
  cesarean section birth and, 89
  congenital heart disease and, 174-175
  pregnancy and, 11
Air leak syndromes, 139-141
  gas exchange and, 140-141
Airway clearance
  choanal atresia and, 158
  cleft lip and, 166
  full-term infant and, 195-196
Anemia, 142-145
  fluid volume deficit and, 143-144
  knowledge deficit and, 145
  signs of, 143
Antepartum, normal, 2-13
Anxiety
  abortion and, 18-19
  bowel obstruction and, 152
  diabetes mellitus and, 55
  intracranial hemorrhage and, 246
  labor and, 98
  necrotizing enterocolitis and, 255
  pregnancy and, 312
  preoperative care and, 263-264
  spinal cord defects and, 290
  tracheoesophageal fistula and, 302
Aortic stenosis, 172t
Apgar scoring system, 128
Aspiration, tracheoesophageal fistula and, 297-298
Atrial septal defect, 172t

B

Ballard Gestational-Age Assessment Tool, 127
Barlow's maneuver, 202
Bathing infant, 328-330
Behavioral assessment of neonate, 131, 132t
Birth trauma, 146-149
  identifying, 147
  knowledge deficit and, 148-149
  supporting recovery from, 147-148
Body image disturbance, pregnancy and, 316

Body temperature, altered, full-term infant and, 196
Bonding, 102
Bottle-feeding infant, 333
Bowel obstruction, 150-153
  congenital abnormalities and, 150-151
  family coping and, 152
  parental anxiety and, 152
Breast engorgement, 113-114
Breast-feeding infant, 330-332
Breathing pattern, ineffective
  diabetes mellitus and, 56
  infectious disorders in infant and, 280
Bronchopulmonary dysplasia, 154-157
  family coping and, 156
  knowledge deficit and, 156-157
  oxygen toxicity and, 155
  respiratory deficiency and, 154-155

C

Caloric needs in infancy, 322
Candidal vaginitis, 81t
Carbohydrate metabolism, diabetes mellitus and, 54-55
Cardiac disease
  cardiac output and, 49-50
  fetal injury and, 51
  maternal injury and, 50-51
  pregnancy and, 48-52
Cardiac output
  congestive heart failure and, 178-180
  labor and, 98
  postoperative care and, 258-259
  pregnancy and, 49-50
CDC. See Centers for Disease Control.
Centers for Disease Control
  AIDS surveillance case definition of, 336
  guidelines for preventing HIV
    transmission in health care settings, 337
  HIV classification system and, 336
  recommendations of, for condom use, 26
Cervical incompetence, signs of, 15
Cesarean section birth, 85-91
  activity intolerance and, 89
  coping with, 85, 87
  fluid volume deficit and, 87-88
  infection and, 88-89
  knowledge deficit and, 90
  nutritional status and, 89-90
  pain related to, 87
  procedures for, 86t
Chlamydia, fetal transmission and, 78
Choanal atresia, 158-159
  airway clearance and, 158
  family coping and, 159
Circumcision, 160-163
  fluid volume deficit and, 162
  infection and, 161-162
  knowledge deficit and, 163
  medical value of, 160
  pain related to, 160-161
Cleft lip, 164-169
  airway clearance and, 166
  family coping and, 167
  knowledge deficit and, 168
  nutrition and, 164-165
  tissue integrity and, 166
Cleft palate, 164. See also Cleft lip.
Clubfoot, 293-296
Coagulopathy, signs of, 17-18
Coarctation of the aorta, 172t
Cold stress, hypothermia and, 229, 232-233

Condom use, CDC recommendations for, 26
Condyloma accuminatum, 81t
Congenital heart disease, 170-176
  activity intolerance and, 174-175
  acyanotic, 172t
  cyanotic, 171t
  grieving related to, 175
  identifying infant at risk for, 173-174
  knowledge deficit and, 175-176
  nutrition and, 174
Congestive heart failure, 177-182
  cardiac output and, 178-180
  family coping and, 181-182
  fluid volume excess and, 180-181
  knowledge deficit and, 182
  nutrition and, 181
Contraceptive methods, 318-320t
Coping, ineffective
  AIDS diagnosis and, 29
  bowel obstruction and, 152
  bronchopulmonary dysplasia and, 156
  cesarean section birth and, 85, 87
  choanal atresia and, 159
  cleft lip and, 167
  congestive heart failure and, 181-182
  drug withdrawal in infant and, 188
  hyaline membrane disease and, 211
  infectious disorders in infants and, 282
  meconium aspiration syndrome and, 249-250
  multiple gestation and, 43
  perinatal complications and, 313
  spinal cord defects and, 291
  talipes deformity and, 294-295
  tracheoesophageal fistula and, 302
Cytomegalovirus, fetal transmission and, 78

D

Depression, postpartum, 313-314
Diabetes mellitus
  anxiety related to, 55
  breathing patterns and, 56
  carbohydrate metabolism and, 54-55
  diagnostic criteria for, using oral glucose tolerance test, 53
  fetal injury and, 56-57
  powerlessness and, 56
  pregnancy and, 53-57
Dietary allowances, maternal, 309t
Discomfort, multiple gestation and, 42
Drug addiction, infant, 183
Drug withdrawal, infant, 183-189
  fluid volume deficit and, 187
  knowledge deficit and, 189
  maternal coping and, 188
  neurologic symptoms of, 184-185
  nutrition and, 186-187
  respiratory state in, 185
  skin integrity and, 188

E

Ectopic pregnancy, 30-33
  fear related to, 33
  fluid volume deficit and, 31
  infection and, 32
  pain related to, 32
  sites of, 30

i refers to an illustration; t, to a table

INDEX

Electrolyte requirements in infancy, 322
Esophageal atresia, 297-302
  family coping and, 302
  fluid volume deficit and, 300-301
  nutrition and, 299-300
  parental anxiety and, 302
  respiratory distress and, 297-298
  skin integrity and, 301
Extracorporeal membrane oxygenation, 249

F

Family assessment, 321
Family planning, methods of, 318-320t
Fear
  abruptio placentae and, 23
  AIDS—infant and, 137
  ectopic pregnancy and, 32
  hyperemesis gravidarum and, 39-40
  placenta previa and, 46
  premature rupture of membranes and, 65
  prolapsed umbilical cord and, 72
Fetal alcohol syndrome, 190-193
  knowledge deficit and, 193
  mental deficiency related to, 190-191
  neurologic state in, 190-191
  nutrition and, 191-192
  parenting and, 192-193
Fetal heart activity, variations in, 95-96t
Fetal injury
  abruptio placentae and, 23
  cardiac disease and, 51
  diabetes mellitus and, 56-57
  maternal well-being and, 8-9
  multiple gestation and, 41-42
  oxytocin-induced labor and, 105
  pregnancy-induced hypertension and, 62
  preterm labor and, 68-69
  prolapsed umbilical cord and, 71-72
  Rh isoimmunization and, 74-76
  vaginal birth and, 101
Fluid requirements in infancy, 322
Fluid volume deficit
  abortion and, 16
  abruptio placentae and, 21-22
  anemia and, 143-144
  cesarean section birth and, 87-88
  circumcision and, 162
  drug withdrawal and, 187
  ectopic pregnancy and, 31
  full-term infant and, 198
  hyaline membrane disease and, 211
  hydatidiform mole and, 34
  hyperemesis gravidarum and, 39
  labor and, 99
  necrotizing enterocolitis and, 253
  placenta previa and, 45
  postoperative care and, 260
  postpartum hemorrhage and, 117-118
  preoperative care and, 264
  preterm infant and, 272
  puerperium and, 109
  thromboembolic disease and, 125
  tracheoesophageal fistula and, 300-301
Fluid volume excess, congestive heart failure and, 180-181
Full-term infant, 194-200
  airway clearance and, 195-196
  body temperature in, 196
  fluid volume deficit and, 198
  infection and, 199
  knowledge deficit and, 200
  metabolic disorders and, 199-200
  nutrition and, 197
  reactivity and, 194
  skin integrity and, 198
Fundal height, landmarks in, 4i, 5

G

Gas exchange
  air leak syndromes and, 140-141
  bronchopulmonary dysplasia and, 154-155
Gastrostomy tube feedings, 300
Genital warts, 81t
Genitourinary function, puerperium and, 108-109
Gonorrhea, fetal transmission and, 78
Grieving
  congenital heart disease and, 175
  hydatidiform mole and, 36
  infant death and, 314-315
  malformation and, 314-315

H

Health maintenance
  hydatidiform mole, 35-36
  prenatal care and, 315
Hematoma formation, puerperium and, 110
Hemorrhage, postpartum, 116-118
  fluid volume deficit and, 117-118
  infection and, 118
Herpes simplex virus type II, fetal transmission and, 78
Hip dysplasia, 201-204
  assessing, 201-202
  knowledge deficit and, 203-204
  skin integrity and, 202-203
  tissue perfusion and, 203
  types of, 201
HIV. See Acquired immunodeficiency syndrome.
Holding infant, 333
Home assessment, 321
Human immunodeficiency virus. See Acquired immunodeficiency syndrome.
Hyaline membrane disease, 205-212
  family coping and, 211
  fluid volume deficit and, 211
  nutrition and, 210
  respiratory insufficiency and, 206-207
  therapy complications and, 208-209
Hydatidiform mole, 34-36
  fluid volume deficit and, 34
  grieving related to, 36
  infection and, 35
  maternal injury and, 35
  metastatic disease and, 35-36
Hydrocephalus, 287. See also Spinal cord defects.
Hyperbilirubinemia, 213-220
  bilirubin level in, 215-218
  exchange transfusion and, 217-218
  knowledge deficit and, 219-220
  parenting and, 219
  phototherapy and, 216-217
Hyperemesis gravidarum, 37-40
  fear related to, 39-40
  fluid volume deficit and, 39
  nutritional status and, 37-38
  pain related to, 40
Hyperglycemia, 225
Hypertension, pregnancy-induced, 58-63
  fetal injury and, 62
  maternal injury and, 58-62
  proteinuria and, 59
Hyperthermia, 229-234
Hypocalcemia, 221-224
  calcium levels in, 222
  infants at risk for, 221
  knowledge deficit and, 223-224
  signs of, 222
  tissue integrity and, 223

Hypoglycemia, 225-228
  glucose levels in, 226-227
  hyperglycemic response and, 227-228
  infants at risk for, 225
  parenting and, 228
  preventing, 227
  prognosis for, 225
  symptoms of, 226
Hypoplastic left heart syndrome, 171t
Hypothermia, 229-234
  cold stress and, 229, 232-233
  core temperature and, 229
  knowledge deficit and, 233
  temperature instability and, 230-232

I

Immune response, puerperium and, 111
Imperforate anus, 150
Infection
  abortion and, 17
  cesarean section birth and, 88-89
  circumcision and, 161-162
  ectopic pregnancy and, 32
  full-term infant and, 199
  hydatidiform mole and, 35
  labor and, 96
  postoperative care and, 259
  postpartum hemorrhage and, 118
  premature rupture of membranes and, 64-65
  preoperative care and, 265
  preterm infant and, 273
  prolapsed umbilical cord and, 72
  puerperium and, 110-111
  sexually transmitted diseases and, 78-79
  spinal cord defects and, 288
Infectious disorders, infant, 276-282
  breathing patterns and, 280
  etiology of, 277t
  maternal coping and, 282
  nutritional deficiency and, 279-280
  preventing, 279, 281
  signs of, 278
Inguinal hernia, 150
Intestinal atresia, 150
Intestinal stenosis, 150
Intracranial hemorrhage, 243-246
  neurologic impairment and, 244-245
  parental anxiety and, 246
  types of, 243
Intrauterine growth-retarded infant, 239. See also Small for gestational age.

JK

Jaundice, types of, 213
Kernicterus, 213
Knowledge deficit
  anemia and, 145
  birth trauma and, 148-149
  bronchopulmonary dysplasia and, 156-157
  cesarean section birth and, 90
  circumcision and, 163
  cleft lip and, 168
  congenital heart disease and, 175-176
  congestive heart failure and, 182
  drug withdrawal in infant and, 189
  fetal alcohol syndrome and, 193
  full-term infant and, 200
  hip dysplasia and, 203-204
  HIV transmission and, 28-29
  hyperbilirubinemia and, 219-220
  hypocalcemia and, 223-224
  hypothermia and, 233
  large for gestational age and, 237
  postoperative care and, 261-262
  pregnancy and, 12-13

Knowledge deficit *(continued)*
  preoperative care and, 266
  preterm infant and, 275
  puerperium and, 114
  small for gestational age and, 241-242
  spinal cord defects and, 291-292
  talipes deformity and, 295-296
  transient tachypnea of the newborn
    and, 304-305

L

Labor, 92-94, 96-99. *See also* Preterm labor.
  anxiety and, 98
  cardiac output and, 98
  fluid volume deficit and, 99
  infection and, 96
  onset of, 93-94
  progression of, 97
  signs of, 92
  stages of, 92-93
Laboratory values for newborn, 323-326t
Large for gestational age, 235-238
  complications of, 236-237
  knowledge deficit and, 237
Low-birth-weight infant, 239. *See also*
    Small for gestational age.

M

Malrotation, 150
Maternal injury
  abortion and, 17-18
  cardiac disease and, 50-51
  hydatidiform mole and, 35
  multiple gestation and, 41-43
  oxytocin-induced labor and, 103-104
  placenta previa and, 46
  pregnancy-induced hypertension and,
    58-62
  vaginal birth and, 101-102
Maternal well-being, fetal injury and, 8-9
Meconium aspiration syndrome, 247-250
  family coping and, 249-250
  respiratory insufficiency and, 249
Meningocele, 287
Metabolic disorders, full-term infant and,
    199-200
Metastatic disease, hydatidiform mole and,
    35-36
Milk products, nutritional content of, 322t
Molar pregnancy, 34-36
Multiple gestation, 41-43
  coping and, 43
  discomfort and, 42
  fetal injury and, 41-42
  maternal injury and, 41-43
Myelocele, 287
Myelomeningocele, 287

N

Necrotizing enterocolitis, 251-256
  bowel involvement in, 252
  complications of, 251, 254-255
  fluid volume deficit and, 253
  nutritional intake and, 252-253
  parental anxiety and, 255
Neonatal behavioral responses, 131, 132t
Neonatal postdelivery assessment, 128
Neonatal reflexes, 129t
Newborn infant assessment guides, 127-
    132
Nonemergency surgery, preparing for, 317
Nursery assessment, 130-131
Nursing diagnoses, taxonomy of, 307-308

Nutrition, altered
  cesarean section birth and, 89-90
  cleft lip and, 164-165
  congenital heart disease and, 174
  congestive heart failure and, 181
  drug withdrawal in infant and, 186-187
  fetal alcohol syndrome and, 191-192
  full-term infant and, 197
  hyaline membrane disease and, 210
  hyperemesis gravidarum and, 37-38
  infancy and, 322
  infectious disorders in infant and, 279-
    280
  necrotizing enterocolitis and, 252-253
  postoperative care and, 259-260
  pregnancy and, 9-11
  preoperative care and, 265
  preterm infant and, 271-272
  tracheoesophageal fistula and, 299-300

OPQ

Oxytocin-induced labor, 103-106
  fetal injury and, 105
  maternal injury and, 103-104
  pain related to, 105
Pain
  abortion and, 18
  abruptio placentae and, 22
  cesarean section birth and, 87
  circumcision and, 160-161
  ectopic pregnancy and, 32
  hyperemesis gravidarum and, 40
  oxytocin-induced labor and, 105
  preterm labor and, 69
  puerperal infection and, 121-122
  puerperium and, 111-112
  urinary tract infections and, 82
  vaginal birth and, 99-100
  vaginal infections and, 83
Parenteral nutrition, types of, 301t
Parenting, altered
  fetal alcohol syndrome and, 192-193
  hyperbilirubinemia and, 219
  knowledge deficit and, 315-316
  postoperative care and, 261
  spinal cord defects and, 292
  vaginal birth and, 102
Parent teaching guides, 328-335
Patent ductus arteriosus, 172t
Peripheral parenteral nutrition, 299, 301t
Periventricular/intraventricular hemorrhage,
    243
Placenta previa, 44-47
  fear related to, 46
  fluid volume deficit and, 45
  maternal injury and, 46
Postoperative care, infant, 257-262
  cardiac output and, 258-259
  fluid volume deficit and, 260
  infection and, 259
  knowledge deficit and, 261-262
  nutritional deficiency and, 259-260
  parenting and, 261
  respiratory compromise and, 257-258
Postpartum exercises, 334-335
Powerlessness, diabetes mellitus and, 56
Pregnancy
  activity intolerance and, 11
  body image disturbance and, 316
  cardiac disease and, 48-52
  discomforts of, 6t
  evidence of, 3t
  immunization and, 9
  knowledge deficit and, 12-13
  nutrition and, 9-11
  physiologic changes of, 3-5, 7

Pregnancy *(continued)*
  sexuality activity and, 12
  substance abuse and, 7t
  urinary tract infection and, 11-12
Premature labor. *See* Preterm labor.
Premature rupture of membranes, 64-66
  fear related to, 65
  infection and, 64-65
Preoperative care, infant, 263-267
  fluid volume deficit and, 264
  infection and, 265
  knowledge deficit and, 266
  nutrition and, 265
  parental anxiety and, 263-264
Preterm infant, 268-275
  apneic episodes in, 270
  complications of, 268
  fluid volume deficit and, 272
  infection and, 273
  knowledge deficit and, 275
  nutritional deficiency and, 271-272
  respiratory distress in, 269-270
  sensory-perceptual alteration in, 274
  skin integrity and, 273-274
  thermoneutral environment and, 270-271
Preterm labor, 67-70
  arresting labor in, 68
  fetal injury and, 68-69
  pain related to, 69
  symptoms of, 67
Proteinuria, pregnancy-induced hyperten-
    sion and, 59
Psychological care, maternal, 312-316
Puerperal infection, 119-122
  pain related to, 121-122
  preventing, 120-121
  signs of, 121
Puerperium, 108-115
  breast engorgement and, 113-114
  fluid volume deficit and, 109
  genitourinary function and, 108-109
  hematoma formation in, 110
  immune response and, 111
  infection and, 110-111
  knowledge deficit and, 114
  normal findings in, 110
  pain related to, 111-112
  urinary elimination and, 112-113
Pulmonic stenosis, 172t

R

Reflexes, neonatal, 129t
Respirator lung disease, 154-157
Respiratory distress syndrome
  type I, 205-212
  type II, 303-305
Rh isoimmunization, 74-76
  fetal injury and, 74-76
  prevention of, 74-76
Rubella, fetal transmission and, 78

S

Sensory-perceptual alteration, preterm in-
    fant and, 274
Sepsis neonatorum, 276-282
Sexuality patterns, altered, pregnancy and,
    12
Sexually transmitted diseases, 77-79
  infection and, 78-79
Skin disorders, 283-286
  assessing, 284
  preventing, 285-286
  skin integrity and, 284

Skin integrity
drug withdrawal in infant and, 188
full-term infant and, 198
hip dysplasia and, 202-203
preterm infant and, 273-274
skin disorders and, 284
spinal cord defects and, 288-289
talipes deformity and, 294
tracheoesophageal fistula and, 301
Small for gestational age, 239-242
complications of, 240-241
knowledge deficit and, 241-242
Spina bifida occulta, 287
Spinal cord defects, 287-292
complications of, 289-290
family coping and, 291
infection and, 288
knowledge deficit and, 291-292
parental anxiety and, 290
parenting and, 292
skin integrity and, 288-289
types of, 287
Spiritual distress, abortion and, 19
Subarachnoid hemorrhage, 243
Subdural hemorrhage, 243
Substance abuse, maternal implications of, 7t
Syphilis, fetal transmission and, 78

T

Talipes deformity, 293-296
circulatory impairment and, 294
family coping and, 294-295
knowledge deficit and, 295-296
skin integrity and, 294
treatment of, 293
types of, 293
Teratogenic substances, 310-311t
Tetralogy of Fallot, 171t
Thermoneutral environment, preterm infant and, 270-271
Thromboembolic disease, 123-125
fluid volume deficit and, 125
sites of, 123
tissue perfusion and, 123-124
Tissue integrity
cleft lip and, 166
hypocalcemia and, 223
Tissue perfusion
hip dysplasia and, 203
thromboembolic disease and, 123-124
TORCH conditions, 77. *See also* Sexually transmitted diseases.
Total parenteral nutrition, 299-300, 301t
Toxoplasmosis, fetal transmission and, 78
Tracheoesophageal fistula, 297-302
family coping and, 302
fluid volume deficit and, 300-301
nutrition and, 299-300
parental anxiety and, 302
respiratory distress and, 297-298
skin integrity and, 301
Transient tachypnea of the newborn, 303-305
knowledge deficit and, 304-305
respiratory distress and, 303-304
Transport of sick infant, 327
Transposition of the great vessels, 171t
Trichomonal vaginitis, 81t
Tricuspid atresia, 171t
Truncus arteriosus, 171t

U

Umbilical cord, prolapsed, 71-73
fear related to, 72
fetal injury and, 71-72
infection and, 72

Universal precautions for blood and body fluid, 337
Urinary elimination
puerperium and, 112-113
vaginal birth and, 99
Urinary tract infections, 80, 82
pain related to, 82
potential for, 80, 82
pregnancy and, 11-12

VWXYZ

Vaginal birth, 92. *See also* Labor.
fetal injury and, 101
maternal injury and, 101-102
pain related to, 99-100
parenting and, 102
urinary elimination and, 99
Vaginal infections, 80, 81t, 83
pain related to, 83
types of, 81t
Ventricular septal defect, 172t
Vital signs, infant assessment of, 323t
Volvulus, 150

i refers to an illustration; t, to a table